NEUROANATOMY

Development and Structure of the Central Nervous System

PROF. DR. P.F.A. MARTINEZ MARTINEZ

Professor of Anatomy and Embryology
University of Groningen
Groningen, The Netherlands

1982   W. B. SAUNDERS COMPANY

PHILADELPHIA/LONDON/TORONTO/MEXICO CITY/RIO DE JANEIRO/SYDNEY/TOKYO

W. B. Saunders Company: West Washington Square
Philadelphia, PA   19105

1 St. Anne's Road
Eastbourne, East Sussex BN21 3UN, England

1 Goldthorne Avenue
Toronto, Ontario M8Z 5T9, Canada

Apartado 26370—Cedro 512
Mexico 4, D.F., Mexico

Rua Coronel Cabrita, 8
Sao Cristovao Caixa Postal 21176
Rio de Janeiro, Brazil

9 Waltham Street
Artarmon, N.S.W. 2064, Australia

Ichibancho, Central Bldg., 22-1 Ichibancho
Chiyoda-Ku, Tokyo 102, Japan

Library of Congress Cataloging in Publication Data

Martinez Martinez, P. F. A.

Neuroanatomy, development and structure of the central
nervous system.

Bibliography: p.

Includes index.

1. Central nervous system—Anatomy.   2. Neuroanatomy.
   I. Title. [DNLM: 1. Central nervous system—Anatomy and
   histology.   2. Central nervous system—Embryology.
   WL 300 M385n]

| QM455.M38 1982 | 599.04′8 | 81–40617 |
| ISBN 0–7216–6147–5 | | AACR2 |

Neuroanatomy: Development and Structure of the
Central Nervous System   ISBN   0-7216-6147-5

Last digit is the print number: 9   8   7   6   5   4   3   2   1

Preface

The compression of anatomy courses into ever briefer periods of instruction in recent years may have reached a natural limit. Still, the amount of information to be dealt with in the medical curriculum demands efficient and effective presentation in lectures and textbooks. This book results from the expansion and differentiation of a syllabus used at the University of Groningen and is intended as a concise textbook for medical students and graduate students and as a quick reference and review for junior residents. It is hoped that the presentation will serve efficiently and effectively.

Efforts have been made throughout to keep the length of the text in control without detracting from the necessary clarity. The chapters on macroscopic anatomy are as brief as possible, but the blood supply of the nervous system is discussed in some detail because of its clinical significance. Anatomy and physiology are so intimately linked that it is impossible to understand the one without at least an elementary knowledge of the other. Accordingly the text offers basic discussion of some important aspects of nervous system function. These judgments will in turn be judged. Despite the greatest care, disorders of growth seem virtually unavoidable in the evolution of a book. Therefore, I welcome the constructive critical remarks of readers. It will be a pleasure to make use of such remarks if another edition is to be prepared.

Writing an extensive text in a language that is not my own was not the easiest part of my task. I therefore owe a special debt of gratitude to my friend and colleague Professor A. G. deWilde, who corrected numerous errors of grammar and oddities of syntax in the original Dutch manuscript.

The illustrations were made with expertise and patience by Miss A. Mutsaars, and I thank her for her valuable contribution to this book. The photographs that illustrate the text were made by H. de Weerd and B. Deddens. Mrs. G. Hoogenberg did a vast amount of work to prepare the manuscript for publication. My thanks go to them all.

Finally I would like to thank the publisher, Wetenschappelijke Uitgeverij Bunge, for the pleasant collaboration in the production of this book.

P. F. A. MARTÍNEZ MARTÍNEZ
Groningen, 1980

iii

Preface

Contents

INTRODUCTION

The nervous system ensures the integration of the various organ systems (cardiovascular, respiratory, muscular, digestive systems) in the functional unit we call "organism." Without a nervous system, the independent activities of the various organ systems would be counterproductive to the maintenance of the entire organism. Such a situation would soon lead to functional changes in the internal environment, and finally to death.

Anatomically, the nervous system is divided into the central and the peripheral nervous systems. The former comprises the brain and the spinal cord, contained in the skull and in the vertebral canal, respectively. The latter comprises the afferent and efferent nerves as well as the peripheral autonomic nervous system (sympathetic trunk, prevertebral and paravertebral ganglia, intramural ganglia) and their fiber connections.

That part of the nervous system that serves in the integration of organ systems is known as the autonomic nervous system; its localization is partly central (hypothalamus, reticular formation, segments of the cranial nerves, the lateral horn of the spinal cord) and partly peripheral (sympathetic trunk, paravertebral ganglia). Vegetative integration, however, is not the only function of the nervous system. Each organism lives within a specific part of the outside world; most animals, moreover, are organized in small or large groups, which in turn must live together with other animal species. The nervous system responsible for adequate interaction between the organism and its environment is called the so-matic nervous system and, anatomically, constitutes by far the largest part of the central nervous system. The somatic and the autonomic nervous systems are closely linked and function as a unit.

The somatic nervous system can be regarded as an information-processing system that can register, interpret, store, assess, and combine data from the outside world (or from the body itself). Messages on the various situations in which the body is placed are constantly coming in. These data are assessed, decisions are made, and instructions are sent to alter the tension in certain muscle groups or to cause them to contract. In somatic terms, the activity of the nervous system focuses on regulation of the contraction of the numerous muscles involved in the execution of coordinated movements.

Information from the environment or from the body itself takes the form of nerve signals generated in sense organs or in the sensory nerve endings (skin sensors or propriosensors). These signals must be transmitted to the central nervous system. The codified flow of information takes its course through certain channels, the so-called afferent fibers. The cells to which these fibers belong are localized in the spinal ganglia (or cranial nerve ganglia). The instructions sent by the somatic nervous system to the skeletal muscles pass through the efferent motor fibers, which are extensions of cells localized in the anterior horn of the spinal cord or in the brain stem.

The central, information-processing part of the nervous system constitutes the necessary link between the sensory and motor systems. The sensory and motor systems are by no means independent: it will be shown in subsequent chapters that cell nuclei that function as wayside stations in a given sensory pathway are often influenced by "motor" systems via collateral axon branches. In this way afferent and efferent pathways are linked to form regulatory circuits that provide the anatomic substrate for the negative feedback mechanism; the amount of information allowed to pass on to higher integrating centers can thus be controlled. Motor and sensory functions are governed by numerous regulatory circuits, and consequently the meaning of the terms "motor" and "sensory" soon fades above the spinal level.

1

The nervous system of humans differs from that of the higher mammals in the number and relative spatial arrangement of neurons. The neurons are interconnected and determine each other's pattern of activities. The abundant ramifications of the dendrites and the innumerable synaptic contacts enable the nervous system to establish neuronal circuits of astonishing complexity. And these neuronal circuits are not established "once and forever": they can change, become more complex, or even disappear. The plasticity of the nervous system ensures that the composition and complexity of the neuronal circuits are adapted to the requirements of varying situations. It is even conceivable that protracted training in intellectual activities can permanently change the connection pattern of many neuronal circuits.

Part I

Development of the Central Nervous System

Chapter 1

The Neural Tube and the Neural Crest

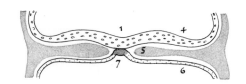

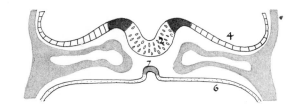

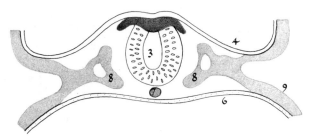

The neural tube develops from a thickened strip of ectoderm, the so-called *neural plate*. After determination of the neural plate, the ectoderm can be divided into a lateral part, from which the epidermis and its derivatives (hair, nails, lactiferous glands, etc.) develop, and a thickened medial part from which the nervous system develops. Differentiation of the original ectoderm to neural plate is caused by induction by the underlying notochord (Fig. 1–1A). This induction requires direct contact between the ectoderm and the notochord; if this contact is prevented, the development of the nervous system fails. The inductors are chemical substances of largely unknown composition. The induced tissue (ectoderm) in turn has to be "competent," that is, able to react to the presence of the inductors by formation of nerve tissue.

Figure 1–1 Cross-sections through an embryo in three successive stages of development. A, neural plate; B, neural groove; C, neural tube.

1. neural groove
2. neural banks
3. neural tube
4. ectoderm
5. mesoderm
6. endoderm
7. notochord
8. somite
9. splanchnopleure

Closure of the Neural Tube

The neural plate is originally localized between Hensen's node and the precordal plate (Fig. 1–2). This zone is histologically characterized by columnar epithelium.

At the start of the third week a shallow median groove (neural groove) appears in the neural plate; this groove deepens and its lateral edges grow toward each other. These edges (neuroectodermal transitions) are slightly elevated in relation to the surface ectoderm and called "neural banks." In the neuroectodermal transition there are groups of fairly large cells (primordium of the neural crest) which, after closure of the neural tube, detach themselves from the ectoderm and migrate to either side of the neural

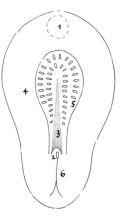

Figure 1–2 The dorsal surface of an embryonic disk of about 17 days. The notochord extension grows between the ectoderm and the entoderm in the direction of the prechordal plate.

1. buccopharyngeal membrane
2. Hensen's node
3. notochord
4. ectoderm
5. neurectoderm
6. primitive streak

5

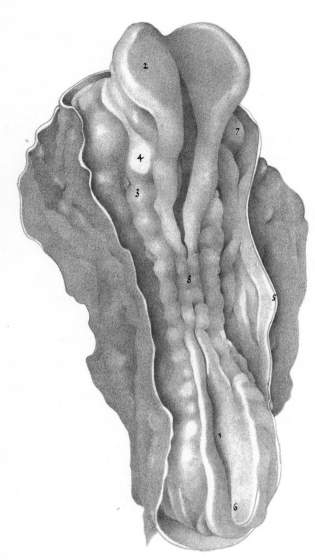

Figure 1–3 Human embryo of seven somites (according to Payne). Closure of the neural canal; the brain primordium is still wide open, and the caudal part of the spinal cord is not yet closed.

1 open neural groove
2 prosencephalon
3 first somite
4 otic placode
5 cut surface of amnion
6 Hensen's node
7 pericardial swelling
8 roof plate of closed neural tube

tube, where the spinal ganglia are ultimately formed. The neural banks grow closer and closer together and finally unite. In this way the groove closes to become the neural tube. Dorsal to the tube, the surface ectoderm arranges itself into a continuous layer of tissue that is initially the floor of the amniotic cavity (Fig. 1–1C).

The closure of the groove begins at the level of the fourth somite and continues both cranially and caudally, thus forming a tube with open ends where the tube lumen communicates with the amniotic cavity (Fig. 1–3). The area cranial to the fourth somite (brain primordium) is from the start broader and more massive than the more caudal area (spinal cord primordium). The latter shows rapid longitudinal growth. In embryos of about 20 days, the caudal end of the neural groove is attached to Hensen's node; as a result of caudad migration of this node, the caudal end of the neural groove moves farther and farther caudally. Finally the neural groove grows past Hensen's node, which remains enclosed within the neural banks.

The open anterior end of the tube (anterior neuropore) closes in the 20-somite stage in the area of the future lamina terminalis. The caudal end (posterior neuropore) closes slightly later, in the 26-somite stage. The closed neural tube rapidly increases in length; the cell population in the wall doubles every eight hours. This rapid cellular proliferation is the cause of expansion of the central nervous system in the cranial and caudal directions. Moreover, this increase in length causes a curvature of the neural tube, which is most pronounced in the area of the brain primordium.

The Neural Crest and the Sensory Ganglia

The neural crest becomes visible as a group of large cells localized at the transition from neural plate to surface ectoderm. These cells soon detach themselves from the ectoderm and migrate on either side of the neural tube in a ventrolateral direction. They initially form a cellular layer between the recently closed neural tube and the ectoderm above it; later, series of cells develop in a position dorsolateral to the neural tube (Fig. 1–1C).

The neural crest develops from the mesencephalon to the end of the spinal cord; distinction is therefore made between a cranial part (cerebral neural crest) and a spinal part (spinal neural crest). The spinal neural crest is soon subject to a process of segmentation that divided the original continuous strand of cells into 30 to 35 cell groups localized between the somites and the ventrolateral aspect of the spinal cord (Fig. 1–4). Among other structures, the sensory ganglia of the spinal nerves develop from these cell groups (His, 1887). The sensory ganglia of the cranial nerves, however, develop both from the cerebral neural crest and from the placodes (see below).

The segmental arrangement of the sensory ganglia is dependent on the segmentation of the paraxial mesoderm. Extirpation of a few somites reduces the number of sensory ganglia; on the other hand, transplantation of extra somites leads to formation of more sensory ganglia.

DIFFERENTIATION OF THE CELLS IN THE SENSORY GANGLIA

The neural crest cells that are to form sensory ganglia first assume a bipolar shape, with the short extension (axon) penetrating the dorsal part of the spinal cord and the long extension (dendrite) uniting with the anterior radix to form a spinal nerve and, via this, reaching the terminal region (trunk, extremities). Subsequently the two extensions fuse and the cell becomes "pseudo-unipolar," with a T-shaped extension that divides into a short central axon and a long peripheral dendrite.

Autonomic Ganglia

Many neuroblasts from the neural crest migrate past the sensory ganglia to the region of the aorta, where a chain of segmentally arranged cell aggregates develops. These cell aggregates are linked by longitudinal nerve fibers, thus forming the sympathetic trunk. Some neural crest cells migrate farther and form ganglia around the main branches of the aorta (preaortic ganglia). Other sympathetic neuroblasts reach the heart, lungs, and intestinal wall, where intramural nerve plexuses can form.

The thoracic ganglia are arranged segmentally. In the cervical region some ganglia fuse so that only three ganglion groups are present. At the level of the brain primordium, too, cells of the cerebral neural crest migrate to form the autonomic ganglia of the cranial nerves (ciliary, sphenopalatine, otic, sublingual, and submandibular ganglia).

The autonomic ganglia are controlled by the central nervous system (CNS). The fibers extending from the spinal cord to the sympathetic trunk are called preganglionic fibers; they synapse with the multipolar nerve cells localized in the ganglion. The fibers that leave the sympathetic trunk after synapsing are known as postganglionic fibers. In many cases they join the spinal nerve to innervate blood vessels, hairs, and sudoriferous glands; other postganglionic fibers extend to the heart, lungs, and digestive tract.

The Cranial Part of the Neural Crest

The cerebral neural crest develops from the neural folds of the two inferior brain vesicles, the mesencephalon and the rhombencephalon. Cranial to the mesencephalon the crest is less sharply defined. Recent views hold that crest cells might originate from, among other structures, the edge of the ocular cup and certain local thickenings of the ectoderm (cranial placodes).

Most of the cerebral crest is divided by the otic vesicle into an anterior (preotic neural crest) and a posterior part (postotic neural crest). These parts in turn divide into a dorsal group, from which the sensory elements of the cranial nerves arise, and a ventral group, which migrates to the branchial arches to participate in the formation of the latter's skeleton (mesectoderm, Fig. 1–4).

The ganglia of the cranial nerves develop in part from the cerebral crest and in part from the cranial placodes; the larger sensory cells are believed to arise from the latter, and the smaller cells from the former.

DEVELOPMENTAL POTENCIES OF THE NEURAL CREST

The neural crest can differentiate in many different directions. Apart from the sensory

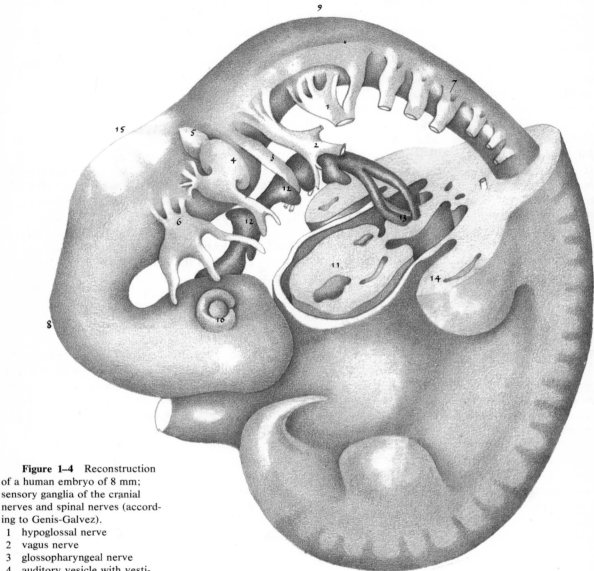

Figure 1–4 Reconstruction of a human embryo of 8 mm; sensory ganglia of the cranial nerves and spinal nerves (according to Genis-Galvez).

1 hypoglossal nerve
2 vagus nerve
3 glossopharyngeal nerve
4 auditory vesicle with vestibulocochlear nerve
5 endolymphatic duct
6 trigeminal ganglion
7 spinal neural crest
8 cranial flexure
9 cervical flexure
10 ocular cup
11 heart primordium
12 pharynx with branchial arches
13 lung primordium
14 primordium of upper extremities
15 roof of the rhombencephalon (rudimentary)

neurons and sympathicoblasts, it provides the following widely diverse end-products:

a) Mesenchymal cells and cartilage cells for certain parts of the skull and branchial arches (trabecula of the skull, palatoquadratum, Meckel's cartilage). The fact that ectodermal cells can produce mesoderm is highly unusual.

b) The Schwann cells (peripheral nerves).

c) The pigment cells of the skin. These highly ramified cells contain pigment inclusions (melanin).

d) Odontoblasts. Like the odontoblasts, the mesenchyma of the dental papilla also originates from the neural crest.

e) The leptomeninges.

This by no means complete enumeration shows how great the developmental potencies of the neural crest are. Differentiation is determined by the induction of the adjacent tissues and by differences in the prospective potencies of the crest cells themselves (Hörstadius, 1950).

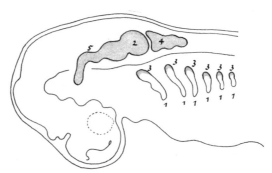

Figure 1–5 Survey of the ectodermal thickenings (placodes) in a fish embryo. Note the dorsolateral and epibranchial placodes. The neural crest is not depicted.

1 branchial clefts
2 otic placode
3 epibranchial placodes
4 postotic placodes
5 pre-otic placodes

Placodes

Placodes are local thickenings of the surface ectoderm from which cells migrate to the underlying mesoderm. Some placodes invaginate and then tie themselves off from the ectoderm to form a closed vesicle (lens placode, auditory placode). Other placodes supply cells that migrate to their ultimate destination.

As a rule neural structures arise from the placodes: sensory neurons for the ganglia of the cranial nerves, the otic vesicle, the gustatory cells of the cranial nerves, and the olfactory epithelium. Mesenchyma develops from the placodes only to a limited extent.

Chapter 2

The Spinal Cord and the Neuroglia

After closure of the neural tube the lateral walls quickly thicken, narrowing the lumen to a slit-like sagittal space. The lateral wall is soon divided by a shallow groove (sulcus limitans) into a ventral, rounded area (basal plate) and a dorsal, somewhat more elongated area (alar plate). The neuroblasts of the basal plate develop into motor neurons and integration neurons; the neuroblasts of the alar plate become neurons involved in the processing of sensory stimuli. The roof and floor plates (Fig. 2–1) contain no neuroblasts but are areas through which nerve fibers cross the midline.

Figure 2–1 Three successive stages of the development of the spinal cord. In stage C, the central canal is partly compressed.

1 sulcus limitans
2 alar plate
3 basal plate
4 roof plate
5 floor plate
6 anterior horn
7 posterior horn
8 marginal zone
9 subventricular zone

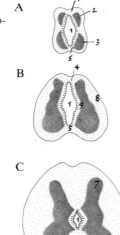

The sulcus limitans is of great theoretical importance because it marks the boundary between the ventral (motor) and the dorsal (sensory) part of the CNS. In the rostral direction, the sulcus limitans can be followed as far as the diencephalon.

The Spinal Cord

HISTOGENESIS

The wall of the neural tube consists of neuroepithelial cells, which extend throughout the thickness of the wall; they have a short, wide peripheral process and extend as far as the lumen. The outer surface of the wall of the neural tube is covered by a basal membrane (external limiting membrane). The thin central processes are interconnected by end-plates ("terminal bars") and end on a basal membrane (internal limiting membrane). The nuclei are located at different levels, hence the designation "pseudo-stratified epithelium."

The neuroepithelial cells undergo certain transformations related to their mitotic divisions. According to recent data, preparations for mitosis (DNA duplication) take place in the most peripheral cell nuclei. After DNA duplication (interphase) the peripheral nuclei migrate toward the lumen. The cells become round, the peripheral process disappears, and the perikaryon is now adjacent to the lumen (Fig. 2–2). Having gone through the metaphase and anaphase, the round cells divide into two daughter cells. Because the mitosis spindle is perpendicular to the longitudinal axis of the spinal cord primordium, one daughter cell loses and the other retains contact with the lumen (Fig. 2–2). The former soon migrates toward the external limiting membrane; the latter slowly extends until the nucleus occupies an intermediate position in the wall, but remains in contact with the lumen through a central process. These cells can divide in turn and repeat the above described cycle; the daughter cells that have come to occupy a central position divide no more. In the rat, the cycle of division lasts about eight hours.

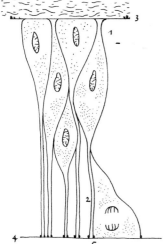

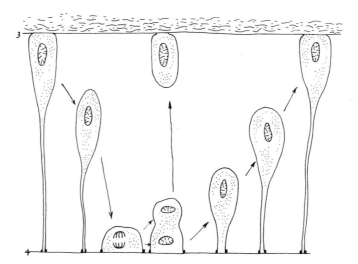

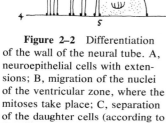

Figure 2–2 Differentiation of the wall of the neural tube. A, neuroepithelial cells with extensions; B, migration of the nuclei of the ventricular zone, where the mitoses take place; C, separation of the daughter cells (according to Hamilton).

1 peripheral extension
2 central extension
3 external limiting membrane
4 internal limiting membrane
5 end-plate

FURTHER DIFFERENTIATION OF THE WALL

The active proliferation of the neuroepithelial cells has its consequences for the structure of the wall. Numerous "free neuroblasts" accumulate beneath the external limiting membrane, where differentiation soon starts. Other cells migrate to well defined sites on their way to their ultimate destination. Initially the neuroblasts are rounded (apolar neuroblasts); shortly after, a central process toward the lumen and a peripheral process develop at opposite sides of the cell. Next, the central process disappears, and the peripheral process grows toward the outer zone of the wall, which assumes a fibrous character as a result of the accumulation of numerous periph-

eral extensions (axons). Finally, new short processes appear (primary dendrites) and a multipolar neuroblast is thus formed (Fig. 2–3). Further cytologic differentiation of perikaryon and extensions gives rise to mature neurons.

During the migration of the neuroblasts, four histologically different layers develop in the wall of the neural tube. Counting from the lumen to the periphery, these layers are: (a) the ventricular zone, where the proliferating neuroepithelial

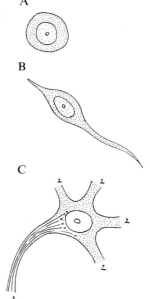

Figure 2–3 Differentiation of the neuroblast. A, apolar neuroblast; B, bipolar neuroblast; C, multipolar neuroblast.

1 axon
2 dendrites

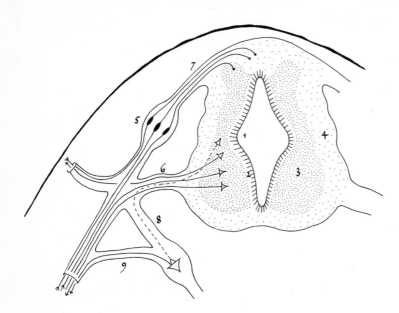

Figure 2–4 Histogenesis of the spinal nerves.

1 sulcus limitans
2 ventricular zone
3 intermediate zone
4 marginal zone
5 spinal ganglion
6 anterior root
7 posterior root
8 white communicating branch
9 gray communicating branch

cells go through the metaphase and anaphase, (b) the subventricular zone, (c) the intermediate zone (previously known as mantle layer, migration layer, or layer of differentiation), and (d) the marginal zone. The intermediate zone gives rise to the gray matter of the spinal cord; the marginal zone initially consists of the cell bodies of the neuroepithelial cells and later of numerous nerve fibers that take a sagittal course. These fibers (axons of the neuroblasts of the intermediate zone) appear fairly early; they are demonstrable as early as the fourth week. Long intersegmental fibers appear in the third month, and corticospinal fibers are demonstrable in the fifth month.

The neuroblasts preferably concentrate in the intermediate zone of the basal plate and the alar plate. The basal plate consequently assumes a rounded, rather massive shape (anterior horn), in which groups of multipolar neuroblasts are soon visible: the motor neurons (α-motoneurons) that innervate the striated muscles. Numerous axons emerge from the ventrolateral part of the spinal cord and penetrate the mesenchyma in quest of the myotomes (Fig. 2–4). These fibers are the precursors of the motor nerves.

The neuroblasts of the alar plate develop slightly later than those of the basal plate. They become neurons that respond to stimuli from the periphery (skin, muscles, joints, and viscera) and to stimuli that reach the alar plate via the axons of the spinal ganglion cells (afferent, "sensory" stimuli). The axons of the alar plate neurons invade the marginal zone, where they either ascend or descend (association fibers). The myelinization of these fibers gives the marginal zone its white color (white matter of the spinal cord).

The neuroblasts of the anterior horn can be divided into a ventral group, which innervate the somatic musculature (skeletal muscles), and a lateral group, which innervate the visceral musculature. The neurons of the lateral group are part of the autonomic nervous system.

THE CAUDAL PART OF THE SPINAL CORD

The caudal part of the spinal cord develops, not from the neural plate but from the so-called tuberculum caudale. The part that originates from the neural plate ends in a funnel-shaped structure called the conus medullaris; the part that develops from the tuberculum caudale forms no nerve cells but a massive strand of cells (filum terminale) with a sac-like terminal dilatation that comes to rest against the ectoderm of the skin in the coccygeal region (Fig. 2–5).

The lumen of the cranial part of the filum terminale, which is adjacent to the conus medul-

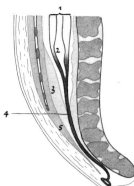

Figure 2–5 Section through the caudal part of the spinal cord in a human embryo of 11 cm (according to Unger-Brugsch).

1 spinal cord
2 terminal ventricle
3 spinal dura mater
4 filum terminale
5 superficial sacrococcygeal ligament

laris, is slightly dilated and can therefore be described as a terminal ventricle. Caudally, the lumen narrows and soon disappears.

When mature, the filum terminale extends from L2 to its insertion on the coccygeal bone. It can be divided into a first, intradural part (as far as S2), which is still surrounded by the roots of the cauda equina, and a second, extradural part which ends on the coccygeal bone.

From the third month on, the vetebral column grows faster than the spinal cord. Consequently the level of the conus medullaris is raised higher and higher. At birth, it has reached the level of the third lumbar vertebra; in adults, the spinal cord terminates at the level of L1. This apparent shortening (ascensus medullae) causes the spinal roots to assume an ever more oblique course on their way to the corresponding intervertebral foramina. The entire structure of spinal roots from L2 to their exits is known as the cauda equina (horsetail).

CONGENITAL MALFORMATIONS

The spinal cord is characterized by its situation within the vertebral canal, which can be compared to an osteofibrous shaft (vertebral

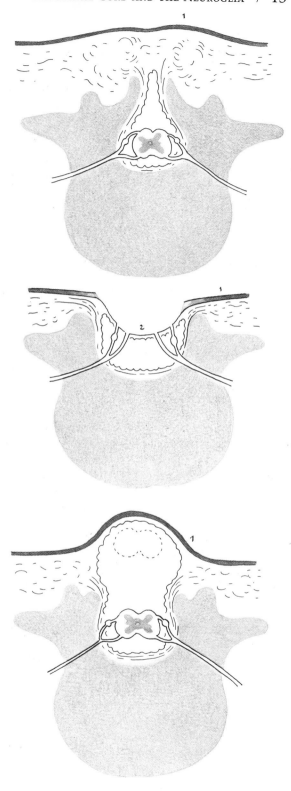

Figure 2–6 Three different types of spina bifida. A, spina bifida occulta; B, spina bifida aperta; C, meningocele (according to Tuchmann-Duplessis).

1 skin
2 neural tube (open)

arches and ligamenta flava). As a result of various disorders the dorsal part of one or several vertebral arches can fail to develop, leaving the vertebral canal partly open (rachischisis). The term spina bifida occulta applies to these cases; the spinal cord itself is normal and the defect is not visible on the surface, although the overlying skin can show changes at the lumbar or sacral levels of the vertebral column. In other cases the meninges protrudes from the aperture in the vertebral canal, a herniation of meninges known as meningocele. In the case of a meningomyelocele the nerve roots and the spinal cord are attached to the inside of the meningeal protrusion; the lumen of the spinal cord is markedly dilated and the dorsal areas of the cord may show signs of degeneration. In still more serious cases (spina bifida aperta) the neural tube has failed to close in the area of the vertebral defect (myeloschisis); the neural banks are attached to the skin and the CNS is exposed because the defect is not covered by skin (Fig. 2–6).

Development of the Neuroglia

When the production of neuroblasts has ended, the neuroepithelial cells begin to form glioblasts. The glioblasts initially have long processes that bridge the entire distance between the two limiting membranes. Later, the central process loses contact with the internal limiting membrane and the cells become astrocytes (fibrous or protoplasmic astrocytes). In mature stages the fibrous astrocytes provide a link between the blood capillaries and the perikarya of neurons, thus forming a "nutritional bridge" between the cytoplasm of the nerve cells and the blood stream.

Other glioblasts (ependymoblasts) usually lose their peripheral extension and finally form the boundaries of the central canal of the spinal cord and of the cerebral ventricles. In later stages numerous cilia grow from the ventricular surface of the ependymal cells in the lumen of the neural tube. Astrocytes and oligodendrocytes together constitute the macroglia. From the third month of the development on, a new type of glia cell is demonstrable in the CNS, the so-called microglia. The origin of these cells remains obscure. Del Rio-Hortega maintains that they originate from the mesodermal lining of the blood vessels at the surface of the nervous system, whence they invade the system. Other investigators, however, postulate that the microglia originate from the neural crest. Be this as it may, it is a fact that microglia can change their position (wandering cells) and scavenge degenerated tissues.

TYPES OF NEUROGLIA

The following types can be distinguished on morphologic grounds.

Astroglia. These cells have highly ramified extensions that fill even the smallest intercellular spaces. Some investigators hold that the cytoplasm of the astrocytes could be regarded as the actual intercellular space in the physiologic sense. Astroglia are divided into fibrous and protoplasmic astrocytes. The fibrous astrocytes have long, virtually cylindrical processes (Fig. 2–7). Many astrocytes have a thicker extension with a terminal button (end-foot) on the wall of an adjacent capillary. The nuclei of the fibrous astrocytes are usually oval, containing little chromatin and no nucleolus. The cytoplasm contains a network of filaments with a diameter of about 80Å, which extends throughout the cytoplasm and the processes. Bundles of these filaments (gliofibrils) can be visualized by light microscopy.

The protoplasmic astrocytes are localized in the gray matter; they have many radiating leaf-like processes localized between the cellular components of the neuropil. Protoplasmic astrocytes also cover the cellular surface of the neurons between the synapses (see Fig. 20–3). The cytoplasm of these cells contains filaments.

The processes of the astrocytes form a limiting membrane against the connective tissue that envelops brain and spinal cord, and against the pial tissue that accompanies the blood vessels in the nerve tissue.

Oligodendroglia. The term oligodendroglia (cells with few dendrites) was introduced in 1921 by Del Rio-Hortega to indicate cells with a round, readily stainable nucleus and few, short processes. These cells often surround the neurons (satellite cells). They are involved in the formation and maintenance of the myelin sheath

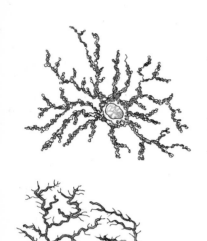

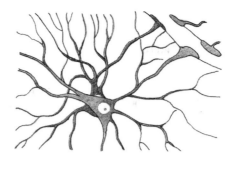

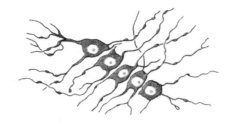

Figure 2–7 Different types of neuroglia cells. A, protoplasmic astrocyte; B, fibrous astrocyte; C, microglia; D, oligodendroglia (according to Rio-Hortega).

of the central axons; the myelin of the peripheral nerves is formed by the lemnoblasts (Schwann cells).

Microglia. Del Rio-Hortega divided the so-called third element of the neuroglia (Cajal, 1913) into oligodendroglia and microglia. The microglia have an irregular cytoplasm with three or more thick, ramified processes that take an erratic course and always end freely. These cells are found all though the gray and white matter. Cammermeyer (1970) demonstrated them in the brain in germ-free rats, and they can therefore not be regarded exclusively as "reactive cells." They are distinguished not only by their shape but also by their ability to change this shape, to migrate, and to exert phagocytic action. In le-

sions of the nerve tissue the ramified microglia change into round, ameboid elements (reactive cells) that act as scavenger cells.

Ependyma. The ependyma line the lumen of the CNS, forming a cell layer whose free surface is covered with microvilli or cilia. The underside of these cells gives rise to a fairly long extension which, in early stages of development, traverses the entire thickness of the wall of the neural tube to the external limiting membrane. In the course of development the ependymal cells lose their peripheral extension, with the exception of a few small areas (circumventricular organs) where the original situation persists. Ependyma that retain their peripheral extension are known as tanycytes.

Chapter 3

Spinal Nerves; Dermatomes and Myotomes; Plexus Formation

blasts of the spinal ganglia. After reaching the marginal zone, the fibers divide into a long, ascending and a short, descending branch (see Fig. 22–5). Both branches synapse at different levels with cells of the gray matter of the cord (see below). Some of the ascending fibers end in the nucleus cuneatus or in the nucleus gracilis of the medulla oblongata (see page 79).

The peripheral processes (dendrites) of the spinal ganglion cells unite with the anterior roots and then form a spinal nerve. The dendrites use this nerve as their "guide" to the terminal area, where they disperse as free or encapsulated nerve endings. These fibers conduct afferent impulses from the skin, joints, muscles, or viscera. In adults, the posterior roots comprise about three times as many fibers as the anterior roots.

The axons of large motor neurons of the basal plate grow in a ventrolateral direction, leave the spinal cord, and invade the adjacent tissue on the way to their destination (muscle tissue of the somite). The direction of growth of these axons is determined, not by specific chemical substances but by the submicroscopic orientation of the molecules of the intercellular matrix. The fibers destined for one particular myotome form the anterior root (radix anterior) of a spinal nerve; they conduct motor impulses from the spinal cord to the muscles.

The posterior roots (radices posteriores) arise from the central processes of the neuro-

Spinal Nerves

FUNCTIONAL COMPONENTS

The spinal nerves are mixed nerves, which is to say that they are made up of motor and sensory components (see Fig. 2–4). These components can in turn be divided, according to the structures they innervate, into somatic and visceral components (Table 3–1).

In connection with the development of the sense organs and the musculature of branchial origin, three other types of fiber may be present in the cranial nerves (see page 27).

Table 3–1 SPINAL NERVES

Motor Fibers General Somatic Efferent (GSE)	Innervation of the skeletal muscles
General Visceral Efferent (GVE)	Innervation of the smooth muscles, the heart muscle, and the glands
Sensory Fibers General Somatic Afferent (GSA)	Conduction of impulses from the skin, skeletal muscles, and joints to the CNS
General Visceral Afferent (GVA)	Conduction of impulses from the viscera to the CNS

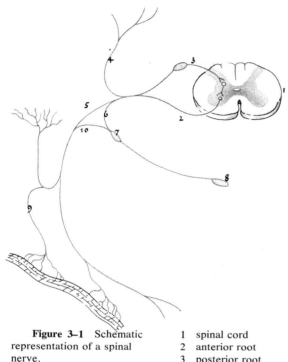

Figure 3–1 Schematic representation of a spinal nerve.

1	spinal cord
2	anterior root
3	posterior root
4	dorsal branch
5	ventral branch
6	white communicating branch
7	sympathetic trunk
8	preaortic ganglion
9	lateral branch
10	gray communicating branch

DISTRIBUTION

Spinal nerves result from the union of posterior and anterior roots (Fig. 3–1), which takes place slightly past the spinal ganglion. Both the ganglion and the beginning of the spinal nerve are localized outside the lining of the dura mater. The trunk of the spinal nerve is very short; the nerve has hardly emerged from the intervertebral foramen when it produces the following branches:

Meningeal Branch (Sensory and Vasomotor). This innervates the dura mater of the spinal cord and, via the intervertebral foramen, the blood vessels of the vertebral canal.

Dorsal Branch (Mixed). This is smaller than the ventral branch. The motor fibers innervate the unmigrated dorsal musculature (erector trunci); the sensory fibers innervate the back from the midline to a line that extends from the occipital protuberance to the acromion and from there to the midiliac crest.

The dorsal branch of the first cervical nerve is purely a motor branch and innervates the short cervical muscles between the skull and the upper cervical vertebrae (m. rectus capitis, m. obliquus capitis). The dorsal branch of the second cervical nerve is largely a sensory branch (n. occipitalis major) and innervates the skin of the occiput.

Ventral Branch (Mixed). This is the largest part of the spinal nerve. It innervates the ventral musculature of the trunk and the *entire* musculature of the extremities. In the thorax, the ventral branches retain their original segmental distribution and largely confine themselves to innervating the still segmentally arranged intercostal muscles. The ventral branch produces a (sensory) lateral branch (Fig. 3–1), which innervates the skin of the ventrolateral part of the thorax. The remainder of the nerve continues to the lateral edge of the sternum and terminates in skin branches on that side of the midline. The ventral branches of the cervical and the lumbosacral regions are linked to form a network (cervical, brachial, lumbosacral plexus) from which branches arise that unite to become separate nerves.

Communicating Branch. This detaches itself from the spinal nerve and extends to a ganglion of the sympathetic trunk. Through the communicating branch pass preganglionic (myelinated) fibers that originate from the lateral horn of the spinal cord. Some of these fibers end in the corresponding ganglion, where they synapse with sympathetic cells. Others pass through the sympathetic trunk and then synapse with cells at a higher or a lower level. The axons of the sympathetic cells are *postganglionic* (postsynaptic) fibers and remain unmyelinated. They extend via the gray communicating branch to the spinal nerve (Fig. 3–1), and from there to their final peripheral destination (blood vessels, sudoriferous glands, hair). The communicating branch is sometimes divided into a white communicating branch, which comprises preganglionic fibers, and a gray communicating branch, which comprises postganglionic fibers. The two branches are usually united to form a single nerve branch.

Other preganglionic fibers leave the sympathetic trunk and do not synapse until they have entered the prevertebral ganglia; the fibers reach these ganglia via the nn. splanchnicus major and minor, which pass through the diaphragm.

Dermatomes and Myotomes; Plexus Formation

The paraxial mesoderm on either side of the neural tube is divided into several segments (somites). These somites, in turn, induce the formation of the spinal ganglia from the neural crest, and thus cause the spinal nerves to be arranged segmentally. During the fourth week of development the somite differentiates into a ventromedial part (sclerotome) and a dorsolateral part (myotome). Each myotome provides the muscle tissue of its own segment. The remainder of the dorsolateral part of the somite (dermatome) then spreads beneath the surface ectoderm and forms the dermis (mesodermal part of the skin).

Each somite is originally innervated by a single spinal nerve. The motor fibers of the nerve innervate the corresponding myotome, while the sensory fibers innervate the dermatome. In early stages these nerves are strictly metamerous; this also applies to the muscles of the extremities. The upper limb bud appears at the level of segments C4 to T2; the lower limb bud lies at the level of L3 to S3. The nerves of these segments invade the limb bud and ramify in the mesenchyma as if the future muscles of the extremity originated from the myotomes. The skin of the limb bud, too, is segmentally innervated.

As development progresses, this situation becomes more complicated. In view of the mechanical demands made by future life, the muscles extend to remote areas of the skeleton, and this often requires fusions of material from several myotomes. Such muscles are called *polymerous* (dimerous, trimerous, etc.). Most muscles of the extremities are polymerous (more specifically, dimerous), and this is of great advantage in the development of polyarticular mus-

cles, which can control the movements of a chain of joints comprising several elements.

Polymerous muscles are innervated by as many segmental nerves as myotomes are involved. This means that the innervating branches that enter the muscle contain fibers from two or more segmental nerves. This situation necessitates a previous exchange of fibers (plexus formation) between the segmental nerves involved.

Segmental nerves destined for the extremities form a plexus as a result of intensive interweaving of their fibers; from this plexus arise the fasciculi that produce the branches that extend to the muscles. The cause of plexus formation, therefore, lies not in the nature of the development of the peripheral nervous system as such but in the polymerous composition of the muscles of the neck and extremities. According to Bolk (1910), the nerves that innervate an extremity form a plexus that extends from their exits in the vertebral column to their terminations in the muscle fibers. Three areas can be distinguished in this plexus: the peripheral area (intramuscular nerve tangles), the central area (nerve trunks like the n. medianus), and the proximal area, which is the plexus proper (brachial plexus, etc.).

The muscular system of the extremity divides early into a ventral and a dorsal layer, initially separated by the primordium of the skeleton. Consequently the segmental nerves are divided into ventral and dorsal branches. Because there are no communications between the ventral and the dorsal branches, the entire plexus is divided into a ventral and a dorsal layer. This means that both the brachial plexus and the lumbosacral plexus have two levels: from the ventral level arise the ventral nerve trunks for the ventral muscles, while from the dorsal level the dorsal nerves for the (topographically) dorsal muscles arise.

SEGMENTAL INNERVATION OF THE SKIN

The skin area for which sensory innervation is provided by a single posterior root is called a *dermatome*. Originally, the dermatomes succeeded each other in a regular

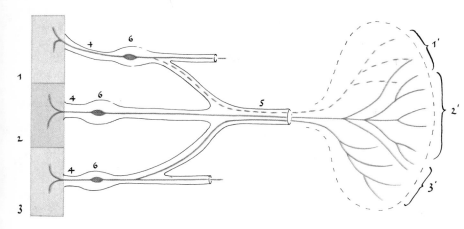

Figure 3–2 The sensory innervation of the skin. Each dermatome is innervated by three successive posterior roots: the dermatome's own posterior root, the one cranial to it, and the one caudal to it.

1,2,3   spinal cord segments
4   posterior root
5   peripheral nerve
1', 2', 3'   dermatomes
6   spinal ganglion

series of superposed zones. This is most apparent in the thorax, where each spinal nerve innervates the musculature and skin area of its own segment. The development of the extremities causes changes in the positions of the dermatomes, with consequent complications.

The dermatomes are not sharply separated. At the boundary between two dermatomes, fibers from the innervating posterior roots become entangled (Fig. 3–2). Total anesthesia of a dermatome, therefore, requires severance (or anesthesia) of at least three consecutive posterior roots.

Dermatomes of the Cervical Region

The first cervical dermatome does not exist, because C1 comprises exclusively motor fibers. The dermatome of C2 (Fig. 3–3) is a long strip that extends along the edge of the jaw to the

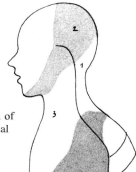

Figure 3–3 Distribution of the dermatomes in the cervical and the occipital regions.

1   boundary between dorsal and ventral regions
2   dermatomes of C2
3   dermatomes of C3

pinna of the ear and the lateral part of the occiput. The dermatome of C3 extends obliquely from the external occipital protuberance to the manubrium sterni. The dermatome of C4 corresponds to the area of the trigonum colli laterale and further extends over the curvature of the shoulder.

Dermatomes of the Upper Extremity

The first indication of the upper extremity is a flat bulge at the level of the lowest four cervical and highest two thoracic segments. As this limb bud grows, the respective dermatomes elongate (Fig. 3–4). The limb bud has dorsal and ventral aspects and cranial, caudal, and lateral margins. The dorsal and ventral aspects of the dermatomes merge along the lateral margin. As the limb bud becomes larger (Fig. 3–4B), the seventh and eighth dermatomes migrate laterally and their place on the trunk is taken by the sixth and ninth dermatomes, which consequently come closer together. Further growth of the limb bud (Fig. 3–4C) causes further migration of the seventh and eighth dermatomes, bringing them entirely into the area of the free extremity. The fifth and tenth dermatomes are "drawn" into the root of the extremity, and the sixth and ninth dermatomes come together. Further migration of the sixth and ninth dermatomes into the free extremity produces a line (axial line) along which the successive dermatomes are placed after their migration from the trunk. In this way the mature situation is approached, in which the fourth cervical dermatome is adjacent to the second

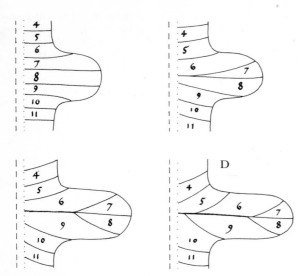

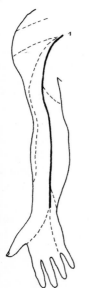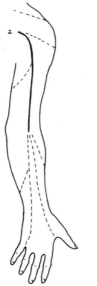

Figure 3–4 Migration of the dermatomes of the upper extremity and formation of the axial line (according to Bolk).

Figure 3–5 Boundaries between the dermatomes of the upper extremity. The black line indicates the axial line; there is but little overlap of the dermatomes along this line (according to Gray).

1 axial line (ventral)
2 axial line (dorsal)

thoracic dermatome, while the dermatomes that originally lay between them have migrated entirely to the free extremity. The seventh and eighth are the smallest dermatomes and are found in the distal part of the upper extremity (Fig. 3–4D).

The distribution of the dermatomes is shown in Figure 3–5. The overlap between the dermatomes is minimal along the axial line.

Dermatomes of the Lower Extremity

The primordium of the lower extremity fluctuates between L1-S2 and L2-S3; the difference in level can amount to more than one segment in

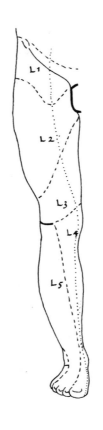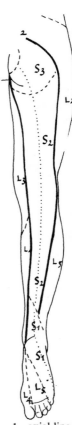

Figure 3–6 Distribution of the dermatomes in the lower extremity (according to Gray).

1 axial line (ventral)
2 axial line (dorsal)

some cases. The migration of the dermatomes is analogous to that described for the upper extremity. However, the distribution of the dermatomes seems more complicated as a result of the characteristic torsion to which the lower extremity is subject during development. This torsion so influences the distribution of the dermatomes as to give them the appearance of a spiral arrangement (Bolk, 1910).

The boundaries of the dermatomes in the mature lower extremity are a matter of some controversy. Figure 3–6 presents a generally accepted diagram of the distribution of the dermatomes.

Chapter 4

Development of the Brain

The development of the brain differs markedly from that of the spinal cord. In the brain the irregular growth of the wall is a conspicuous feature; it leads to local dilatations in the lumen of the neural tube (formation of brain vesicles). Another factor is the early occurrence of curvatures in the longitudinal axis. Moreover, some parts of the wall are reduced to epithelial lamellae (roof of the third and fourth ventricles). In later phases of development the shape of the brain is determined largely by the growth of the hemispheres, which almost completely cover other parts of the brain.

The Phase of Three Brain Vesicles and Two Curvatures

At about the ten-somite stage, a ventral bend occurs in the anterior part of the brain, called the cephalic flexure. As a result of this curvature the brain can be divided into an anterior part rostral to the bend (the prosencephalon), a slightly narrowed midportion that coincides with the curvature (the mesencephalon), and a wide posterior part at the level of the otic placode (the rhombencephalon), which merges into the spinal cord at the level of the fourth cervical somite (Fig. 4–1).

The second brain curvature (cervical flexure) appears in embryos of about 26 days at the boundary between the rhombencephalon and spinal cord. At the same time, a shallow transverse groove is seen in the roof of the tube at the level of the cephalic flexure (see Fig. 4–4). This groove (rhombencephalic isthmus) is the boundary between the mesencephalon and the rhom-

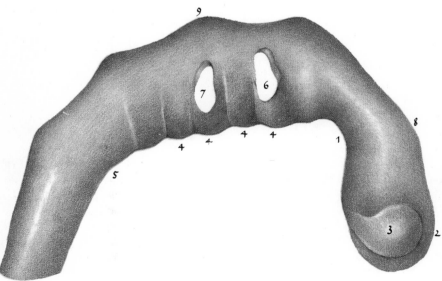

Figure 4–1 Brain of a human embryo of 3.5 mm (according to Hochstetter).

1 cephalic flexure
2 prosencephalon
3 ocular cup
4 rhombomeres
5 cervical flexure
6 ganglion of the 5th cranial nerve
7 ganglion of the 7th and 8th cranial nerves
8 mesencephalon
9 rhombencephalon

22

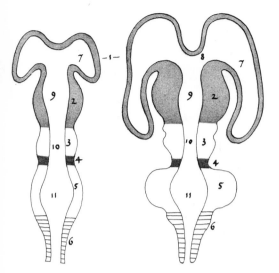

Figure 4–2 The brain vesicles in two phases of development. In Figure 4–5 the diencephalon is more and more covered by the dorsally developing hemispheres.

1 telencephalon
2 diencephalon
3 mesencephalon
4 isthmus
5 metencephalon
6 myelencephalon
7 lateral ventricle
8 interventricular foramen (foramen of Monro)
9 third ventricle
10 cerebral aqueduct (Sylvian aqueduct)
11 fourth ventricle

The Phase of Five Brain Vesicles and Three Curvatures

In embryos of about 6 mm, changes occur that give the brain an entirely different shape. On either side of the prosencephalon, the ocular cup grows toward the epidermis (Fig. 4–3). In the prosencephalon a feeble bulge ventral to the ocular cup heralds the development of the hemispheric vesicle (Fig. 4–3). The hemispheric vesicle is separated from the diencephalon by a deepening groove, the telediencephalic sulcus. The prosencephalon can now be divided into a posterior part (diencephalon) and an anterior part, which comprises a midportion (telencephalon medium) and two lateral parts (hemispheric vesicles).

The lumina of the hemispheric vesicles (lateral ventricles) communicate with the third ventricle via an initially wide passage, the foramen of Monro. In the course of development the foramen of Monro becomes smaller and smaller as a result of the growth of structures like the corpus striatum, the white matter of the hemisphere, and the fornix.

In the diencephalon the communication between the ocular cup and the lateral wall of the diencephalon (eye pedicle) elongates and can now be called fasciculus opticus. Behind the exit sites of the optic fasciculi the primordium of the neurohypophysis is seen as a thickening of the floor, and soon after as a depression, the recessus infundibuli. The wall of the recess (infundibulum) is from the start in direct contact with the anterior part of the wall of Rathke's pouch, from which the adenohypophysis develops. (The neurohypophysis develops from the infundibulum.)

The distance between recessus infundibuli and recessus mamillaris (Fig. 4–3) gradually increases; this means that the diencephalon is subject to significant longitudinal growth. A small outpouching on the superior aspect of the diencephalon marks the position of the epiphysis cerebri (pineal body). Ventral to the epiphysis cerebri, the habenular commissure develops; dorsal to it, the posterior commissure lies at the boundary between the diencephalon and the mesencephalon.

bencephalon. The boundary between the prosencephalon and the mesencephalon on the basal side is the primordium of the mamillary eminence.

The lumen of the brain primordium initially shows two dilatations that coincide with those of the diencephalon and rhombencephalon. The lumen of the rhombencephalon is called the fourth ventricle, whereas the lumen of the diencephalon is known as the third ventricle. The two ventricles communicate via the lumen of the mesencephalon which, as a result of the marked thickening of its walls, is compressed to a narrow canal, called the cerebral aqueduct or aqueduct of Sylvius (Fig. 4–2). The cerebrospinal fluid can circulate freely between the prosencephalon and the spinal cord.

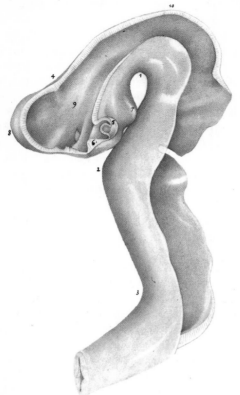

Figure 4–3 Brain of a human embryo of about 7 mm (according to His). The ocular cup communicates with the third ventricle via a wide eye pedicle.

1 cephalic flexure
2 pontine flexure
3 cervical flexure
4 sulcus telediencephalicus
5 ocular cup
6 lamina commissuralis
7 mamillary eminence
8 telencephalon
9 diencephalon
10 mesencephalon

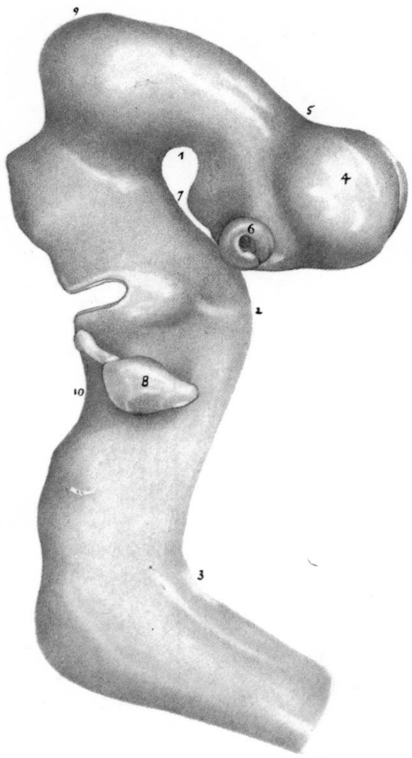

Figure 4–4 Brain of a human embryo of about 9 mm (according to Hochstetter); phase of five brain vesicles and three curvatures.

1 cephalic flexure
2 pontine flexure
3 cervical flexure
4 telencephalon
5 sulcus telediencephalicus
6 ocular cup
7 mamillary eminence
8 otic vesicle
9 mesencephalon
10 rhombencephalon

MESENCEPHALON

The mesencephalon grows more slowly than the prosencephalon. At about the stage of 10 to 14 mm the cephalic flexure becomes even sharper, and consequently the diencephalon and mesencephalon come closer together. The cephalic flexure persists and this is why, in maturity, the telencephalon and diencephalon are perpendicular to the longitudinal axis of the rhombencephalon.

RHOMBENCEPHALON

The changes in the rhombencephalon are substantial. In embryos of about 9 mm the rapid longitudinal growth gives rise to a (compensatory) ventral curvature that soon deepens (pontine flexure). As a result, the dorsal part of the rhombencephalon, specifically the roof plate, elongates and the two alar plates diverge (Fig. 4–4).

The elongated roof plate persists as a thin,

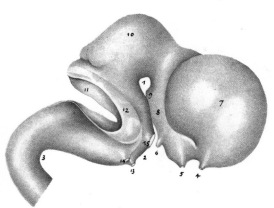

Figure 4–5 Brain of a human embryo of 27 mm (according to Hochstetter); phase of five brain vesicles and three curvatures.

1 cephalic flexure
2 pontine flexure
3 cervical flexure
4 olfactory bulb
5 optic nerve
6 infundibulum
7 hemispheric vesicle
8 hypothalamus
9 mamillary eminence
10 mesencephalon
11 cerebellum
12 roof of fourth ventricle
13 facial nerve
14 vestibulocochlear nerve
15 trigeminal nerve

but tangles of capillaries covered with a layer of ependyma and facing the ventricular cavity.

At this time the lumen of the brain is well differentiated and comprises two lateral ventricles, the third ventricle, the cerebral aqueduct, and the fourth ventricle. In embryos of about 60 mm, a few small areas in the roof of the fourth ventricle degenerate. Through the resulting apertures the cerebrospinal fluid escapes from the cerebral ventricles into the subarachnoid space. The three apertures are the foramen of Magendie in the middle and the foramina of Luschka in the lateral recesses of the fourth ventricle (see Fig. 17–4).

Rhombomeres. In the floor of the wide fourth ventricle there are several transverse bulges called rhombomeres (Fig. 4–1). These segmentally arranged cell aggregates disappear at about the 14 mm stage; their significance is obscure.

Structure of the Rhombencephalon. After the formation of the pontine flexure the rhombencephalon can be divided into a ventral part (metencephalon), which is separated from the mesencephalon by an isthmus, and a caudal part (myelencephalon), which is continuous with the spinal cord. The tela choroidea of the fourth ventricle merges into the thickened lateral edges of the rhomboid fossa; these edges are known as rhombic lips (labia rhombencephali). On the ventral side, the roof is attached to a ridge that protrudes into the fourth ventricle (Fig. 4–5). The floor of the ventricle is diamond-shaped (rhomboid fossa).

In embryos of 12 mm, a transverse groove is visible in the floor of the ventricle. This is the sulcus transversus, which marks the boundary between a cranial (metencephalic) and a caudal (myelencephalic) region.

slightly protruding membrane (lamina choroidea epithelialis) that forms the roof of the widened lumen (fourth ventricle). This layer is covered by the highly vascularized mesenchyma of the pia mater. The mesenchymal layer and the epithelial layer together form the tela choroidea. Numerous blood vessels of the pia mater cause the ventricular lumen to bulge in and form the choroid plexus. These structures, which govern the production of cerebrospinal fluid, are nothing

Chapter 5

The Rhombencephalon

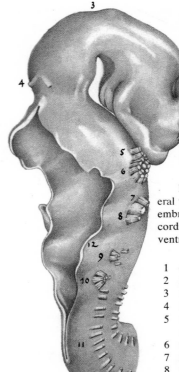

Figure 5–1 Dorsolateral view of the brain of an embryo of about 10 mm (according to His); the fourth ventricle is wide open.

1 optic nerve
2 hemispheric vesicle
3 mesencephalon
4 trochlear nerve
5 motor root, 5th cranial nerve
6 trigeminal nerve
7 facial nerve
8 vestibulocochlear nerve
9 glossopharyngeal nerve
10 vagus nerve
11 accessory nerve
12 cut edge of the roof of the fourth ventricle

Structural Design of the Rhombencephalon

After the formation of the fourth ventricle, the rhombencephalon and the spinal cord seem totally different structures (Fig. 5–1). The principal causes of the increasing complexity of the rhombencephalon are (a) the lateral "eversion" of the lateral walls of the rhombencephalon, (b) the development of the reticular formation, and (c) the development of numerous long nerve pathways that cross the midline. The gross lines of the design of the spinal cord, however, are not lost altogether; this is most evident in the ventricular floor, where the sulcus limitans still marks the boundary between the medial basal plate (motor) and the lateral alar plates (sensory). This is the region of the nuclei of origin of the cranial nerves (Fig. 5–2). In accordance with the specific developmental history of the head, the "somatic" nuclei of the cranial nerves become less important, whereas the "visceral" and "special visceral" nuclei take prominence.

At some distance from the ventricular floor is found a new structure in the myelencephalon, the *reticular formation*. This structure is morphologically characterized by irregularly distributed large neurons that show no tendency to form nuclei or to arrange themselves in layers. This basal region is commonly called tegmentum; in it, phylogenetically new nuclei without equivalents in the spinal cord develop (olive, lateral vestibular nucleus).

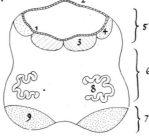

Figure 5–2 Schematic representation of the structure of the rhombencephalon. Three levels are distinguished: ventricular floor, tegmentum, and base.

1 sulcus limitans
2 roof plate (roof of fourth ventricle)
3 basal plate
4 alar plate
5 ventricular floor
6 tegmentum
7 base
8 olive
9 corticospinal tract

26

Through the most ventral area of the rhombencephalon pass the long suprasegmental tracts (corticospinal tract, pontocerebellar fibers), which have developed prominently only in the higher mammals (Fig. 5–2).

In summary, three different levels can be distinguished in the rhombencephalon: (a) the ventricular floor, which comprises the phylogenetically old nuclei of origin of the cranial nerves; this level can be compared to an opened-out spinal cord; (b) the tegmentum, which consists of the reticular formation and the special nuclei contained in it (olive, vestibular nucleus); and (c) the level of the long fiber systems, which take a sagittal or transverse course (such as the corticospinal tract).

Development of the Ventricular Floor

The rhombencephalon gives rise to the so-called branchial arch nerves (trigeminal, facial, glossopharyngeal, vagus, and accessory) and a few somatomotor nerves (abducens, hypoglossal), whose nuclei of origin are localized in the basal plate. The sensory cells of the branchial arch nerves are localized in the corresponding ganglia; their relay nuclei are found lateral to the sulcus limitans (Fig. 5–3).

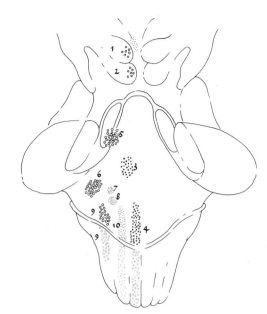

Figure 5–3 Efferent nuclei of the cranial nerves. The somatomotor (GSE) nuclei are indicated by black points, and the general visceral efferent (GVE) nuclei by gray points. Circles indicate the special visceral efferent (SVE) nuclei.

1	oculomotor nucleus
2	trochlear nucleus
3	abducens nucleus
4	hypoglossal nucleus
5	masticatory nucleus
6	facial nucleus
7	superior salivatory nucleus
8	inferior salivatory nucleus
9	ambiguous nucleus
10	dorsal nucleus of vagus nerve

BASAL PLATE

The somatomotor nuclei of the cranial nerves can be regarded as the cranial continuation of the large multipolar anterior horn cells; they innervate striated muscles that originate from the myotomes. These nuclei form a "somatic efferent column," which extends from the myelencephalon to the mesencephalon. The myelencephalon contains the nucleus of origin of the hypoglossal nerve (12th cranial nerve). The metencephalon contains the abducens nucleus (6th cranial nerve). Both nuclei are localized close to the midline; functionally they are pure motor nuclei and their nerve fibers are general somatic efferent (GSE) fibers (Fig. 5–3).

Other efferent nuclei are the so-called general visceral efferent (GVE) nuclei, such as the dorsal nucleus of the vagus nerve, the inferior salivatory nucleus (glossopharyngeal nerve) and, in the metencephalon, the superior salivatory nucleus (facial nerve). The fibers that arise from these nuclei (GVE fibers) are part of the autonomic nervous system and innervate smooth muscles, the heart muscle, and glands. Characteristic features of the rhombencephalon are a new kind of efferent nuclei (not present in the spinal cord), which are involved in the innervation of skeletal muscles of branchial origin. These are the special visceral efferent (SVE) nuclei. Examples are the nucleus ambiguus, the nucleus of the facial nerve, and the motor nucleus of the trigeminal nerve (the last two in the metencephalon). Special visceral efferent (branchiomotor) fibers arise from these nuclei (Fig. 5–3).

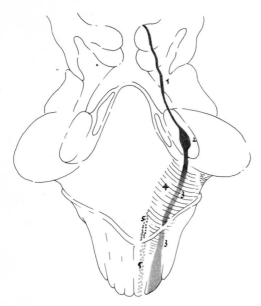

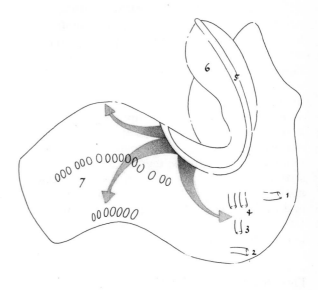

Figure 5–4 Afferent nuclei of the cranial nerves. The relay nuclei of the trigeminal nerve are indicated in solid black (GSA), the vestibular and the acoustic area (SSA) are hatched, and the solitary nucleus (GVA and SVA) is indicated by small circles.

1 nucleus of mesencephalic tract of trigeminal nerve
2 principal nucleus of trigeminal nerve
3 nucleus of spinal tract of trigeminal nerve
4 vestibular area
5 solitary nucleus

Figure 5–5 Migration of neuroblasts from the rhombic lip.

1 trigeminal nerve
2 abducens nerve
3 facial nerve
4 vestibulocochlear nerve
5 insertion of tela choroidea of fourth ventricle
6 cerebellum
7 myelencephalon

ALAR PLATE

In the alar plate the sensory relay nuclei of the branchial arch nerves are found lateral to the sulcus limitans. Examples are the solitary nucleus, where sensory fibers from the viscera (GVA fibers) and gustatory fibers of the tongue and palate (SVA fibers) terminate (Fig. 5–4). Lateral to the solitary nucleus, the nucleus of the spinal tract of the trigeminal nerve develops, where sensory fibers from the facial region (GSA fibers) terminate. Quite lateral in the alar plate, beneath the lateral recess of the fourth ventricle, the relay nuclei of the vestibulocochlear nerve arise, where afferent fibers from the vestibular and cochlear ganglia terminate (special somatic afferent, SSA fibers).

Migration of Neuroblasts

It has been known since His published his findings (1890) that the neuroblasts migrate during ontogenesis. According to Hamburger and Levi-Montalcini (1950), three types of cell migration can be distinguished: (a) migration of undifferentiated neuroblasts to the ventricular zone (preparatory to mitosis), (b) migration of neuroblasts from the ventricular to the intermediate zone, and (c) migration of young neurons to their final position.

The development of the olivary nuclei (myelencephalon) and the pontine nuclei (metencephalon) is a good example of cell migration. The cells from which these nuclei arise are originally localized in the area of the myelencephalic rhombic lip, that is, within the angle between the edge of the lateral recess of the fourth ventricle and the insertion of the tela choroidea (Fig. 5–5). From this site, the cells arrange themselves to form a thin layer immediately beneath the surface. Next, they migrate to the pontine flexure but retain their superficial position (Essick,

1912). At the level of the trigeminal nerve (Fig. 5–5) the two streams of migrating cells curve to the midline and unite. These cells form the pontine nucleus. The olivary nucleus complex likewise arises from cells that originate in the rhombic lip of the myelencephalon.

Differentiation of the Metencephalon

The metencephalon differs from the myelencephalon in the marked development of the dorsolateral parts of the alar plates (rhombic lip), from which the cerebellum is to develop. Another difference lies in the formation of a large system (middle cerebellar peduncle or brachium pontis) of transverse fiber bundles in the basal part of the tegmentum. These pontocerebellar fibers form a new system, which is superimposed beneath the phylogenetically older tegmental tracts.

DEVELOPMENT OF THE CEREBELLUM

In embryos of about 8 mm, the cerebellum is indicated by a bilateral thickening of the rostral edges of the rhomboid fossa (Fig. 5–6). As the curvature of the pontine flexure becomes more acute, these edges ("labia metencephali"*) assume a more and more transverse position. They are initially separated by the marginal incisure (Fig. 5–6), but soon the medial parts of the labia come closer together until they fuse in the midline. The metencephalic edge of the rhomboid fossa now forms a transverse ridge (cerebellar plate). The lateral parts of the labia grow so fast that their inside seems to turn out (eversion of the cerebellum). In relation to the insertion of the tela choroidea, the cerebellar plate can now be divided into an intraventricular and an extraventricular part (Fig. 5–7). The latter grows much faster and consequently the entire

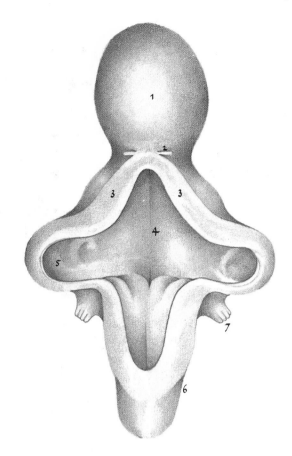

Figure 5–6 Dorsal view of the rhomboid fossa in a human embryo of 14 mm (according to Hochstetter).

1 mesencephalon
2 trochlear nerve
3 labium metencephali
4 fourth ventricle
5 lateral recess
6 medulla oblongata
7 facial nerve and vestibulocochlear nerve

cerebellar primordium turns downward on its transverse axis. The insertion of the tela choroidea changes its position: it now attaches to the undersurface of the cerebellar plate, the future inferior medullary velum.

Two phases are distinguished in the development of the cerebellum: the phase of the cerebellar plate and the phase of cerebellar fissuration. In the first phase the cerebellum consists of a transverse bank with a narrow central part (the vermis) and two slightly thickened lateral parts (the future hemispheres). At this

---

*The designation "labium metencephali" ("rhombic lip," "Rautenlippe") is rather confusing. We define the term as denoting the dorsolateral edge of the neuroepithelial layer of the alar plate, quite near the transition to the tela chorioidea.

fissure separates the nodulus from the uvula and the flocculus from the hemisphere (Fig. 5–8).

The region cranial to the posterolateral fissure constitutes by far the largest portion of the cerebellum in primates. In embryos of about 70 mm, a transverse groove appears in the corpus cerebelli, dividing it into anterior and posterior lobes. This groove (primary fissure) becomes the deepest fissure of the adult cerebellum. Soon afterward other grooves appear in the surface and divide the corpus cerebelli into a number of lobules. All of these grooves make their first appearance in the medial (vermian) region, gradually extending laterally into the hemispheres.

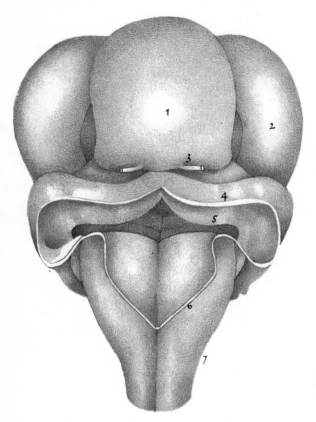

Figure 5–7 Reconstruction of cerebellum and fourth ventricle of an embryo of about 27 mm (according to Hochstetter). The cerebellar plate covers most of the rhomboid fossa in the metencephalon.

1 mesencephalon
2 hemispheric vesicle
3 trochlear nerve
4 extraventricular part of cerebellar plate
5 intraventricular part of cerebellar plate
6 cut edge of roof of fourth ventricle
7 medulla oblongata

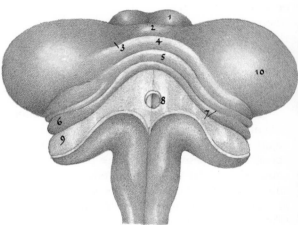

Figure 5–8 Roof of the fourth ventricle in a fetus of about 120 mm (according to Hochstetter). Start of cerebellar fissuration; the cerebellar hemispheres are well developed.

1 tectum
2 culmen
3 primary fissure
4 pyramid
5 uvula
6 flocculus
7 posterolateral fissure
8 foramen of Magendie (median aperture of fourth ventricle)
9 lateral recess of fourth ventricle
10 cerebellar hemisphere

time the entire structure shows a smooth surface. Cerebellar fissuration starts in the fourth month with a transverse groove known as the posterolateral fissure. This fissure separates the thickened rhombic lip (future flocculus) from the rest of the cerebellum (corpus cerebelli). Fusion of both flocculi at the median line gives rise to the nodulus. The two flocculi and the nodulus together with the rostrally growing fibers of the vestibular nerve constitute the flocculonodular lobe, phylogenetically the oldest part of the cerebellum with mainly vestibular connections. The posterolateral

Histogenesis of the Cerebellar Cortex

During the second month of development the primordium of the cerebellum consists of a ventricular, an intermediate, and a marginal zone. After the 14th week, mitotic activity in the ventricular zone diminishes. In fetuses of 19 weeks, the cerebellar cortex has an outer granular layer followed by a poorly cellularized zone (Fig. 5–9A), which can be regarded as the primordium of the future molecular layer. Beneath this primordium there is a dense population of cells that is not readily separable from the intermediate zone.

In fetuses of 21 weeks, the cerebellar cortex consists of five layers. The principal changes occur in the densified area beneath the molecular layer. As a result of the formation of a new acellular zone (Hayashi's lamina dissecans), a new layer of cells is separated from the intermediate zone (Fig. 5–9B). The sequence of layers at this time is (1) outer granular layer, (2) molecular layer, (3) dense layer of cells above the lamina dissecans, (4) lamina dissecans, and (5) intermediate zone. In later stages, the third layer becomes the Purkinje cell layer and the fifth layer broadens.

Factors contributing to the formation of the definitive cerebellar cortex include migration of cells from the outer granular layer and regression of the lamina dissecans. The cells of the outer granular layer migrate to deeper levels and pass the layer of Purkinje cells; this migration starts at about the 17th week. During migration the granular cells are fusiform. The cell nucleus is guided by the radial processes of Bergmann's glial cells. Several granular cells slide in succession down the same glial process to the level of the nucleus of the glia cell, where they leave their "slide path" and settle in the new inner granular layer. After the migration of the granular cells, a poorly cellularized molecular layer remains. The lamina dissecans consists of a rich plexus of terminal axons and primitive dendrites of immature Purkinje cells. The regression of this layer causes the Purkinje cells to come into contact with the new inner granular layer.

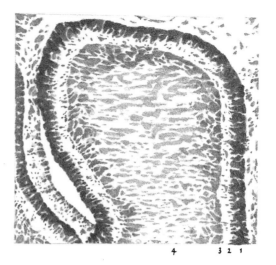

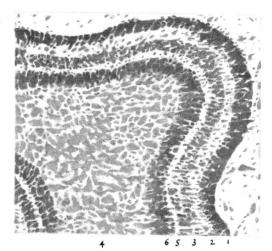

Figure 5–9 Composition of the cerebellar cortex. Cortical layers in a fetus of 19 weeks (A) and one of 21 weeks (B) (according to Rakič-Sidman).

1   outer granular layer
2   poorly cellularized zone
3   densified outer surface of the intermediate zone (future layer of Purkinje cells)
4   intermediate zone
5   lamina dissecans
6   new inner granular layer

Ontogenesis of the Cerebellar Nuclei

The cerebellar nuclei (dentate, globose, fastigial, and emboliform) arise from the intermediate zone. These nuclei differentiate earlier than the cells of the cortex. The cerebellar nuclei give rise to most of the efferent fibers of the cerebellum.

Chapter 6

The Mesencephalon

Ontogenetically, the mesencephalon can be regarded as a continuation of the rhombencephalon. However, the alar plates do not evert laterally and the roof plate is not elongated. The walls are markedly thickened and consequently the lumen is reduced to a narrow canal, the aqueduct of Sylvius. The marginal layer of the basal plate expands grossly as a result of the development of the long nerve pathways. These systems, macroscopically visible in humans, can be observed in the most ventral part of the mesencephalon, where they form the crura cerebri.

The basal plate and alar plate are readily identifiable in cross-sections. The aqueduct is surrounded by the central gray matter, a layer of small fusiform cells with many unmyelinated fibers.

Basal Plate.   Immediately next to the midline, the column of somatic efferent cells (trochlear nerve, oculomotor nerve) consists of cells that innervate the extrinsic striated ocular muscles. Lateral to it is the column of general visceral efferent nuclei from which parasympathetic fibers arise to innervate the intrinsic ocular muscles (Fig. 6–1). Other neuroblasts of the basal plate develop into neurons of the reticular formation of the tegmentum. Some nuclei (red nucleus) are regarded as partly derived from ventrally migrated cells of the alar plate. The development of the substantia nigra is still unclear.

The fibers of the oculomotor nerve pass through the red nucleus and through the medial part of the substantia nigra and, via the medial surface of the crura cerebri, leave the mesencephalon. The fibers of the trochlear nerve, however, circumvent the cerebral aqueduct and leave the CNS on its *dorsal* surface. The exceedingly strange course of the fibers is still an enigma.

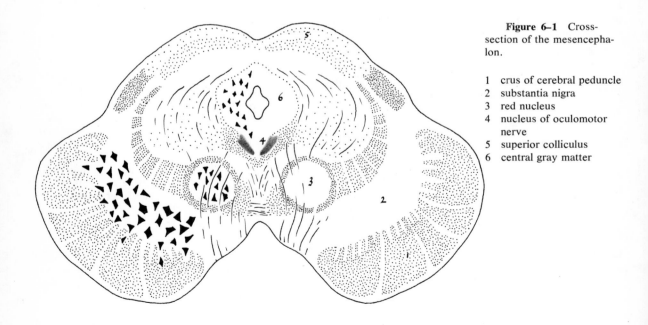

Figure 6–1 Cross-section of the mesencephalon.

1   crus of cerebral peduncle
2   substantia nigra
3   red nucleus
4   nucleus of oculomotor nerve
5   superior colliculus
6   central gray matter

Alar Plate. From the alar plate, the tectum develops and, as a result of the irregular proliferation of cells, is soon divided into the superior and inferior colliculi (Fig. 6–1). The superior colliculi are centers with a layered structure because the neuroblasts that have migrated from the ventricular zone arrange themselves in layers (the deeper layers being formed first). The inferior colliculi are less distinctly stratified; these nuclei serve as synaptic stations for the auditory reflexes. The superior colliculi are subcortical centers of integration for the visual system.

Chapter 7

The Prosencephalon

After closure of the anterior neuropore (see Fig. 4–3), the structure of the prosencephalon does not differ much from that of the remainder of the neural tube. A transverse section shows fairly thick lateral walls connected by the much thinner roof plate and floor plate. On the outside one observes the ocular cup, attached to the prosencephalon by the ocular pedicle (Fig. 4–3). This simple configuration, however, soon changes as a result of the development of the hemispheric vesicles (page 40).

The hemispheres are already clearly distinguishable in embryos of 12 mm. The caudal part of a hemispheric vesicle is continuous with the diencephalon (hemispheric pedicle); in dorso-cranial direction the hemisphere is separated from the diencephalon by the telediencephalic sulcus (see Fig. 4–4). In mediorostral direction the hemispheric vesicles merge into the telencephalon medium.

The anterior neuropore closes rostral to the primordium of the hemispheres. The anterior wall of the third ventricle, rostral to the interventricular foramen, is therefore regarded as part of the telencephalon medium. The space of the unpaired telencephalon medium is the ventriculus impar. The mature third ventricle comprises the ventriculus impar and the original third ventricle.

The Dorsal Wall of the Prosencephalon

The roof of the third ventricle becomes a thin epithelial membrane, the lamina choroidea epithelialis of the third ventricle. This membrane

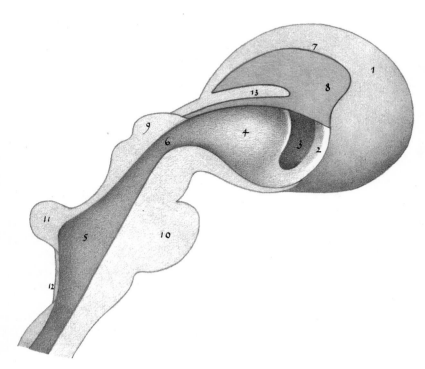

Figure 7–1 Schematic representation of the left cerebral hemisphere of a human embryo (according to Tandler, modified).

1 hemispheric vesicle
2 telencephalon medium
3 interventricular foramen
4 third ventricle
5 fourth ventricle
6 cerebral aqueduct
7 tenia fornicis
8 lamina chorioidea epithelialis of lateral ventricle
9 tectum
10 pons
11 cerebellum
12 lamina choroidea of fourth ventricle
13 lamina choroidea of third ventricle

continues above the interventricular foramen along the medial wall of the hemispheres, thus giving rise to a swallow-shaped weak spot in the roof of the prosencephalon (Fig. 7–1). The lines of attachment of the epithelial layer to the thicker wall of the prosencephalon are called teniae.

The anterior boundary of the lamina choroidea epithelialis of the third ventricle is determined by the paraphysis. From this point, the lamina extends as far as the habenular commissure (see Fig. 9–8).

The Rostral Wall of the Telencephalon

The rostral wall of the telencephalon medium (see Fig. 9–8) is the anterior boundary of the ventriculus impar. This median area extends between the plate of the chiasm and the paraphysis. Like His (1904) and Rakič and Yakovlev (1968), we distinguish a ventral lamina terminalis and a rapidly thickening dorsal lamina reuniens (Fig. 9–8), which is of great importance for the development of the cerebral commissures.

Histogenesis of the Diencephalon

The division of the diencephalon into a basal plate and an alar plate is a subject of scientific discussion. The question of whether the sulcus limitans continues in the diencephalon is controversial (Richter, 1965). There are indeed grooves in the wall of the third ventricle (median and ventral diencephalic sulci), but the significance of these grooves is uncertain.

Studies by Herrick (1910, 1933), Kuhlenbeck (1929, 1930), Richter (1965), and others have revealed that the diencephalon comprises several superimposed levels. The boundaries between these areas are indicated by structural changes related to the mitotic activity of the ventricular zone; laterally, these boundaries gradually become less sharply defined (Fig. 7–2). In any case, the aforementioned sulci indicate the boundaries of the various parts of the ventricular zone fairly accurately.

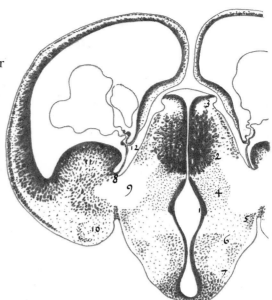

Figure 7–2 Transverse section through the prosencephalon of an embryo of about 37 mm (12 to 13 weeks). Note the marked proliferation of cells of the dorsal thalamus; the mitotic activity in the subthalamus and the ventral thalamus has already taken place and is now minimal (according to Richter).

1	hypothalamic sulcus
2	dorsal thalamus
3	epithalamus
4	ventral thalamus
5	external pallidum
6	subthalamus
7	hypothalamus
8	terminal sulcus
9	internal capsule
10	amygdala
11	striatum
12	choroid fissure

STRUCTURAL DIVISION

Five "levels" are distinguishable in the diencephalon.

Hypothalamus. This area is characterized by a thin ventricular zone. Mitotic activity and migration of neuroblasts are moderate.

Subthalamus. This level shows a ventricular zone with numerous mitoses; large numbers of neuroblasts migrate early to the intermediate zone. The subthalamus gives rise to the corpus subthalamicum, the nucleus entopeduncularis, and the pallidum.

Ventral Thalamus. This area is localized between the ventral diencephalic sulcus (hypothalamic sulcus) and the median diencephalic sulcus. The migration of neuroblasts attains its

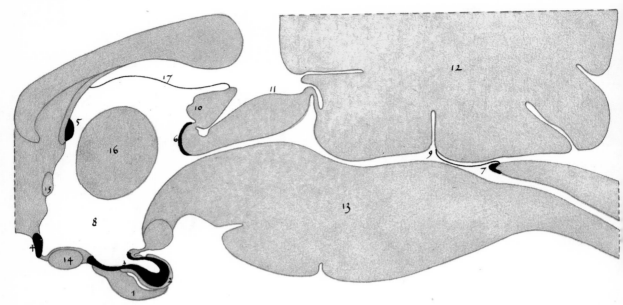

Figure 7–3 Median section through the brain of a mature cat *(Felix domestica);* localization of the circumventricular organs (according to Duvernoy).

1 adenohypophysis (pars distalis)
2 pars intermedia
3 neurohypophysis
4 vascular organ lamina terminalis
5 subfornical organ
6 subcommissural organ
7 area postrema
8 third ventricle
9 fourth ventricle
10 pineal body (epiphysis cerebri)
11 mesencephalic tectum
12 cerebellum
13 brain stem
14 optic chiasm
15 anterior commissure
16 connexus interthalamicus (massa intermedia)
17 roof of third ventricle

maximum during the seventh week. After the migration, the ventricular zone remains fairly thick. The ventral thalamus gives rise to the lateral reticular nucleus and the lateral geniculate body.

Dorsal Thalamus. This is what is usually meant by "thalamus." The migration of neuroblasts starts late (14th week) but is very extensive. This area will show the strongest growth and exceed all other levels in size.

Epithalamus. The highest level in the diencephalon remains almost rudimentary. The ventricular zone shows few mitoses; this area gives rise to the habenular nucleus, localized quite near the attachment of the pineal body. This pineal body (epiphysis cerebri) and two commissures — the habenular and the posterior commissure — also develop in the epithalamic area (see Fig. 9–8).

This outline of the structural design of the diencephalon applies particularly to the early stages of development. In the course of the third month, important changes occur as a result of the further development of the migrated cell populations. The subthalamus is gradually detached from the ventricular wall and assumes a position lateral to the hypothalamus. The derivatives of the ventral thalamus also lose contact with the ventricular wall. By the fourth month, the structural pattern has changed entirely and already closely resembles that of the mature diencephalon.

MORPHOLOGY OF THE CIRCUMVENTRICULAR ORGANS

The circumventricular organs (Hofer, 1958) are small, well defined areas of the wall of the

ventricles, distinguished by a particular structure. These organs have some structural characteristics in common and can therefore be brought
under a common denominator (Fig. 7–3). The
circumventricular organs include the following
structures: neurohypophysis, pineal body, vascular organ of the lamina terminalis, subfornical
organ, subcommissural organ, and area postrema. The area postrema is localized in the fourth
ventricle, whereas all other circumventricular
organs are found in the third ventricle.

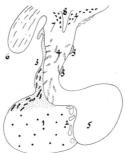

Figure 7–4 Sagittal section through a human hypophysis.

1 adenohypophysis
2 pars intermedia
3 pars tuberalis
4 infundibulum
5 infundibular process
6 optic chiasm
7 infundibular nucleus
8 infundibular recess

Neurohypophysis

The neurohypophysis arises from a morphologically specialized area of the floor of the
diencephalon. In embryos of about four weeks,
that part of the floor that is intercalated between
the plate of the chiasm and the premamillary area
is a fairly thin, inactive area (Fig. 7–4). This area
is characterized by close contact with a part of
the ectoderm of the primitive oral roof that lies
immediately rostral to the buccopharyngeal
membrane. Owing to several factors (such as
pressure from the rapidly proliferating
chiasmic plate, and formation of the cephalic
flexure), the inactive area is passively stretched
to form a funnel-shaped evagination in the
surrounding mesenchyma, the infundibulum.

In early stages, no mesenchyma is admitted
between the infundibulum and oral roof ectoderm. The lack of mitoses in the infundibulum
does not inhibit its growth; this is insured by
migration of cells from adjacent areas and in-
growth of axons from the so-called hypophyseal
nuclei (see page 271).

The lumen of the infundibular recess extends to the midportion of the infundibulum.
Consequently a proximal, hollow part (pars cava
infundibuli) and a distal, solid part (pars compacta infundibuli) can be distinguished. The infundibular process of the neurohypophysis develops
from the distal part. .

Adenohypophysis

The adenohypophysis arises from Rathke's
pouch, an ectodermal evagination of the primitive oral roof (Fig. 7–4). In embryos of about 12

mm, this pouch extends between oral roof and
infundibulum; in embryos of about 22 mm, the
communication with the oral roof is lost. In some
cases a small part of the pouch persists in the
pharyngeal wall.

The cells of the anterior part of the pouch
show more marked proliferation than those of
the other parts and form the anterior lobe (pars
distalis). As the anterior lobe grows, the lumen of
the pouch is virtually obliterated. The posterior
wall of the pouch, which has always been in
contact with the infundibulum, develops to become the pars intermedia. From the rostral part
of the pars distalis, an extension grows around
the pedicle of the infundibulum; this is the pars
tuberalis in which the capillaries of the primary
plexus are localized (see page 276).

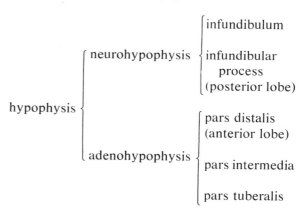

Almost the entire circumference of the
neurohypophysis is covered by parts of the adenohypophysis: the infundibulum by the pars tuberalis, and the infundibular process by the pars
intermedia (which in humans is not highly developed).

Pineal Body

The pineal body (epiphysis cerebri) begins as a thickening of the most caudal part of the roof plate of the diencephalon (see Fig. 9–8), and in maturity becomes a small solid organ lying on the roof of the mesencephalon. The surface turned to the third ventricle (Fig. 9–8) is lined with highly ciliated ependyma. Within the pineal body, septa of connective tissue divide it into follicles. The specific cells of the follicles are the pinealocytes (probably modified neurons); astroglia are found as well. Typical neurons (apart from a few stray autonomic nerve cells) are absent.

The pineal body is regarded as an endocrine organ involved in the regulation of gonadal functions. In adults, calcareous concretions (acervulus cerebri or brain sand) form in the pineal body; these concretions are roentgenographically visible.

Vascular Organ of the Lamina Terminalis

The lamina terminalis is a thin triangular plate closing the third ventricle; it is localized between the anterior commissure and the optic chiasm. The anterior side of the layer is covered by the anterior communicating artery and is in contact with the pia mater. The posterior side has an ependymal lining. Histologically, a distinction is made between the outer (superficial) and the inner (deep) lamina terminalis; the latter consists of glia fibers. A characteristic feature is the vascular plexus (vascular organ) of the lamina terminalis, which consists of a superficial and a deep network of capillaries. The superficial network receives blood from arterial branches of, among other vessels, the anterior communicating artery. This blood is then drained to the deep network, from which it reaches the anterior cerebral veins (Fig. 7–5). Many capillaries have an endothelium with pores.

Subfornical Organ

The subfornical organ is a hemispheric evagination of the wall of the third ventricle, localized between the fornix columns at the level of the interventricular foramen. Its ventricular surface is, for the most part, lined with ependymal cells that have many microvilli.

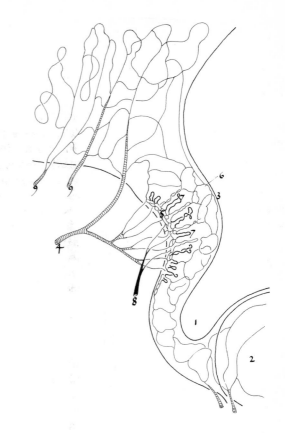

Figure 7–5 Vascularization of the vascular organ of the lamina terminalis (according to Duvernoy).

1. supraoptic recess
2. optic chiasm
3. lamina terminalis
4. preoptic artery
5. superficial capillary network
6. deep capillary network
7. long capillary loops
8. preoptic vein
9. anteromedial arteries

The organ comprises several types of nerve cells, glia cells, and special ependymal cells (tanycytes) that have a long peripheral extension. The subfornical organ is presumably involved in mechanisms of osmoregulation.

Area Postrema

This is a small area in the myelencephalic part of the fourth ventricle, immediately rostral to the obex (see Fig. 7–3). It consists of modified neurons, glia cells, and a complicated network of wide capillaries. The area postrema receives afferent fibers, which probably arise from the solitary nucleus. The functional significance of this area is still obscure; some investigators suggest that it may be involved in the vomiting reflex circuit.

General Characteristics of the Circumventricular Organs

All circumventricular organs have a few characteristics in common and thus seem to be components of a functional system rather than a group of separate, unrelated structures. These common characteristics are the following:

a) Special vascularization: Besides their own separate plexus, these organs have simple or complex capillary loops to which the peripheral processes of the tanycytes (see page 15) are attached.

b) The blood-brain barrier is absent: Substances injected into the blood stream very quickly enter the intercellular space of the circumventricular organs. This is probably explained by the fact that these capillaries have pores.

c) All circumventricular organs are immediately adjacent to the CSF.

d) Part of the ependyma of these organs consists of specialized ependymal cells (tanycytes), which could function as a "bridge" between the CSF and the blood that circulates in the capillary network.

Chapter 8

The Telencephalon

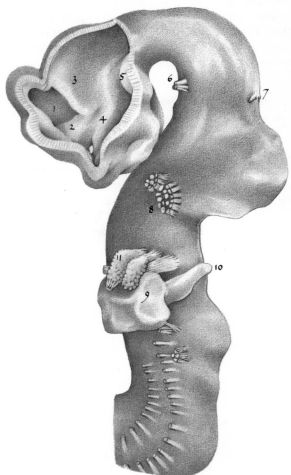

During the sixth week the hemispheric pedicle (transition between the thalamus and the basal part of the hemispheric wall) rapidly thickens to form the corpus striatum. The increase in volume of the corpus striatum makes an important contribution to the reduction in size of the interventricular foramen (Fig. 8–1). The remainder of the wall of the brain vesicle initially remains thin (pallium). From this, the major part of the cerebral cortex (isocortex) develops. The pallium expands eccentrically in relation to the hemispheric pedicle; the cortex on the lateral side of the corpus striatum (the insula of Reil) does not expand and is later covered by adjacent cortical areas (the frontal and the temporal opercula). These opercula completely hide the insula from view by the time of birth.

In the rapidly growing pallium, an anteriorly oriented part (frontal lobe) can be distinguished from a superiorly oriented part (parietal lobe) and a posteriorly oriented part (occipital lobe and temporal lobe) (Fig. 8–2). The diencephalon, and later the mesencephalon, is completely covered by the hemispheres. The occipital lobe (part of the temporal lobe) comes to lie above the cerebellum, from which it is separated by a duplicature of the pia mater, the tentorium cerebelli, to which the falx cerebri attaches.

Figure 8–1   Lateral view of the brain of a human embryo of 11 mm (according to Hochstetter).

1	interventricular foramen
2	corpus striatum
3	thalamus
4	para optica hypothalami
5	pars mamillaris hypothalami
6	oculomotor nerve
7	trochlear nerve
8	trigeminal nerve
9	otic vesicle
10	endolymphatic duct
11	acoustic ganglion

40

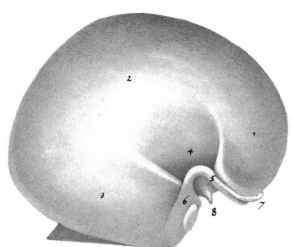

Figure 8–2 Lateral surface of the right hemisphere in a fetus of about 100 mm; the opercula overgrow the insula of Reil (according to Hochstetter).

1	frontal lobe
2	parietal lobe
3	temporal lobe
4	insula
5	olfactory tract
6	lateral olfactory stria
7	olfactory bulb
8	optic nerve

TENIAE AND LAMINA AFFIXA

The choroid area can be easily excised, leaving a mural defect that is demarcated by two parallel cut edges. The upper edge follows the underside of the hippocampus (tenia fornicis), while the lower one follows the medial boundary of the caudate nucleus (tenia choroidea). The two teniae merge posteriorly. The tenia choroidea continues through the interventricular foramen as tenia thalami (Fig. 8–3). In later stages the tenia fornicis attaches to the lateral, fairly sharp margin of the fornix (Fig. 8–3). The tenia choroidea moves medially until it is localized on the dorsal surface of the thalamus (Fig. 8–4). This is achieved in that a part of the rudimentary wall medial to the sulcus terminalis (infrachoroid layer) is everted and adheres to the dorsal surface of the thalamus (lamina affixa). This displacement is largely a result of the growth of the thalamus.

Choroid Fissure

As already mentioned, one part of the medial wall of the hemisphere remains restricted to a layer of ependymal cells, covered on the outside with mesenchyma (choroid area). This rudimentary part of the wall continues at the level of the interventricular foramen into the roof of the third ventricle (see Fig. 7–1).

Owing to the posterior growth of the hemisphere, the choroid area is extended posteriorly and ultimately forms parts of the medial wall of the inferior horn of the lateral ventricle. The choroid area is invaginated by highly vascularized mesenchyma so that the capillary villi appear to become localized inside the lateral ventricles. The double line along which this mesenchyma has entered is the *choroid fissure*.

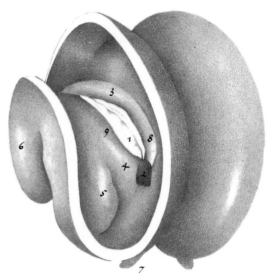

Figure 8–3 Dorsal view of the striatum in a fetus of 46 mm; the suprastriatal part of the cortex has been removed (according to Hochstetter).

1	lamina choroidea
2	interventricular foramen
3	hippocampus
4	medial corpus striatum
5	lateral corpus striatum
6	lateral fissure
7	olfactory bulb
8	tenia fornicis
9	tenia choroidea

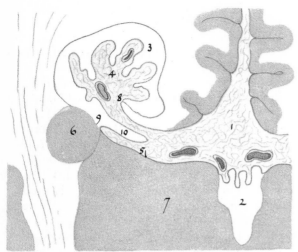

Figure 8–4 Formation of the lamina affixa. The lamina infrachoroidea is everted and fuses with the upper surface of the thalamus.

1	velum interpositum
2	third ventricle
3	lateral ventricle
4	choroid plexus
5	future tenia choroidea
6	caudate nucleus
7	thalamus
8	tenia fornicis
9	sulcus terminalis (original tenia choroidea)
10	lamina infrachoroidea

CHOROID PLEXUS

The plexus of the lateral ventricle extends from the interventricular foramen to the inferior horn of the lateral ventricle. The anterior and posterior horns are free from plexus. The interventricular foramen connects this plexus to that of the third ventricle. The CSF produced in the lateral ventricles flows through the interventricular foramen and, together with the CSF produced in the third ventricle, passes through the aqueduct to the fourth ventricle and hence, through the apertures in the roof, to the subarachnoid space.

Development of the Corpus Striatum: Caudate Nucleus and Putamen

In embryos of about 15 mm, the dorsocaudal part of the hemispheric pedicle rapidly thickens. Soon, the thickened part protrudes into the lumen of the lateral ventricle and into that of the interventricular foramen. This part is the corpus striatum, in which two (more anteriorly, three) striatal ridges are distinguishable, the medial and the lateral corpus striata. The entire structure grows quickly and, as a result of the posterior curving of the hemisphere, assumes a horseshoe shape (Fig. 8–3). Medially, the sulcus terminalis marks the boundary between thalamus and corpus striatum.

As a result of the growth of the hemispheric vesicle posteriorly and laterally around the interventricular foramen, the corpus striatum is extended and bent (Fig. 8–3). The elongated caudal area of the caudate nucleus changes its position in relation to the inferior horn of the lateral ventricle: at the interventricular foramen its position is ventrolateral, whereas in the temporal lobe it is dorsomedial to the ventricular space.

At the level of the interventricular foramen (Fig. 8–5), the striatum is divided by an increasing number of nerve fibers (internal capsule) into a dorsomedial (caudate nucleus) and a ventrolateral (putamen) part during the seventh week. A thin layer of nerve fibers (external capsule) separates the putamen from the claustrum on the lateral side. Anteriorly, the caudate nucleus and the putamen remain in part joined because the fibers of the internal capsule do not extend so far rostrally.

The amygdaloid body and the tail of the caudate nucleus arise from the lateral corpus striatum; the head of the caudate nucleus and the putamen develop from the three anterior parts of the corpus striatum (Hewitt, 1961).

INTERNAL CAPSULE

The medial and the lateral corpus striata continue down the depth of the hemispheric pedicle as the medial and the lateral layers of cells (Fig. 8–5B). The fibers of the internal capsule first appear in embryos of 15 mm as a small bundle near the medial layer. In embryos of 35 mm, the capsule has grown to become a thick fibrous layer that traverses the lamellae to the diencephalon. The internal capsule contains an enormous number of afferent and efferent fibers that connect the cerebral cortex with the lower parts of the CNS.

MIGRATIONS OF STRIATAL CELLS TO THE DIENCEPHALON

Studies by Rakič and Sidman (1969) have shown that the striatal primordium can be regarded as a highly mitotic area from which cells migrate to the thalamus. The stream of migrating cells dips around the floor of the sulcus terminalis and extends to its final destination in the pulvinar of the thalamus. This means that the thalamus should in part be of telencephalic origin.

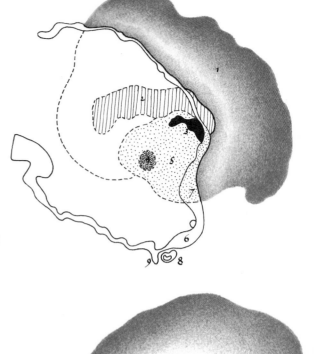

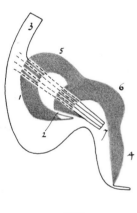

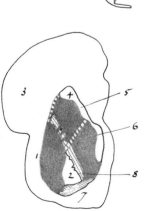

Figure 8–5 Schematic representation of the early development of the internal capsule (according to Hewitt). The medial and the lateral corpus striatum continue down as lamina medialis and lamina lateralis. The laminae are cut off by the ingrowing fibers of the internal capsule.

A
1 putamen
2 pallidum
3 cerebral cortex
4 thalamus
5 lateral corpus striatum
6 medial corpus striatum
7 internal capsule

B
1 putamen
2 pallidum
3 cerebral cortex
4 lateral ventricle
5 lateral corpus striatum
6 medial corpus striatum
7 anterior commissure
8 internal capsule

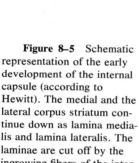

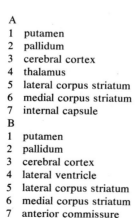

Figure 8–6 Reconstruction of the prosencephalon. The left hemisphere is seen from the inside; the hemispheric pedicle has been cut. Note the development and migration of the fibers of the internal capsule. A is 24 mm, B is 41 mm (according to Sharp).

1 hemispheric vesicle
2 epithelial choroid area
3 interventricular foramen
4 internal capsule
5 hemispheric pedicle
6 optic chiasm
7 lamina terminalis
8 adenohypophysis (Rathke's pouch)
9 infundibulum

GROWTH OF THE HEMISPHERIC PEDICLE

The increase in size of the hemispheric pedicle required to allow the passage of the increasingly numerous fibers of the internal capsule may be achieved either by fusion of the medial wall of the hemispheric vesicle with the lateral wall of the diencephalon (see Fig. 4–2) or by thickening of the transition zone between the diencephalon and telencephalon without fusion.

Studies by Sharp (1959) have confirmed the old hypotheses advanced by Schwalbe (1880) and Hochstetter (1895), postulating that no fusion occurs; the rapid growth of the surface of the hemispheric pedicle does coincide with the first appearance of the fibers of the internal capsule. This is an argument in favor of Hochstetter's view, for otherwise the superficial growth should precede the development of the fibers (Fig. 8–6)

Chapter 9

Histogenesis of the Cerebral Cortex

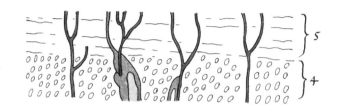

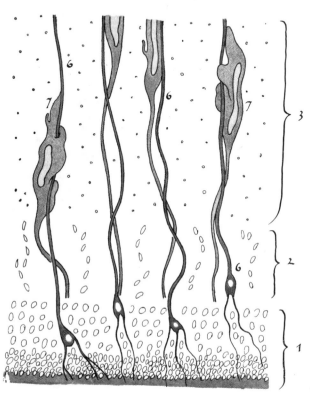

The histogenesis of the cerebral cortex shows distinct similarities to that of the cerebellum and is characterized by frequent migrations of cells. In early stages the wall of the telencephalic vesicle consists of a pseudostratified neuroepithelium; the cells are oblong and extend throughout the thickness of the wall.

Migration of the Neuroblasts

Cell divisions take place in the ventricular and later in the subventricular zone, as in the spinal cord. According to Berry and Rogers (1965) the daughter nucleus, after mitosis, migrates within the cytoplasm of the neuroepithelial parent cell toward the pial surface, where *cytoplasmic* division occurs. The migrating neuroblasts accumulate in a layer parallel to the pial surface (cortical plate). This cortical plate appears at about the seventh week and constitutes the primordium of the *isocortex* (Fig. 9–2). After the tenth week the first wave of migration from the ventricular zone ceases. At the same time, numerous nerve fibers appear in the intermediate zone, which thickens markedly.

A second long wave of migration begins between the 13th and the 15th week. These cells originate probably in the zona subventricularis. This time, the immature neuroblasts en route to

Figure 9–1 Migration of neuroblasts to the outer surface of the brain vesicle, guided by the extensions of glia cells.

1 ventricular zone
2 subventricular zone
3 intermediate zone
4 cortical plate
5 marginal zone
6 extensions of glia cells
7 migrating neuroblasts

the cortical plate need the assistance of long, radially arranged processes of glia cells because they must go a much longer way through the strongly thickened intermediate zone. At these late stages the neuroblasts migrate indeed in contact with long processes of glia cells (Fig. 9–1), which they use as pathways of ascent.

45

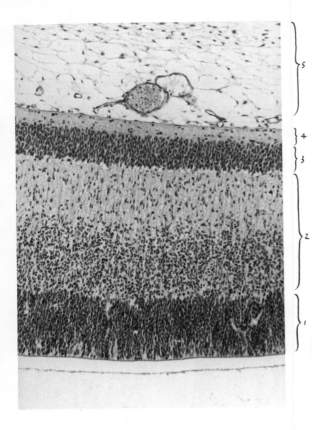

After the 18th week the ventricular zone has been exhausted and is reduced to a thin epithelial lining of the ventricular space. The cortical layer, on the other hand, has become much thicker and shows distinct stratification. The original marginal zone becomes the molecular (plexiform) layer of the definitive cortex; layers 2 through 5 develop from the cortical plate itself. The sixth cortical layer develops from the outside of the intermediate zone. The intermediate zone is occupied by numerous afferent and efferent fibers that connect the cortex to other regions of the CNS (white matter of the hemisphere).

Regional Structural Differences in the Cerebral Cortex

The above described developmental mechanisms lead to the formation of a cortical plate from which a six-layered structure develops (the

Figure 9–2 Suprastriatal part of the cortex in an embryo of 30 mm. The cortical plate is well developed and the ventricular zone very active (magnification, 141 ×).

1 ventricular and subventricular zone
2 intermediate zone
3 cortical plate
4 marginal zone
5 pia mater

These glial processes can be used simultaneously by several successive neuroblasts.

Neuroblasts that have arrived via a particular glial process remain arranged in vertical columns; this applies especially to the "sensory" areas of the cerebral cortex. The late neurons slide past the already present neurons of the cortical plate and ultimately arrange themselves peripheral to their predecessors. The neurons that arrive in the cortex first are displaced to deeper levels by those that arrive later. The cortical plate thickens owing to the constant migration of neuroblasts and sharply demarcates itself from the adjacent marginal zone.

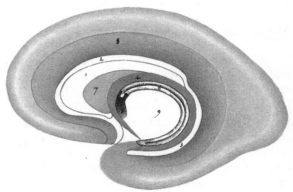

Figure 9–3 Medial aspect of the hemisphere in an embryo of about 65 mm; topography of the archicortex (according to Tandler).

1 corpus callosum
2 indusium griseum (supracallosal gyrus)
3 dentate gyrus
4 hippocampus and fornix
5 interventricular foramen
6 choroid area (fissure)
7 septum pellucidum
8 cingulum
9 wall of third ventricle (edges not shown)

isocortex). This is localized in the suprastriatal part of the hemisphere and encompasses about 94 per cent of the cortex in the adult brain. Other parts of the cortex more or less differ from the isocortex in structure and developmental history; these parts are collectively known as *allocortex*. There are two main types: the archicortex and the paleocortex. Both show a similar two-layered structure with a superficial fibrous layer (stratum moleculare) and a deep layer of pyramidal cells, which is often divided into two sublayers. The entire structure is arranged as follows:

lamina I	1	stratum moleculare
lamina II	2	stratum pyramidale (layer of pyramidal cells)
	3	stratum multiforme (layer of polymorphic cells), which continues in the underlying white matter

ARCHICORTEX

The archicortex is the first part of the cerebral cortex to differentiate. It is localized in the medial wall of the hemisphere, between the choroid fissure and the hippocampal sulcus (sulcus of the corpus callosum). As the hemispheric vesicle grows posteriorly, the archicortex migrates farther and farther through the medial wall to the inferior horn of the lateral ventricle.

In the superior and anterior parts of the archicortex, and especially in the area above the corpus callosum (supracallosal gyrus), regressive changes occur. The caudal part (Fig. 9–3) differentiates to hippocampus (horn of Ammon), dentate gyrus, and subiculum. The hippocampus is the major structure of the archicortex. In the course of development it evaginates into the space of the temporal horn of the lateral ventricle and disappears from view in the depth of the hippocampal fissure (Fig. 9–3). The subiculum is the area of transition between the hippocampus and the parahippocampal gyrus.

In summary, the archicortex is a phyloge-

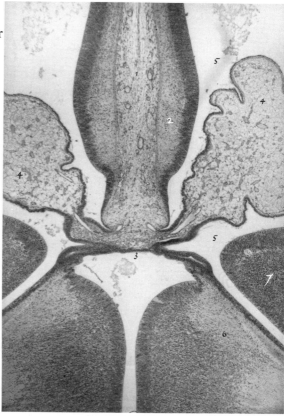

Figure 9–4 Floor of the longitudinal cerebral fissure and formation of the commissural mass in an embryo of 30 mm (magnification, 33.5 ×).

1 longitudinal cerebral fissure
2 hippocampus
3 roof of third ventricle (rostral part)
4 choroid plexus of lateral ventricle
5 lateral ventricle
6 thalamus
7 corpus striatum

netically old part of the cerebral cortex which develops around the choroid fissure. Histologically the archicortex consists of two layers of cells; the cranial part is rudimentary and forms a thin layer of gray matter above the corpus callosum. Rostrally, the supracallosal gyrus continues in the subcallosal gyrus and, via this gyrus, in the diagonal band of Broca. This diagonal band in turn continues in Giacomini's band (see Fig. 11–2), thus closing the archicortical ring. The

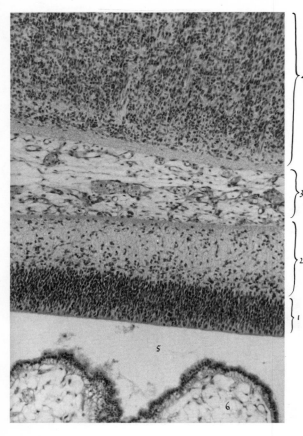

4

3

2

1

5

6

Figure 9–5 Allocortex in an embryo of 30 mm; note the absence of the cortical plate (magnification, 141 ×).

1 ventricular and subventricular zone
2 intermediate zone
3 pia mater
4 thalamus
5 lateral ventricle
6 choroid plexus

dentate gyrus extends around the splenium corporis callosi and finally merges into the supracallosal gyrus (indusium griseum) (Fig. 9–3).

Regarding the development of the archicortex it should be noted that the cortical plate does not appear until the fourth month, that is, three weeks later than in the isocortex. Moreover, the cortical plate is less rich in cells and less sharply defined from the intermediate zone. It is therefore not entirely comparable with the cortical plate of the isocortex (Fig. 9–4).

PALEOCORTEX

The primordium of the paleocortex lies in the area adjacent to the corpus striatum, in the basal wall of the hemispheric vesicle. The boundaries of the paleocortex are a controversial subject. It is generally assumed that the so-called primary olfactory cortex (prepiriform area and periamygdaloid area) is, in any case, part of the paleocortex.

Embryologically, the paleocortex is characterized by the *absence* of a cortical plate. This phylogenetically oldest type of cortex therefore differs maximally from the isocortex (Fig. 9–5).

DEFINITION OF A CORTEX

There are marked structural differences in the wall of the hemisphere, and it is therefore desirable to know which criteria must be fulfilled for any part of the brain shell to be defined as "cortex." According to Pigache (1970), the following criteria might be postulated: (1) the part should be composed of at least three layers: an outer fiber layer and two successive layers of cells; (b) the layers should be connected by radially arranged cell processes (columnar organization); and (c) there should be tangential as well as radial connections.

The purpose of the perpendicularly arranged types of connection is to organize the cells in vertical columns and to integrate the columns into a larger structure. Acceptance of this definition implies that a distinction be made between "mantle of the hemisphere" and "cortex": the mantle of the hemisphere is the shell of gray matter that lines the surface of the cerebrum; the cortex is gray matter structured in accordance with certain principles. Some areas of the olfactory part of the brain (rhinencephalon) do not have the structure of a "cortex" and should be regarded simply as superficial gray matter.

TOPOGRAPHY OF THE DIFFERENT CORTICES

A transverse section through the prosencephalon of a macrosmatic mammal (marsupial)

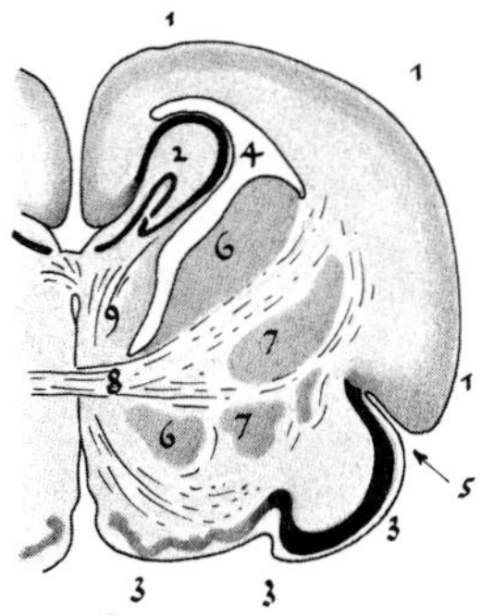

Figure 9–6 Topography of the three main constituents of the brain shell in the marsupial *Hyposiprimnus rufescens*. Note the absence of the corpus callosum (according to Beccari).

1 neopallium (neocortex)
2 archicortex, consisting of hippocampus (lateral) and dentate gyrus (medial)
3 paleopallium (piriform area)
4 lateral ventricle
5 rhinal sulcus
6 caudate nucleus
7 putamen
8 anterior commissure
9 septum

provides a survey of the localization of the three principal types of cortex.

The paleocortex occupies an important part of the ventrolateral area of the cerebral cortex (Fig. 9–6). Here, olfactory fibers that originate from the olfactory bulb and olfactory tubercle synapse and reach the paleocortex via the lateral olfactory stria. The rhinal sulcus separates the paleocortex from the isocortex (Fig. 9–6). The isocortex (neocortex, neopallium) is localized dorsolaterally, between the rhinal sulcus and the hippocampal sulcus. This part receives afferent fibers from the thalamus. The archicortex (hippocampal formation) forms a ring of gray matter around the choroid fissure on the medial side of the brain (Fig. 9–6). The hippocampal sulcus is adjacent to the isocortex.

Even in anosmatic mammals (whales) the hippocampal formation is well developed. This is one of several facts that warrant the conclusion that this structure can have little to do with the sense of smell.

Cerebral Commissures

Commissures are bundles of fibers that connect symmetric parts of the brain across the midline, ensuring the integration of the two hemispheres in a functional unit. The commissures of the telencephalon are the anterior commissure, the commissure of the fornix (fornical commissure), and the corpus callosum. The only site at which fibers from the telencephalon can cross the midline is the telencephalon medium with its derivatives, the lamina terminalis and the lamina reuniens (page 35). The former is a rather inactive, thin wall; the latter, localized rostral to the paraphysis, comprises a much thicker layer of cells that has been subjected to significant changes (such as formation of the commissures and development of septal nuclei).

The cells of the lamina reuniens form the structure through which the decussating fibers pass. The anterior commissure is the first commissure to develop. Its fibers cross the midline in the lower part of the lamina reuniens (septal area) in embryos of about 40 mm. The fibers of the hippocampal commissure and the corpus callosum cross the midline in the dorsal part of the lamina reuniens. In embryos of about 55 mm, decussating fibers can be observed in the floor of the longitudinal fissure, between the right and the left primordium of the fornix; these fibers constitute the fornical commissure.

In embryos of about 30 mm, morphologic changes in the dorsal part of the lamina reuniens begin to prepare for the development of the corpus callosum. The lamina is divided into two halves by a narrow median groove filled with mesenchymal tissue (Fig. 9–4). The walls of this groove (median sulcus of the telencephalon medium) fuse to form the "commissural mass," the area through which the fibers of the corpus callosum will pass. The commissural mass appears first in the dorsal area of the lamina reuniens, immediately anterior to the paraphysis. The medial walls of the hemispheres are therefore not involved in the formation of the commissural mass, but the walls of the lamina reuniens (telencephalon medium) are.

The corpus callosum is the principal commissure of the cerebral cortex; it connects the nonolfactory areas of the right cortex with those of the left. In embryos of 55 mm, the first fibers cross the midline via the commissural mass. The constant growth of the cerebral cortex causes the corpus callosum to expand rapidly, particularly

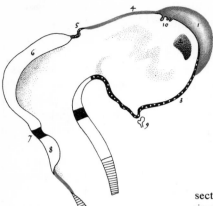

Figure 9–7 Sagittal section through the brain of an embryo of 9 mm.

1 hemispheric vesicle
2 interventricular fora-
men
3 lamina terminalis
4 roof of third ventricle
5 pineal body
6 mesencephalon (tec-
tum)
7 isthmus
8 metencephalon
9 hypophysis
10 paraphysis

Figure 9–8 Sagittal section through the brain of an embryo of 65 mm.

1 hemispheric vesicle
2 hippocampal sulcus
3 roof of third ventricle
4 habenular commissure
5 posterior commissure
6 pineal body
7 mesencephalon
8 corpus callosum
9 hippocampal commis-
sure
10 septum pellucidum
11 anterior commissure
12 interventricular fora-
men
13 optic chiasm
14 metencephalon
15 thalamus
16 lamina terminalis

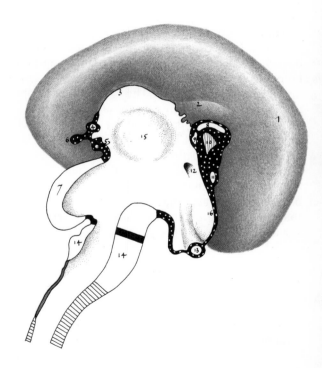

in a posterior direction where it overgrows the thin roof of the third ventricle (Fig. 9–8). This expansion of the corpus callosum reduces the commissural mass to a thin membrane, the septum pellucidum, which extends between the for-nix (below) and the corpus callosum (above). The space between the two leaves of the membrane is quite variable but certainly does not communicate with the ventricular system proper.

Chapter 10

Metabolic Factors in the Development of the Central Nervous System

The complex phenomena of differentiation and migration that characterize the development of the CNS presuppose a normal composition of the interior environment. Metabolic disorders such as malnutrition and hormonal dysfunctions might generally be expected to exert an unfavorable influence on development. Psychological studies in fact indicate that the intellectual achievements of children subjected to malnutrition in the first years of life are markedly diminished. Animal experiments have demonstrated with certainty that the CNS is extremely sensitive to metabolic disorders, especially during the first four weeks after birth. After this vulnerable period the effect of these disorders is less pronounced.

Various investigations have revealed that proliferation and differentiation of neuroblasts continue after birth, particularly in areas like the hippocampus, neocortex, and cerebellum, where vast numbers of young neurons develop. The migration and differentiation of these late neuroblasts could easily be influenced by malnutrition and hormonal disorders.

Malnutrition

It has been demonstrated in experiments on rats that, in malnutrition, the duration of DNA synthesis (S-phase), which precedes mitosis, is increased. This increase is largely canceled out, however, by a reduced duration of the G1-phase (period between the end of mitosis and the start of DNA synthesis), and consequently the total duration of the cycle of division remains virtually unchanged. In undernourished rats, the aforementioned reduction of the duration of G1-phase is especially marked on the first, sixth, and twelfth days after birth. According to Lewis et al. (1975), drastic reduction of this phase can have untoward consequences for the differentiation of the neurons. But malnutrition can also have another untoward effect on the development of the CNS. Calculations of the DNA content in the subventricular zone of the rat have shown that, in undernourished animals, the cell population in this zone was reduced by about 1.5 per cent on the sixth and the twelfth days after birth. The reduction in the cerebellum was even more marked (10 to 20 per cent of the cells of the outer granular layer).

The various cell types in the cerebellar cortex develop in a particular sequence: Golgi cells appear at about the time of birth, basket cells by about the sixth day, and star cells by about the twelfth day after birth; subsequently, large numbers of granular cells develop (about 50 per cent of the total). When malnutrition prevails during the first two weeks, it is in particular the inhibitory cortical cells (Golgi, basket, and star cells) that are affected; in more protracted malnutrition the (excitatory) granular cells are most affected. Consequently the neuronal circuits in the cerebellar cortex cannot develop normally.

It can be stated in summary that malnutrition during the first two weeks after birth causes not only a reduction of the number of proliferating cells but also a delay of the DNA synthesis of the cells that are preparing themselves for mitosis. These disorders lead to a reduction of the neuron population and to corresponding abnormalities in the configuration (or structure) of neuronal circuits.

Influence of Hormones

Experimental studies of the rat cerebellum have yielded new data on the influence of hormones on the development of the CNS. The cerebellum of young rats with thyroid deficiency contains fewer cells during the second week after birth than it normally does. The principal causes of this reduction in cell population are diminution of the number of neuroblasts in the outer granular layer and increased degeneration of cells. A few weeks later the disturbed balance is restored in that the outer granular layer continues to produce neuroblasts ten days longer than in normal rats. This ensures a degree of compensation in the number of cells but not in the structure of synaptic circuits. Studies by Rebière and Legrand (1972) have shown that the dendritic tree of the Purkinje cells in young rats with thyroid deficiency grows more slowly and ultimately remains hypoplastic. Owing to delays in the migration of granular cells and the abnormal dendritic ramifications, normal synaptic circuits cannot develop. In rats with thyroid deficiency, motor coordination is disturbed.

Thyroxine has proved to be of decisive importance for the development of the cortex during the first ten days after birth. Animals deprived of adequate amounts of thyroxine during this period developed neurologic disorders that could not be remedied by subsequent administration of the hormone. In humans the association of cretinism (hypothyroidism) and mental deficiency has long been known. Large doses of corticosteroids cause marked inhibition of the mitotic activity of the brain. According to Howard (1968), the DNA content of the cerebrum of animals given large doses of corticosterone (0.08 to 0.06 mg day) from the second day after birth is 18 per cent lower than that in controls. Discontinuation of corticosteroid medication failed to improve the condition of the cerebrum or the cerebellum.

Of the sex hormones, testosterone is the only androgen formed by the fetal testes in humans. Testosterone induces development of the epididymis, vas deferens, and seminal vesicles. Another androgen, dihydrotestosterone, initiates development of the external genitalia. Sex hormones are also bound by specific areas in the brain (hypothalamus, area septalis, hippocampus) that influence sexual behavior and release of gonadotropin from the hypophysis. The neurons responsible for male behavior differentiate under the influence of testosterone in such a way that the structure of some hypothalamic regions (nucleus preopticus) is different in both sexes.

Blood levels of testosterone increase at birth in the male. Under influence of this hormone, the hypothalamus is sensitized for further action of the hormone in the brain. Testosterone levels decrease after birth and rise again at puberty. The testosterone receptors of the hypothalamus at puberty are able to effectively bind testosterone and activate the neural mechanisms that result in masculine behavior.

Neonatal blood contains an estrogen-binding protein that prevents estrogen from entering the brain. The female hypothalamus develops in the absence of any influence by such hormones. It seems that the typical cyclic pattern of gonadotropin secretion in the female results from this absence.

Part II

Gross Anatomy of the
Central Nervous System

Chapter 11

External Configuration of the Cerebrum

The CNS comprises the brain (encephalon), which is contained in the cranial cavity, and the spinal cord (medulla spinalis), which is localized in the vertebral canal. The boundary between cerebrum and spinal cord is the site of exit of the first spinal nerve, which leaves the vertebral canal between the atlas and occipital bone.

The cerebrum has three distinguishable main components: the hemispheres, the brain stem, and the cerebellum. The hemispheres are well developed and cover large parts of the brain stem and the cerebellum (Fig. 11–1). Only on the basal side of the brain (basis cerebri) can the brain stem and cerebellum be accurately examined.

The totality of the mature brain is egg-shaped, with the longitudinal axis in the sagittal direction and the most massive part in the occipital region. The dorsal surface of the brain is convex and exactly follows the inside of the skull; a cast of the cranial cavity gives a good impression of the shape and position of the principal convolutions of the surface of the brain. Despite this proximity there is no site of contact between brain tissue and cranium. Throughout, the delicate brain tissue is separated from the hard skull by a continuous space (subarachnoid space) that is filled with cerebrospinal fluid. On the basal side of the brain, where the shape of the brain surface deviates significantly from that of the base of the skull, there are consequently large spaces (cisterns) with a relatively large amount of CSF. Because the specific gravity of the CSF slightly exceeds that of the brain tissue, the brain is "supported" by the surrounding fluid and its weight is therefore evenly distributed over the entire skull. On the other hand, changes in brain volume can to some extent be compensated for by diminution or enlargement of the CSF-filled spaces.

The weight of the adult brain is 1200 to 1500 gm, depending on body size and sex. The neonatal brain weight is 10 per cent of the total body weight. No organ grows more rapidly than the brain during the first five years of life: The neonatal brain weight of 400 gm is doubled after a year and trebled after three years.

External Configuration of the Cerebral Hemispheres

The cerebral hemispheres are on the whole horseshoe-shaped, with the inferior part (Fig. 11–1) showing a slight lateral deviation and the midportion producing a posterior outgrowth (occipital lobe) that covers the cerebellum. Each hemisphere can be divided into a frontal pole, a posterior (occipital) pole, and an inferior, anteriorly directed (temporal) pole. The frontal pole rests on the orbit, the occipital pole rests on the cerebellar tentorium, and the temporal pole lies in the middle cranial fossa.

The hemispheres are separated by the longitudinal fissure, in which the falx cerebri is located. The floor of the fissure consists of the corpus callosum. Posteriorly, the hemispheres are separated from the cerebellum by the transverse fissure, in which the cerebral tentorium is located.

The surface of the hemisphere has many deep and very variable grooves (sulci). Primary and secondary sulci can be distinguished. Some primary sulci are interrupted by a so-called transitional gyrus. These gyri are localized between the sulci; about two-thirds of the cerebral cortex lie hidden in the depth of the sulci. The pattern of gyri and sulci are far from constant.

Each cerebral hemisphere has a convex surface, which faces the inner surface of the cranium, a medial surface, and a basal surface.

CONVEX SURFACE

The numerous gyri and sulci of the surface are a characteristic feature of the lateral aspect of the hemispheres. The variability of the gyri is so pronounced that no two hemispheres are entirely identical. This variability applies in particular to the so-called secondary and transitional gyri; the primary sulci, however, can always be traced.

The two principal sulci of the convex surface are the lateral (sylvian) sulcus and the central (rolandic) sulcus. The lateral sulcus forms because the striatal part of the cortex does not participate in the general growth of the pallium and is gradually overgrown and covered by the adjacent cortex (see Fig. 13–2). This sulcus rostrally separates the temporal from the frontal lobe and dorsally separates the temporal from the parietal lobe. Parts of these three lobes constitute "opercula," which cover the insula.

The central sulcus extends from the approximate center of the upper margin of the hemisphere, obliquely down and anteriorly, almost as far as the lateral sulcus. It separates the frontal from the parietal lobe.

The *frontal lobe* is relatively more developed in humans than in other mammals and constitutes about 36 per cent of the total surface of the hemisphere. On its convexity one finds one vertical and two horizontal grooves (Fig. 11–1), namely:

a) Precentral Sulcus. This begins near the margin of the hemisphere and extends down parallel to the central sulcus. Between the central and the precentral sulci, the precentral gyrus constitutes the primary motor area.

b) Superior Frontal Sulcus. From the precentral sulcus, this sulcus extends parallel to the upper margin of the hemisphere.

c) Inferior Frontal Sulcus. This sulcus extends parallel to the superior frontal sulcus.

There are three gyri between these sulci: the superior, the middle and the inferior frontal gyri. The inferior frontal gyrus is divided by two sulci ascending from the lateral sulcus into an orbital, a triangular, and an opercular part (Fig. 11–1). The so-called speech center is localized in the triangular and the opercular parts of the dominant hemisphere.

The principal sulci of the *parietal lobe* are: the postcentral sulcus, which parallels the central sulcus, and the interparietal sulcus (Fig. 11–1). The demarcation from the occipital lobe is visible only on the medial side (parietooccipital sulcus). The postcentral gyrus extends parallel to the central sulcus. Between the two sulci, the primary somatosensory area is localized. In the inferior parietal gyrus, the convolution that surrounds the end of the lateral sulcus is called the supramarginal gyrus, whereas that which surrounds the end of the superior temporal gyrus is called the angular gyrus.

In the *temporal lobe,* the superior, middle, and inferior temporal gyri are separated by sulci of the same designation. The inferior temporal sulcus is often interrupted and is less well defined. Part of the superior temporal gyrus that bounds the lateral sulcus shows a few transverse convolutions (Heschl's transverse gyri), where the cortical acoustic area is localized. The inferior temporal gyrus rests largely on the basal surface of the hemisphere.

The *insula* is a hidden triangular area with the base of the triangle on top of the apex (limen insula) pointing caudally and rostrally. On the surface, the short gyri are visible in the anterior and the long gyrus is seen in the posterior part.

The *occipital lobe* tapers down in a posterior direction, with the lateral occipital gyri on the lateral side.

MEDIAL SURFACE

A section through the midline reveals first a peripheral area that is the medial surface of the hemisphere (Fig. 11–2). Toward the center are the large commissures of the telencephalon cut perpendicularly; in the most central position lies the third ventricle, with its complete lateral wall and part of the rostral, basal, and cranial walls.

The corpus callosum is separated from the medial cortex of the hemisphere by the callosal sulcus. This sulcus circumvents the splenium of the corpus callosum and extends on the mediobasal surface as a groove between the dentate gyrus and the hippocampus (hippocampal sulcus). The cingulate sulcus extends parallel to the anterosu-

Figure 11–1 Configuration of the brain surface; sulci and gyri of the convex surface.

1 central sulcus
2 lateral sulcus
3 superior frontal sulcus
4 inferior frontal sulcus
5 precentral sulcus
6 anterior branch of lateral sulcus
7 superior branch of lateral sulcus
8 postcentral sulcus
9 pars orbitalis
10 pars triangularis
11 pars opercularis
12 interparietal sulcus
13 angular gyrus
14 precentral gyrus
15 postcentral gyrus
16 superior temporal gyrus
17 middle temporal gyrus

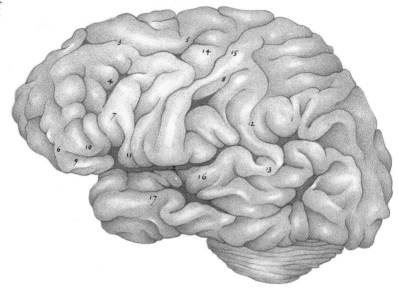

Figure 11–2 Medial aspect of the hemisphere.

1 corpus callosum
2 lateral ventricle
3 septum pellucidum (torn edge)
4 parahippocampal gyrus
5 uncus (uncinate gyrus)
6 intralimbic gyrus
7 band of Giacomini
8 entorhinal area
9 collateral sulcus
10 calcarine sulcus
11 lingual gyrus
12 fusiform gyrus
13 foramen of Monro

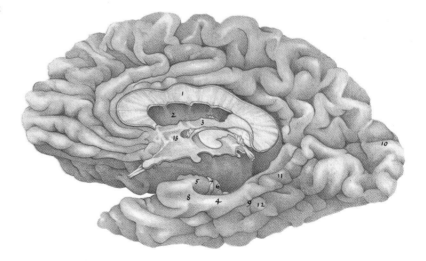

perior margin of the corpus callosum. This sulcus begins beneath the rostrum of the corpus callosum (Fig. 11–2) and takes a rather irregular course as far as the cuneus, where it bifurcates and ends. Between the callosal sulcus and the cingulate sulcus lies the cingulate gyrus, a part of the so-called limbic lobe (see below).

The parietooccipital sulcus is localized behind the splenium of the corpus callosum; it extends ventrally and caudally from the margin of the hemisphere. At the level of the inferior margin of the splenium it unites with the calcarine sulcus (Fig. 12–2), which terminates quite near the hippocampal sulcus. The calcarine sulcus is a deep groove that extends occipitally from the parietooccipital sulcus to the occipital pole. The triangular area between the two sulci is the cuneus; the more quadrangular area between the parietooccipital sulcus and the cingulate sulcus is the precuneus.

Beneath the calcarine sulcus lies the collateral sulcus, a long but shallow groove that runs parallel to the parietooccipital sulcus. The collateral sulcus is usually interrupted by transitional gyri. The most rostral part of the sulcus is known as the rhinal sulcus. The convolution between the inferior temporal and the collateral sulci is the fusiform gyrus (Fig. 11–2). Medial to the collateral sulcus lies the lingual gyrus, which continues anteriorly into the parahippocampal gyrus. The parahippocampal gyrus is localized between the hippocampal and the collateral sulci. Posteriorly, the parahippocampal gyrus continues in the cingulate gyrus and the lingual gyrus; anteriorly it ends in the uncus (Fig. 11–2), which is part of the piriform lobe (see pages 48, 49, and 62 and Fig. 9–6).

BASAL SURFACE

The basal aspect shows structures that have developed from each of the five brain vesicles. Topographically, three levels can be distinguished: an anterior level (frontal lobe), which rests in the anterior cranial fossa; a middle level (temporal lobe), which lies in the middle cranial fossa; and a posterior level (cerebellum and brain stem), which remains enclosed in the posterior cranial fossa. The anterior aspects of the medulla oblongata and pons (rhombencephalon) lie against the clivus (Fig. 11–3).

Along the midline is found the longitudinal cerebral fissure, which separates the hemispheres (Fig. 11–3). The fissure can be followed as far as the lamina terminalis, behind which the optic chiasm is located. It is here that we distinguish between the optic nerve and the optic tract. The fibers of the optic tract extend laterodorsally to the thalamus but are soon hidden from view by the temporal lobes of the brain. On the lateral side of the chiasm is found an area that is perforated by numerous small blood vessels; this is the anterior perforated substance, superior to the middle cerebral artery (Fig. 11–3).

Behind the chiasm lies the tuber cinereum, which is a gray elevation that forms part of the floor of the third ventricle and ends conically in the infundibulum. From this, the hypophysis is suspended, which lies in the sella turcica of the sphenoid bone. Further dorsally, two rounded white elevations are visible — the mamillary bodies, which are part of the hypothalamus and form the rostral boundary of the interpeduncular fossa. The floor of the fossa is perforated by many small blood vessels (posterior perforated substance). The interpeduncular fossa is bounded laterally by the crura cerebri (mesencephalon). From the medial margin of the crus cerebri the oculomotor (third cranial) nerve emerges, whereas the trochlear (fourth cranial) nerve extends laterally around the crus cerebri.

The pons is a massive bridge of transverse fibers, which continues laterally as the middle cerebellar peduncle. This massive bundle of fibers enters the cerebellum (Fig. 11–3). The surface of the pons is transversely grooved by bundles of transverse fibers. Along the midline is found the median sulcus, against which the basilar artery is located. The trigeminal nerve exits in the lateral part of the pons (Fig. 11–3).

The medulla oblongata is located caudal to the pons. It extends from the inferior margin of the pons to the level of the foramen magnum; the demarcation from the spinal cord is indicated on the ventral surface by fibers of the corticospinal tract. These fibers cross the midline and thus interrupt the ventral median fissure (pyramidal decussation). The decussating fibers are some-

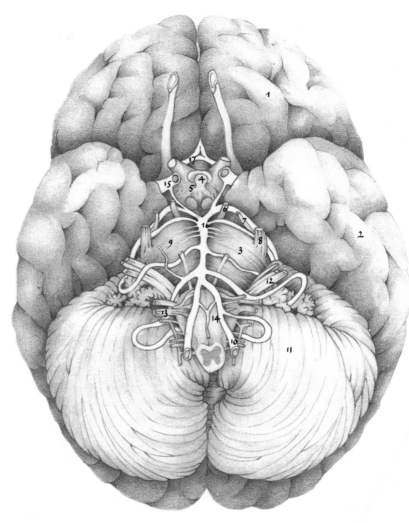

Figure 11–3 Basal aspect of the cerebrum with the exits of the cranial nerves.

1 frontal lobe
2 temporal lobe
3 brain stem (pons)
4 neurohypophysis
5 tuber cinereum
6 oculomotor nerve
7 trochlear nerve
8 trigeminal nerve
9 abducens nerve
10 vertebral artery
11 cerebellum
12 vestibulocochlear nerve
13 hypoglossal nerve
14 medulla oblongata
15 middle cerebral artery
16 basilar artery
17 anterior communicating
   artery

times localized deep in the fissure, which may therefore appear uninterrupted.

On either side of the ventral median fissure is found a pyramid, a rounded mass made up of numerous corticospinal fibers that have assumed a superficial position. Lateral to the pyramid lies an oval elevation called the olive, beneath which the inferior olivary nucleus is located. Between the pyramid and olive (ventrolateral sulcus), the roots of the hypoglossal (twelfth cranial) nerve leave the medulla oblongata.

The cerebellum is situated on either side of the brain stem. The cerebellar surface shows numerous transverse, more or less parallel grooves that divide the surface into narrow convolutions. These grooves are of variable depth; because a median section shows a pattern reminiscent of a tree the area is sometimes described as an "arbor vitae."

THE RHINENCEPHALON

This is a complex of more or less heterogeneous areas of gray matter that are functionally involved in olfaction. Like Brodal (1969), we define the following structures as parts of the rhinencephalon: olfactory bulb, olfactory tract and anterior olfactory nucleus, olfactory trigone with the medial and lateral olfactory striae, anterior perforated substance and olfactory tubercle, prepiriform cortex (prepiriform area and periamygdaloid area), and the corticomedial group of nuclei of the amygdala.

All of these structures are allocortical, which means that the six-layered structural pattern that characterizes the isocortex is not seen in them. Many parts of the rhinencephalon, in fact, cannot be regarded as cortex because they do not fulfill the pertinent criteria (see page 46). Some parts (anterior olfactory nucleus, olfactory trigone, and corticomedial nuclei of the amygdala) have an irregular structure and sometimes a lamination that cannot be compared with that of isocortex or allocortex.

Olfactory Bulb. This is an oval structure on either side of the longitudinal fissure on the undersurface of the frontal lobe. The olfactory nerves (fila olfactoria) of the neuroepithelium of the nasal mucosa enter the cranial cavity via the lamina cribrosa and penetrate the olfactory bulb.

Olfactory Tract. This is a bundle of fibers that arise from the cells of the bulb and extend posteriorly (see Fig. 14–1). The tract ends in a thickened area (olfactory trigone) from which two delicate streaks of white matter arise, the medial and lateral olfactory striae. Both the tract and the striae are bundles of fibers accompanied by cortical convolutions that have become rudimentary (anterior olfactory nucleus with the tract, and lateral and medial olfactory gyri with the respective striae). Between the medial and lateral olfactory striae on the one hand and the diagonal band of Broca on the other, the anterior perforated substance is localized. In some animals the rostral part of this substance shows a distinct elevation (olfactory tubercle).

Lateral Olfactory Stria. This stria and the corresponding lateral gyrus extend laterally in the direction of the apex of the insula (limen insulae), at which point they suddenly change direction and approach the uncus of the hippocampus. The stria ends in a slightly raised area of gray matter (semilunar gyrus), which is bounded on the inferior side by the uncus. The lateral olfactory gyrus continues along with the gyrus ambiens (see Fig. 40–1). The semilunar gyrus and the underlying corticomedial nuclei of the amygdala gradually merge at deeper levels.

Medial Olfactory Stria. This stria and its accompanying gyrus extend to the medial side of the hemisphere and are lost in the parolfactory area of Broca (subcallosal gyrus).

Anterior Perforated Substance. This is an area caudal to the bifurcation of the olfactory tract. Medially, this area continues in the tuber cinereum, from which it is separated by the diagonal band of Broca. Numerous blood vessels perforate this area, and consequently removal of the pia mater exposes numerous delicate apertures (see Figs. 14–1 and 40–1).

Uncus of the Parahippocampal Gyrus. The anterior end of the parahippocampal gyrus curves back sharply over the hippocampal sulcus to form the uncus which, together with the gyrus ambiens and semilunar gyrus (see Fig. 40–1) belongs to the paleopallium. The area of the parahippocampal gyrus beneath the uncus (Fig. 11–2) is known as entorhinal area. The uncus marks the end of the dentate gyrus and the hippocampal fimbria. Giacomini's band (continuation of the dentate gyrus) divides the medial surface of the uncus into the uncinate gyrus and the intralimbic gyrus (Fig. 11–2). Against the lateral aspect of the uncus the gyrus ambiens and semilunar gyrus are clearly visible, especially in the fetal stages (Fig. 40–1). These areas are part of the actual olfactory regions of the cerebral cortex.

Chapter 12

Internal Configuration of the Cerebrum

The internal configuration of the cerebrum can be studied without difficulty on the basis of horizontal and frontal sections. Plastic reconstructions and gross specimens are of great importance for a good understanding of the three-dimensional relations of the internal structures.

White Matter

The white matter enclosed by the cortex (Fig. 12–1) comprises an enormous number of myelinated fibers with blood vessels and neuroglia. The fibers belong to one of the three following categories: projection fibers, commissural fibers, or association fibers.

PROJECTION FIBERS

Projection fibers are afferent or efferent fibers that conduct stimuli to or from the cortex, respectively; many of these fibers connect the thalamus and the cerebral cortex (reciprocal connections). The radiating projection fibers (see Fig. 33–2) constitute the corona radiata. Other projection fibers connect the cortex with nuclei of the brain stem and spinal cord (corticopontine tract, corticospinal tract). These long fibers converge from extensive areas of the cortex to a region between the caudate nucleus and thalamus on the one hand, and the lentiform nucleus on the other (internal capsule). The long projection fibers thus leave the diencephalon and extend to the crura cerebri of the mesencephalon.

Internal Capsule. The fibers that connect the cortex with lower levels of the CNS make their way to their final destination through the original hemispheric pedicle (see page 158). These fibers divide the corpus striatum into caudate nucleus and putamen. Extirpation of the lentiform nucleus exposes the internal capsule as a distinctly striated, thick layer of myelinated fibers curving to the midline (Fig. 12–2). In a superior direction the fibers radiate to the cortex; in an inferior direction they are closely packed. In horizontal sections the fibers form a wide angle opening laterally, in which we distinguish

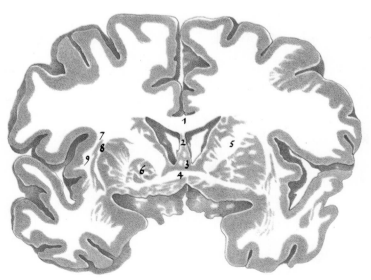

Figure 12–1 Frontal section through the cerebrum at the level of the anterior commissure.

1 corpus callosum
2 septum pellucidum
3 septal area
4 anterior commissure
5 internal capsule
6 pallidum
7 claustrum
8 external capsule
9 extreme capsule

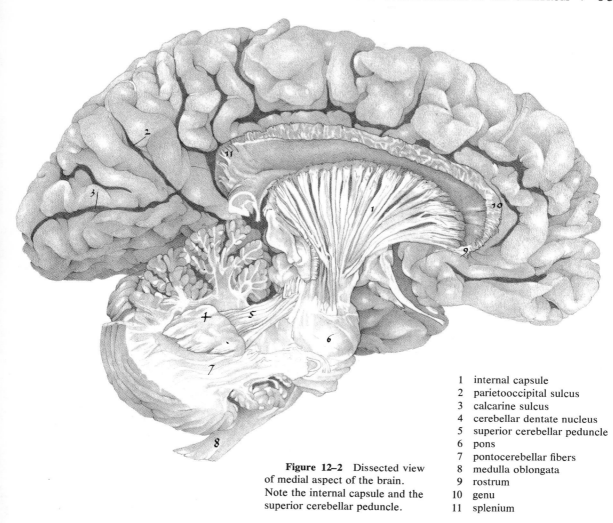

Figure 12–2 Dissected view of medial aspect of the brain. Note the internal capsule and the superior cerebellar peduncle.

1 internal capsule
2 parietooccipital sulcus
3 calcarine sulcus
4 cerebellar dentate nucleus
5 superior cerebellar peduncle
6 pons
7 pontocerebellar fibers
8 medulla oblongata
9 rostrum
10 genu
11 splenium

the following: an anterior part (anterior crus), a sharp kink pointing to the sulcus terminalis (genu), a larger posterior part (posterior crus), and a smaller posterior part localized behind the lentiform nucleus (retrolenticular part; see Fig. 26–2). In a frontal section the internal capsule forms a sharp angle that likewise opens laterally (Fig. 12–1). A horizontal, smaller posterior leg of the capsule is known as the sublenticular part.

COMMISSURAL FIBERS

These fibers are components of the large commissures of the telencephalon. They cross the midline and connect corresponding areas of the two hemispheres.

Corpus Callosum. This is the largest commissure of the telencephalon (about 10^8 fibers). In specimens cut through the midline (Fig. 12–2) we distinguish an initial part (rostrum), which extends as far as the anterior commissure, the genu (that is, the site at which the commissure curves dorsally), the trunk which gradually extends occipitally, and finally the splenium or thickened end of the corpus callosum at the level of the pineal body.

The fibers of the corpus callosum connect symmetric areas of the hemispheres and nonhomologous areas of the two hemispheres. Only a few cortical areas (area 17; parts of the temporal lobe) are not connected with each other by callosal fibers. The fibers of the splenium curve occipitally and form a strong U-shaped bundle (forceps major) that connects the occipital lobes with each other. In the genu the fibers curve anteriorly and radiate in the frontal lobe (forceps minor).

The dorsal surface of the corpus callosum is covered by a thin layer of gray matter (indusium griseum); this structure is part of the hippocampal formation (see below). On either side of the indusium, two fiber bundles extend: the medial stria and the lateral longitudinal stria (of Lancisi).

Anterior Commissure. In a midline section the anterior commissure is visible as a perpendicularly cut fiber strand on the boundary between the rostrum of the corpus callosum and the lamina terminalis. Between the anterior commissure and the interventricular foramen (Fig. 12–1) the fornix column curves toward the mamillary body. Laterally, the commissure extends on either side along the undersurface of the lentiform nucleus, where the fibers leave a groove. The commissure connects certain areas of the temporal lobes (fusiform gyri) with each other. In lower mammals a distinction is made between an anterior part (chiefly olfactory) and a posterior part; the anterior part is not well developed in man.

Fornix Commissure. Most of the fibers of this commissure connect the two fornicles where they diverge beneath the splenium of the corpus callosum. Resection of the splenium reveals a triangular plate of transverse fibers (see Fig. 12–7).

ASSOCIATION FIBERS

These fibers connect areas within the same hemisphere. There are short and long association fibers: The short fibers extend between adjacent gyri, whereas the long fibers connect various lobes with each other. The long association fibers are arranged in grossly dissectable bundles (uncinate bundle, arcuate bundle, and cingulum). The uncinate bundle (Fig. 12–3) extends beneath the limen insulae and connects the orbital gyri of the frontal lobe with the anterior areas of the temporal lobe. The arcuate bundle connects the frontal lobe with the temporal and the occipital lobes. The cingulum is located on the medial surface of the hemisphere (cingulate gyrus) and

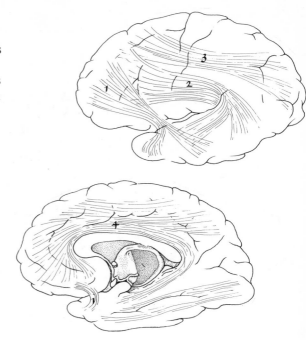

Figure 12–3 The long association fibers of the white matter of the hemisphere. A, Convex surface. B, Medial surface.

1 uncinate bundle
2 arcuate bundle
3 frontooccipital bundle
4 cingulum

serves as a pathway of connection for the limbic system.

Extreme Capsule. Lateral to the claustrum (Fig. 12–1) is found another, narrow layer of fibers that separates the cortex of the insula from the claustrum. The further course of these fibers is unknown.

External Capsule. Between the claustrum and the lateral surface of the putamen, a thin layer of white matter (external capsule) is localized through which fibers extend that connect the cortex with the putamen.

Basal Ganglia

The basal ganglia are large gray nuclei that have assumed a central position in the white matter of the hemisphere. The following nuclei are regarded as basal ganglia: caudate nucleus,

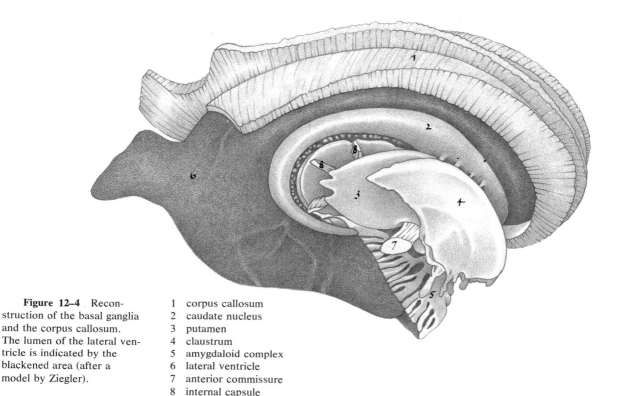

Figure 12–4 Reconstruction of the basal ganglia and the corpus callosum. The lumen of the lateral ventricle is indicated by the blackened area (after a model by Ziegler).

1 corpus callosum
2 caudate nucleus
3 putamen
4 claustrum
5 amygdaloid complex
6 lateral ventricle
7 anterior commissure
8 internal capsule

putamen, pallidum, amygdaloid body, and claustrum. The putamen and caudate nucleus together form the phylogenetically recent corpus striatum. The phylogenetically older pallidum (or globus pallidus) is called paleostriatum. Putamen and pallidum are part of the lentiform nucleus but are very different anatomically and functionally. In model reconstructions it can be seen that the separation between putamen and caudate nucleus has remained incomplete. Anteriorly (Fig. 12–4), the head of the caudate nucleus and the anterior part of the putamen merge; dorsally, however, the caudate nucleus and the putamen are separated from each other by an increasingly large space that is occupied by fibers of the internal capsule. Connections between the two nuclei are established by strips of gray matter that pass right through the internal capsule.

Caudate Nucleus. This is a narrow, horseshoe-shaped mass of gray matter, which protrudes in the wall of the lateral ventricle. This nucleus can be divided into a head, a body, and a tail. The head is continuous with the putamen; the body extends along the dorsolateral margin of the thalamus and, with the latter, forms the terminal sulcus in which the terminal stria and the terminal vein are localized (Fig. 12–4). The tail of the caudate nucleus curves ventrally and forms part of the roof of the temporal horn of the lateral ventricle. The tail extends as far as the amygdaloid body.

Lentiform Nucleus. This nucleus resembles a pyramid, the base of which (putamen) is located laterally; the apex of the pyramid (pallidum) points to the midline. In frontal sections the lentiform nucleus appears to be triangular (Fig. 12–1). A thin layer of fibers (lateral medullary layer) marks the boundary between pallidum (on the medial side) and putamen (on the lateral side). The pallidum in turn is divided by the medial medullary layer into an internal and an external pallidum.

Amygdaloid Body. The amygdaloid body (amygdaloid nucleus) is a complex of nuclei localized within the uncus of the parahippocampal gyrus (see Figs. 12–4 and 38–4). The amygdaloid body is connected with the cortex of the prepiriform area. Anatomically, the amygdaloid body comprises a number of smaller nuclei separated by narrow layers of fibers.

Claustrum. This consists of a layer of gray matter, about 1.5 mm thick, between the lateral surface of the putamen and the cortex of the insula (see Fig. 13–2). The lateral surface of the claustrum is irregular and reflects the cortical gyri of the insula.

The Limbic System

The limbic system comprises the totality of the components of the nervous system involved in experiencing emotions and maintaining the vital drives (libido, sensations of hunger and satiation) as well as in programming the behavior patterns subservient to these drives. In addition, this system exerts a regulatory influence on autonomically innervated organs.

Cortical and subcortical parts of the limbic system are distinguished. The cortical components (limbic lobe) comprise the following areas: subcallosal gyrus, gyrus cinguli, parahippocampal gyrus, dentate gyrus, hippocampus, and indusium griseum (see Fig. 38–4). Structurally, some of these areas are part of the so-called mesocortex (cingulate gyrus and parahippocampal gyrus), whereas other areas (such as the hippocampus) are considered to be part of the allocortex.

Subcortical components are the amygdala (amygdaloid body) and the septum (septal area). In the diencephalon, the principal structures are the hypothalamus and the habenular ganglion; many fibers from the cortical and subcortical structures of the limbic system converge on these diencephalic structures. The limbic system therefore consists of a complex of structurally widely diverse areas. Within these areas, the hippocampal formation is a component with a characteristic structure, which is grossly visible in the wall of the bladder horn of the lateral ventricle.

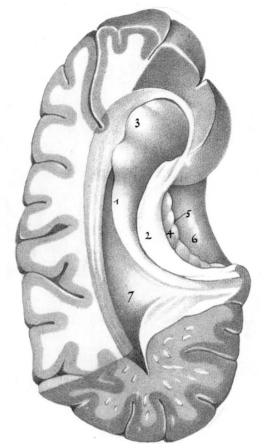

Figure 12–5 Inferior horn of the lateral ventricle, opened: hippocampus, fimbria, and dentate gyrus.

1 hippocampus
2 fimbria
3 pes hippocampi
4 dentate gyrus
5 hippocampal sulcus
6 parahippocampal gyrus
7 lateral ventricle

HIPPOCAMPAL FORMATION

Embryology teaches that the hippocampal formation (archicortex) is originally localized between the choroid fissure and the hippocampal sulcus. The development of the corpus callosum changes this situation because the commissure inserts itself between the fornix and the dorsal part of the archicortex, thus dividing the latter into a superior part (indusium griseum) and an inferior part (fornix).

In maturity, the hippocampal formation is seen as a ring of gray matter on the medial aspect of the hemispheres. Some parts of this formation have evidently regressed (indusium griseum), but the hippocampus has so developed as to become enfolded in the space of the inferior horn of the lateral ventricle, thus disappearing from the cortical surface. The transition between the hippocampus and the cortex of the temporal lobe (parahippocampal gyrus) is known as "subiculum" (Figs. 12–5 and 12–6).

Components

The ring of gray matter is composed of three concentric components: hippocampus and fimbria hippocampi; dentate gyrus; and gyrus fasciolaris. Fimbria and gyrus fasciolaris are separated by the second fimbriodentate sulcus; on the other hand, the first fimbriodentate sulcus marks the boundary between the gyrus fasciolaris and the dentate gyrus (Fig. 12–6). The gyrus fasciolaris is largely rudimentary and grossly visible only in the immediate vicinity of the splenium of the corpus callosum.

Topography

In relation to the corpus callosum we distinguish a pericommissural and a retrocommissural part. The latter comprises the hippocampus, dentate gyrus, gyrus fasciolaris, and subiculum. The hippocampus can be seen only after opening the inferior horn of the lateral ventricle; it is then visible as a sickle-shaped arch (Fig. 12–5). At the level of the uncus the hippocampus shows a few elevations (digitationes hippocampi or pes hippocampi). The hippocampus gradually narrows toward the corpus callosum. Along the superomedial margin of the hippocampus lies the fimbria, a white, flat band of fibers that continues in the crus of the fornix. Numerous fibers from the hippocampus pass through the fimbria.

When the walls of the hippocampal sulcus are pulled slightly apart, the dentate gyrus is seen as a long, narrow, nodular convolution in the upper wall of the groove. The other wall of the sulcus is the subiculum. The hippocampus is consequently not visible on the outside of the brain. The subiculum extends dorsally as far as the level of the splenium of the corpus callosum and ends in the so-called retrosplenial gyri. The

dentate gyrus likewise extends dorsally around the splenium and continues with the indusium griseum. Ventrally, the dentate gyrus extends between the uncus and the parahippocampal gyrus, curves, and continues as Giacomini's band over the outer surface of the uncus. Some authors maintain that Giacomini's band could extend as far as the diagonal band of Broca.

The fornix is the continuation of the fimbria hippocampi. It extends to the splenium (crus of the fornix), then curves ventrally beneath the surface of the splenium (fornix column) and forms the anterior boundary of the interven-

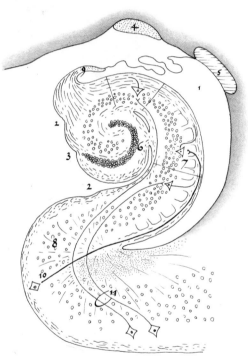

Figure 12–6 Frontal section through the inferior horn of the lateral ventricle.

1 inferior horn (lateral ventricle)
2 (top) second fimbriodentate sulcus; (bottom) hippocampal fissure
3 first fimbriodentate sulcus
4 optic tract
5 tail of the caudate nucleus
6 dentate gyrus
7 hippocampus
8 subiculum
9 fimbria
10 fasciculus alvearis
11 fasciculus perforans

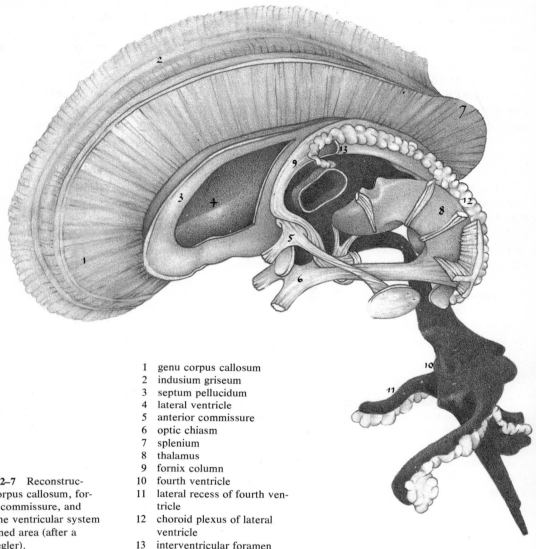

1   genu corpus callosum
2   indusium griseum
3   septum pellucidum
4   lateral ventricle
5   anterior commissure
6   optic chiasm
7   splenium
8   thalamus
9   fornix column
10 fourth ventricle
11 lateral recess of fourth ven-
    tricle
12 choroid plexus of lateral
    ventricle
13 interventricular foramen

Figure 12–7 Reconstruction of the corpus callosum, fornix, anterior commissure, and
optic tract; the ventricular system
is the blackened area (after a
model by Ziegler).

tricular foramen. Between the underside of the
corpus callosum and the fornix column, the
septum pellucidum is located (Fig. 12–7). Here,
the fornix column is localized above the thin
epithelial roof of the third ventricle. The lamina
choroidea of the lateral ventricle attaches to
the lateral margin of the fornix column (tenia
fornicis).

Past the interventricular foramen, the fornix

column descends and crosses the anterior commissure. Here the fornix column divides into a
precommissural part, which extends in front of
the anterior commissure to the septal area, and a
postcommissural part, which, behind the anterior commissure, disappears in the wall of the
third ventricle on its way to the maxillary body,
where most of the fibers synapse (precommissural fornix).

Pericommissural Part

The pericommissural part (indusium griseum) consists of a rudimentary layer of gray matter (continuation of the dentate gyrus) localized above the corpus callosum. Here we find two sagittal fiber bundles (medial and lateral longitudinal striae), between which microscopic strips of gray matter extend. Some of the fibers of the striae originate from the fornix; the other fibers come from the dentate gyrus and the cells of the indusium. The indusium griseum extends ventrally (Fig. 12–7) and follows the corpus callosum as far as the rostrum; it is usually impossible to follow it past the rostrum. According to Gastaut and Lammers (1961), this rostral area consists of a microscopic band of allocortex localized in the floor of the posterior parolfactory sulcus. This band (subcallosal gyrus) connects the indusium griseum with the medial olfactory gyrus. Broca's diagonal gyrus is believed to close the limbic ring of gray matter via the connection between the medial olfactory gyrus and Giacomini's band.

Chapter 13

The Diencephalon

The diencephalon constitutes the wall of the third ventricle. The optic chiasm and the floor of the third ventricle (tuber cinereum) are visible on the outside of the brain; the remaining diencephalon is hidden from view by the hemispheres. Above the diencephalon lie commissural structures (corpus callosum, fornix) and the pia mater of the velum interpositum (Fig. 13–1). Laterally, the sulcus terminalis and the internal capsule mark the boundary of the diencephalon. Caudally, the diencephalon continues as (mesencephalic) tegmentum (subthalamus).

The Dorsal Surface of the Thalamus

The dorsal surface of the thalamus can be brought to view by removal of the corpus callosum and the fornix (Fig. 13–1). At the same time, this exposes the inside of the lateral ventricle, showing the sulcus terminalis enclosing the thalamostriatal vein, and the stria terminalis. The choroid plexus of the lateral ventricle extends parallel to the sulcus terminalis and disappears ventrally through the interventricular foramen.

Between the sulcus terminalis and the tenia choroidea is found the lamina affixa (see page 41), to which part of the dorsal surface of the thalamus adheres. The area medial to the choroid plexus is filled by low-density leptomeningeal tissue (velum interpositum) (Fig. 13–1). Embedded in this connective tissue are the two internal cerebral veins, which unite to form the great cerebral vein. The dorsal surface of the thalamus, the roof of the third ventricle, and the epithalamus are covered by the velum interpositum.

The thin epithelial roof of the third ventricle attaches to the relatively sharp upper margin of the thalamus (tenia thalami), along which the stria medullaris thalami extends (a fiber bundle which connects the septal area with the habenular nucleus). Dorsally, the tenia thalami extends to the habenular trigone (see Fig. 14–2), whereupon it crosses the midline along with the habenular commissure and closes the epithelial roof of the third ventricle. Ventrally, the tenia passes through the foramen of Monro and continues in the tenia choroidea. Behind the habenular commissure lies a small, heart-shaped organ, the pineal body, which is covered by the great cerebral vein. The pineal body rests on the mesencephalic tectum and is connected with the habenular commissure by a short pedicle. The posterior commissure is located immediately beneath this pedicle.

The superior surface of the thalamus extends far dorsally to form the thalamic pulvinar — the largest nuclear complex of the thalamus. On the undersurface are found the lateral and the medial geniculate bodies, which are jointly known as the metathalamus. The former is a small elevation in which the optic tract ends; the latter is connected with the inferior colliculus of the mesencephalon (Fig. 14–2).

The superior surface of the thalamus is covered by a thin layer of white matter (stratum zonale), which gives it a whitish color. The medial surface is partly adherent to that of the contralateral side in about 40 per cent of cases (interthalamic adhesion); this is not a commissure but a mass of gray matter. A layer of myelinated fibers (internal medullary layer) traverses the entire length of the thalamus; in relation to this layer, several groups of nuclei can be distinguished (rostral, lateral, medial, and ventral nuclei).

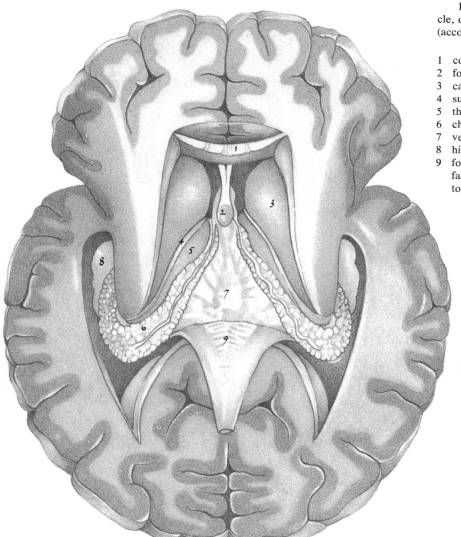

Figure 13–1 Lateral ventricle, opened from the dorsal side (according to Tandler).

1 corpus callosum
2 fornix, columns
3 caudate nucleus
4 sulcus terminalis
5 thalamus (lamina affixa)
6 choroid plexus
7 velum interpositum
8 hippocampus
9 fornix commissure, undersurface (this tissue flap connects to 2 above)

THE SUBTHALAMUS

The subthalamus is an area of transition between the thalamus and the mesencephalic tegmentum. The subthalamic nucleus and the zona incerta are located in this area, which lies ventral to the thalamus and medial to the internal capsule (see Fig. 36–3).

The Hypothalamus

The hypothalamus is located beneath the hypothalamic sulcus and constitutes the inferior part of the lateral wall of the third ventricle. Ventrally, the hypothalamus extends to the preoptic region, the lamina terminalis, and the anterior perforated substance; laterally, it ex-

Figure 13–2 Horizontal section at the level of the pineal body.

1 longitudinal fissure
2 corpus callosum
3 lateral ventricle
4 septum pellucidum
5 crus of the fornix
6 third ventricle
7 pineal body (epiphysis)
8 hippocampus
9 pallidum
10 internal capsule
11 insula
12 caudate nucleus

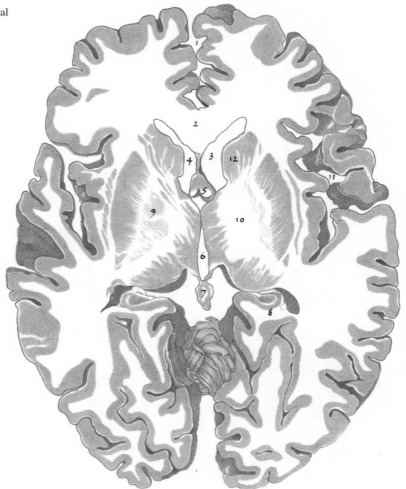

tends to the inferior part of the internal capsule. Its rostrocaudal length is about 12 mm. The hypothalamus is traversed by the fornix; in relation to the plane of the fornix–mamillo-thalamic tract, three zones are distinguishable in the mediolateral direction: periventricular zone, medial layer, and lateral layer. The first is localized between the ventricular wall and the lateral margin of the fornix; the second is a strip of tissue whose width equals that of the fornix; the third is localized lateral to the lateral margin of the fornix (see Fig. 39–3).

The Third Ventricle

The third ventricle is a narrow, midline space bound laterally by the thalamus and hypothalamus. Rostrally, the ventricle is closed by

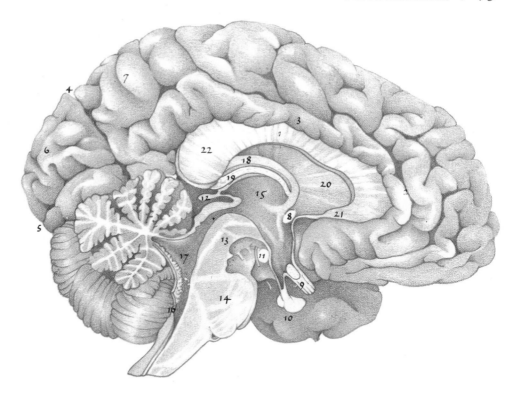

Figure 13–3 Medial aspect of the cerebrum; left hemisphere.

1 corpus callosum
2 cingulate sulcus
3 cingulate gyrus
4 parietooccipital sulcus
5 calcarine sulcus
6 cuneus
7 precuneus
8 anterior commissure
9 optic nerve
10 hypophysis
11 mamillary bodies
12 pineal body
13 mesencephalon
14 pons
15 third ventricle
16 median aperture of the fourth ventricle
17 fourth ventricle
18 fornix
19 choroid plexus of the third ventricle
20 septum pellucidum
21 rostrum of the corpus callosum
22 splenium

the lamina terminalis; its floor is formed by the hypothalamus (tuber cinereum, infundibulum, mamillary bodies). Important evaginations of the ventricular floor are the optic recess and the infundibular recess (Fig. 13–3); the latter is a funnel-shaped space in the infundibulum of the neurohypophysis.

Caudally, the third ventricle continues in the cerebral aqueduct beneath the posterior commissure.

Chapter 14

The Brain Stem

The brain stem comprises derivatives of the mesencephalon and rhombencephalon. Mesencephalon, pons, and medulla oblongata are here regarded as an entity, whereas the cerebellum is considered separately.

The upper boundary of the brain stem can be considered to be marked by a horizontal plane that connects the optic tract with the posterior commissure. The posterior perforated substance, the crura cerebri, and the roof of the aqueduct (tectum) are then components of the upper part of the brain stem (Fig. 14–1). The caudal boundary is the exit of the first spinal nerve, which leaves the vertebral canal between atlas and occipital bone. This caudal boundary is rather arbitrary in neuroanatomic terms, because the transition from the spinal cord to the medulla oblongata is a gradual one. The total length of the brain stem is about 7 cm. Relative to the rostrocaudal axis of the telencephalon, the longitudinal axis of the brain stem describes an angle of about 70°. This is probably due to failure of the cephalic flexure to disappear completely.

As already mentioned on page 27, we distinguish in the brain stem three levels and a central ventricular system. In a ventrodorsal direction, the base, tegmentum, ventricular wall, and roof are the successive structures.

The base consists of long, phylogenetically young fiber systems (crura cerebri, ventral part of the pons, pyramids; Fig. 14–1). The tegmentum is localized between the base and the ven-

tricular system and continues uninterrupted through mesencephalon, pons, and medulla oblongata. This region comprises the reticular formation, the nuclei of origin of the cranial nerves, and specialized nuclei like the olive, red nucleus, and substantia nigra. Moreover, the tegmentum has numerous ascending and descending fiber tracts. The ventricular system comprises the cerebral aqueduct and the fourth ventricle. These spaces are partly enclosed by a central layer of gray matter (central gray substance).

The roof of the brain stem lies dorsal to the lumen. Well developed components of the roof are the mesencephalic tectum and the superior and inferior medullary vela, which cover a large part of the fourth ventricle.

The Mesencephalon

The dorsal part (tectum) is caudally bounded by the superior medullary velum and the brachium conjunctivum. Four round elevations can be distinguished: the two anterior mounds (superior colliculi) are slightly flatter than the two inferior mounds (inferior colliculi). The four elevations are jointly known as the corpora quadrigemina. The superior colliculus is connected with the lateral geniculate body of the thalamus by a fiber bundle called the brachium of the superior colliculus. The inferior colliculus is connected with the medial geniculate body by the brachium of the inferior colliculus (Fig. 14–2). Between the inferior colliculi is found the frenulum of the superior medullary velum, which caudally continues in the superior medullary velum. On either side of this frenulum are found the fibers of the trochlear nerve, the only cranial nerve to leave the brain stem on the dorsal side.

In the ventral part of the mesencephalon the crura cerebri converge toward the midline; the interpeduncular fossa, which lies between the crura (Fig. 14–1), is perforated by numerous delicate blood vessels. After extirpation of the pia mater, the floor of the fossa shows small apertures (posterior perforated substance). The exits of the oculomotor nerve lie against the medial margin of the crus cerebri.

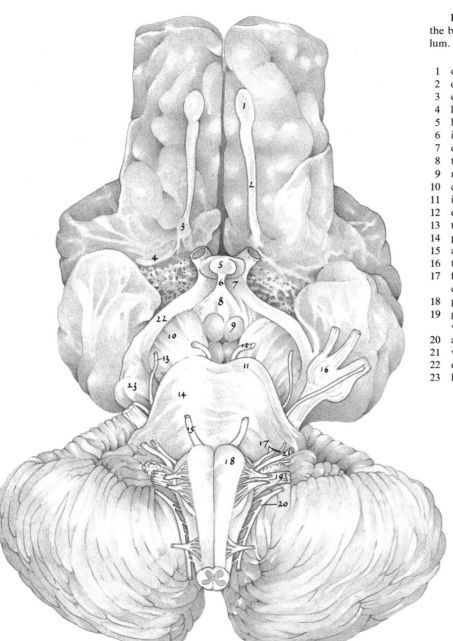

Figure 14–1 Basal aspect of the brain stem and the cerebellum.

1 olfactory bulb
2 olfactory tract
3 olfactory tubercle
4 lateral olfactory stria
5 hypophysis
6 infundibulum
7 optic chiasm
8 tuber cinereum
9 mamillary body
10 crus cerebri
11 interpeduncular fossa
12 oculomotor nerve
13 trochlear nerve
14 pons
15 abducens nerve
16 trigeminal ganglion
17 facial nerve and intermediate nerve
18 pyramid
19 glossopharyngeal nerve and vagus nerve
20 accessory nerve
21 vestibulocochlear nerve
22 optic tract
23 lateral geniculate body

Figure 14–2 Brain stem and rhomboid fossa (fourth ventricle) after removal of the cerebellum.

1   caudate nucleus
2   thalamus (lamina affixa)
3   tenia choroidea
4   posterior commissure
5   pineal body (epiphysis)
6   habenular trigone
7   superior colliculus
8   inferior colliculus
9   crus cerebri
10 medial geniculate body
11 trigeminal nerve
12 superior cerebellar peduncle
13 brachium of the superior
    colliculus
14 frenulum veli
15 middle cerebellar peduncle
16 inferior cerebellar peduncle
17 trochlear nerve
18 medial eminence
19 hypoglossal trigone
20 locus ceruleus
21 striae medullares
22 trigone of vagus nerve
23 vestibular area
24 area postrema
25 accessory nerve
26 choroid plexus
27 first spinal nerve
28 sulcus limitans
29 fasciculus gracilis
30 fasciculus cuneatus

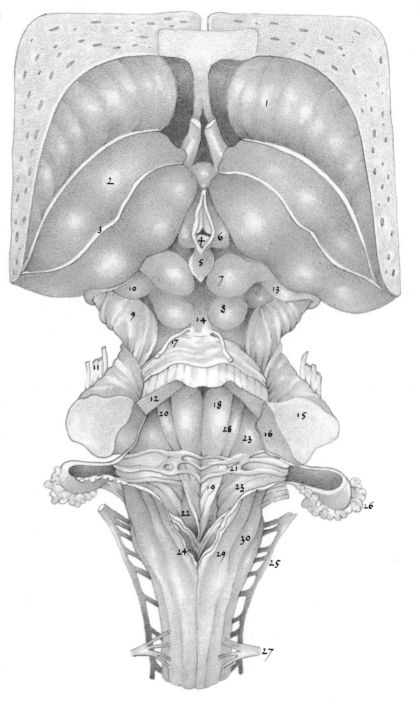

On the lateral side of the mesencephalon is located the trigonum lemnisci, a triangular area in which the fibers of the medial lemniscus (sensory stimuli) and the lateral lemniscus (acoustic stimuli) are located immediately beneath the surface.

INTERNAL CONFIGURATION

The various levels are readily recognizable in a transverse section. Conspicuous nuclei are (1) the substantia nigra, a pigmented layer of gray matter on the boundary between base and tegmentum (see Fig. 31–2) and (2) the red nucleus, a large, slightly reddish nucleus that is round in transverse sections and lies in the tegmentum. The red nucleus is perforated by the fibers of the oculomotor (third cranial) nerve.

The cerebral aqueduct occupies a central position and is enclosed in a layer of gray matter. The colliculi are located dorsal to the aqueduct.

The Pons

The pons is the middle part of the brain stem. Grossly it is a well developed, broad, transverse ridge that encloses the brain stem like a ring. The surface of the pons is slightly grooved by the numerous transverse nerve fibers. Laterally the pons continues in the middle cerebellar peduncle (brachium pontis), which enters the cerebellum. The rostral margin of the ventral surface of the pons is accepted as the boundary between pons and peduncle (Fig. 14–1). This nerve consists of a slender motor root and a much thicker sensory root. On the basal surface is found the median sulcus, in which the basilar artery is located.

The boundary from the medulla oblongata is marked by a sharp transverse groove through which the abducens (sixth cranial) and, more laterally, the facial (seventh cranial) and vestibulocochlear (eighth cranial) nerves leave the brain stem.

The dorsal aspect of the pons constitutes the upper half of the rhomboid fossa (fourth ventricle). Its roof consists of the brachium conjunctivum (superior cerebellar peduncles), between which the superior medullary velum is located (Fig. 14–2).

INTERNAL CONFIGURATION

Base and tegmentum are well developed, whereas the roof lags far behind. The base consists of transverse fiber bundles between which numerous nuclei (pontile nuclei) are localized. These transverse fibers are axons of the cells of the pontile nuclei; they cross the midline and enter the cerebellum (middle cerebellar peduncle or brachium pontis).

In the base of the pons, the pyramidal tract is divided into many bundles that cross the horizontal pontocerebellar fibers. The pyramidal fibers come together again in the medulla oblongata and form the pyramid (Fig. 14–1).

In the dorsal part of the pons, the tegmentum extends to the floor of the ventricle. It is connected with the tegmentum of the mesencephalon and the medulla oblongata. The medial lemniscus marks the boundary between tegmentum and base.

The Medulla Oblongata

The medulla oblongata is the lowest part of the brain stem. Further caudally, it is continuous with the spinal cord. The structure has a conical shape, with a broad upper part and a gradually narrowing lower part. This region can be compared with an unfolded spinal cord in which the dorsal wall has become a thin epithelial wall.

VENTRAL ASPECT

On the ventral side, the anterior median fissure divides the medulla oblongata into two symmetric halves. The fissure ends cranially immediately beneath the margin of the pons in a small depression, the cecal foramen. On either side of this foramen the abducens nerve leaves the brain stem. The median fissure has fibers that decussate in its depth so that the fissure appears to be uninterrupted (Fig. 14–1).

Lateral to the anterior median fissure is found an oblong mass (the pyramid), which is made up of the closely packed fibers of the corticospinal tract. Lateral to the pyramid is seen an oval elevation with a length of 1.5 cm at the cranial end of the medulla; this is the olive, beneath which the inferior olivary nucleus is localized. Between the pyramid and the olive, the anterior lateral sulcus is the cranial continuation of the sulcus of the same name in the spinal cord. The hypoglossal nerve arises from this cranial part of the anterior lateral sulcus and can therefore be compared with the anterior root of a spinal nerve. The root fibers of the accessory nerve (cranial roots), the vagus nerve, and the glossopharyngeal nerve exit through the post-olivary sulcus (Fig. 14–1). Above the olive, at the boundary between pons and medulla, the facial and the vestibulocochlear nerves leave the brain stem.

DORSAL ASPECT

On the dorsal side of the medulla oblongata, the posterior median fissure is closed superiorly by a transverse fiber bundle (the obex) to which the tela choroidea attaches. On either side of the median sulcus is found the posterior funiculi (fasciculus gracilis and fasciculus cuneatus), which are separated by a shallow posterior intermediate sulcus. The cuneate and the gracile fasciculus end in, respectively, the cuneate and gracile tubercles, which are eminences of the nuclei of the same name.

Between the cuneate fasciculus and the roots of the accessory nerve (cranial segment), an oblong darker area is discernible (tuberculum cinereum), which marks the transition of the nucleus of the spinal tract of the trigeminal nerve to the gelatinous substance of the posterior horn of the spinal cord.

THE FOURTH VENTRICLE

The lumen of the brain stem expands markedly in the rhombencephalon and forms the fourth ventricle. Its floor is the rhomboid fossa, which can be divided into a superior, metencephalic and an inferior, myelencephalic area (Fig. 14–2). The rostral margins are formed by the superior cerebellar peduncles, and the caudal margins by the nuclei of the posterior funiculi and the inferior cerebellar peduncles. The ventricle extends laterally as a lateral recess (Fig. 14–2), in which the lateral aperture is localized through which the CSF reaches the subarachnoid space.

Configuration of the Ventricular Floor

The very variable configuration of the floor is caused by local accumulations of gray matter (Fig. 14–2). Most surface configurations are localized on either side of the midline. The rhomboid fossa is divided into two symmetric halves by the median sulcus. Lateral to it, the medial eminence is visible in the metencephalic part. This eminence contains the facial colliculus. The colliculus is the site at which the fibers of the facial nerve curve around the nucleus of origin of the abducens nerve.

Lateral to the sulcus limitans is found the vestibular area, where the nuclei of origin of the vestibular nerve are localized. Slightly cranial to the vestibular area lies the locus ceruleus, a small area that is conspicuous due to its abundance of dark pigment.

On the boundary between the metencephalic and the myelencephalic areas, a number of transverse fiber bundles (striae medullares) extend in the floor from the median sulcus and disappear among the fibers of the inferior cerebellar peduncle.

In the myelencephalic area, a medial trigone of the hypoglossal nerve and a lateral trigone of the vagus nerve are localized above the nucleus of the hypoglossal nerve and the dorsal nucleus of the vagus nerve, respectively. On the caudal side, the trigone of the vagus nerve is adjacent to an oblique, delicate cord that consists of ependyma and neuroglia cells, the funiculus separans.

The area between the funiculus separans and the tenia choroidea is the small, but structurally very interesting area postrema.

The Roof of the Fourth Ventricle

The locally very thin roof of the ventricle covers the rhomboid fossa like a tent. The highest point of the roof (fastigium) lies beneath the central white matter of the cerebellum.

The myelencephalic part of the roof is formed medially by the fastigium, laterally by the inferior medullary velum, and caudally by the lamina choroidea. The inferior medullary velum is a rudimentary part of the cerebellum that extends between the nodulus and the flocculus. The lamina choroidea closes the space between the inferior medullary velum and the lower margin of the rhomboid fossa. Quite near its caudal corner is found the median aperture of the fourth ventricle (foramen of Magendie; see Fig. 17–4).

The lamina choroidea is invaginated by blood vessels and leptomeningeal connective tissue, the choroid plexus of the fourth ventricle. In the dorsal view, the invagination takes the approximate shape of two inverted letters L (ꓶꓤ). The lateral parts of the line of invagination extend as far as the lateral recesses of the ventricle, where a small part of the plexus protrudes into the subarachnoid space.

Chapter 15

The Cerebellum

By virtue of its size and characteristic position in relation to the brain stem, the cerebellum is a special structure within the CNS. Topographically it is located in the posterior cranial fossa and separated from the occipital lobe by the very strong cerebellar tentorium. The brain stem is located on its ventral side (Fig. 15–1); the two structures are connected by three strong fiber bundles: the superior, middle, and inferior cerebellar peduncles. The longest axis of the cerebellum is a transverse line, perpendicular to that of the brain stem. Of great importance for the functional significance of the cerebellum is its position outside the large ascending and descending tracts that connect the cerebral cortex and the spinal cord. In relation to these large tracts (corticospinal tract, medial lemniscus, etc.) the cerebellum is "connected in parallel," so that the signals on their way to the cerebral cortex or the spinal cord can pass unhampered without first having to go to the cerebellum. The location of the cerebellum within a virtually enclosed space is not without clinical implications. Expanding lesions beneath the cerebellar tentorium soon produce symptoms of increased intracranial pressure. This increased intracranial pressure can cause herniation of the cerebellar tonsils through the foramen magnum.

Structural Characteristics

The nerve cells in the cerebellar cortex are arranged in layers. The cortex lies on the outside of the cerebellum and encloses a nucleus of white matter, the corpus medullare. Like the cerebral cortex, the cerebellar cortex has a greatly enlarged surface area as a result of its convolutions. The gyri are separated by numerous transverse grooves that divide the cortex into lobes, lobules, and folia. In a section through the midline, these grooves produce the image of the "arbor vitae" (Fig. 15–1).

Grossly, the cerebellum can be divided into a central vermis and two lateral, much larger hemispheres. The inferior part of the vermis lies deeply enclosed between the hemispheres; the hollow between the hemispheres is called the vallecula cerebelli. The superior aspect of the vermis rises above the hemispheres, from which it cannot be sharply defined.

Superior Surface. The superior surface of the cerebellum is flat. Vermis and hemispheres are not sharply separated (Fig. 15–2A). The dorsal boundary from the inferior surface is marked by a deep transverse groove, the horizontal fissure.

Inferior Surface. The inferior surface is convex and lies in the posterior cranial fossa. The vermis constitutes the floor of the deep vallecula cerebelli and is well-defined from the hemispheres (Fig. 15–2B). The cerebellar tonsils (parts of the hemispheres) are located on either side of the vermis at the level of the foramen magnum.

Structural Development of the Cerebellum

The macroscopic division proceeds from the existence of certain deep transverse grooves that divide the cerebellum into three lobes and nine lobules. The posterolateral fissure separates the flocculonodular lobe from the remainder of the cerebellum (body of the cerebellum). The flocculonodular lobe (archicerebellum) is the phylogenetically oldest part and has mostly vestibular connections.

The cerebellar body is divided by the primary fissure into an anterior lobe (paleocerebellum) and a posterior lobe (neocerebellum). The anterior lobe is connected predominantly with the spinal cord, whereas the posterior lobe is phylogenetically younger and develops in close association with the cerebral cortex.

82

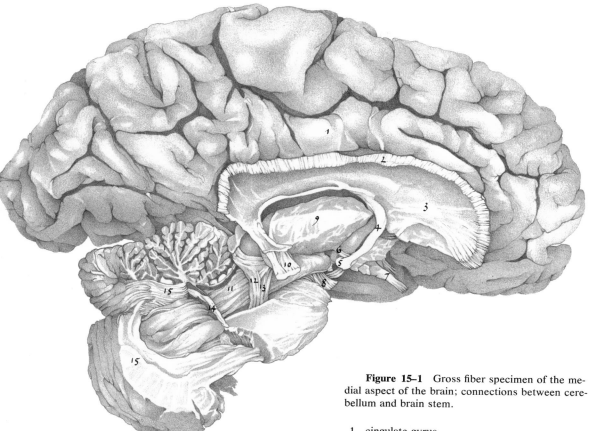

Figure 15–1 Gross fiber specimen of the medial aspect of the brain; connections between cerebellum and brain stem.

1 cingulate gyrus
2 corpus callosum
3 septum pellucidum
4 fornix column
5 mamillary body
6 mamillothalamic fasciculus
7 optic nerve
8 oculomotor nerve
9 thalamus
10 crus of the fornix and hippocampus
11 superior cerebellar peduncle
12 anterior spinocerebellar tract
13 lateral lemniscus
14 posterior spinocerebellar tract and olivocerebellar tract
15 cerebellum

Figure 15–2 Dorsal (A) and ventral (B) aspects of the cerebellum.

A
1 cerebellar vermis (culmen)
2 quadrangular lobule
3 quadrangular lobule (posterior part)
4 primary fissure
5 posterior superior fissure
6 tuber vermis
B
1 nodulus vermis
2 uvula
3 tuber
4 folium
5 tonsil
6 flocculus
7 biventral lobule
8 inferior semilunar lobule

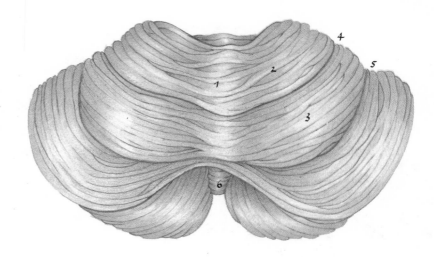

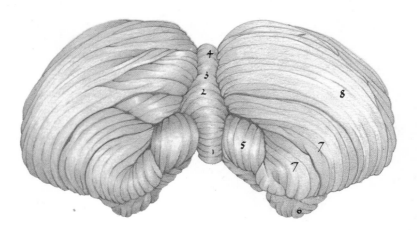

Table 15–1 LARSELL'S DIVISION

Vermis		Hemispheres	
I	Lingula		
II	Central Lobule	Wing of central lobule	
III	Culmen	Quadrangular lobule (anterior part)	Anterior lobe
		Primary fissure	
IV	Declive	Quadrangular lobule (posterior part)	
V	Folium	Superior semilunar lobule	Posterior lobe
		Horizontal fissure	
VI	Tuber	Inferior semilunar lobule	
VII	Pyramis	Biventral lobule	
VIII	Uvula	Cerebellar tonsil	
		Posterolateral fissure	Flocculonodular lobe
IX	Nodulus	Flocculus	

The transverse grooves traverse vermis and hemispheres without interruption, thus outlining horizontal zones whose central part belongs to the vermis, while the lateral parts belong to the hemispheres. Larsell numbered the lobules of the vermis from I to IX in a rostrocaudal direction (Fig. 15–3 and Table 15–1).

Other, more functional divisions are based mainly on the afferent and efferent fiber projections. Three vertical zones are thus distinguished in the cortex: vermis, intermediate zone (one on either side of the vermis), and hemispheres. Each zone seems to be anatomically and functionally related to a particular central nucleus (vermis to fastigial nucleus; intermediate zone to nucleus interpositus; hemisphere to dentate nucleus). The functional division distinguishes the following areas:

1 vestibulocerebellum (flocculonodular lobe)

2 spinocerebellum (anterior lobe, pyramids, uvula)

3 pontocerebellum (hemisphere, declive, folium, tuber)

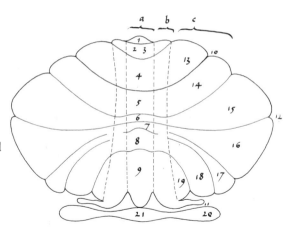

Figure 15–3 Morphologic divisions of the cerebellum.

a	vermis
b	intermediate part
c	hemisphere
1	lingula
2,3	central lobe
4	culmen
5	declive
6	folium vermis
7	tuber vermis
8	pyramis
9	uvula
10	primary fissure
11	posterolateral fissure
12	horizontal fissure
13	quadrangular lobule (anterior part)
14	quadrangular lobule (posterior part)
15	superior semilunar lobule
16	inferior semilunar lobule
17	gracile lobule
18	biventral lobule
19	tonsil
20	flocculus
21	nodulus

Central Nuclei

In each cerebellar hemisphere, four nuclei are located in the white matter: dentate, globose, emboliform, and fastigial nuclei. In many mammals the emboliform and the globose nuclei have fused to form a single nucleus, the nucleus interpositus. The dentate nucleus is the largest and most lateral of these nuclei; it consists of an irregularly coiled gray lamella from which the fibers of the superior cerebellar peduncle arise. Fastigial nuclei are located on either side of the midline in the roof of the fourth ventricle (Fig. 15–4).

Connections with the Brain Stem

It is clearly seen that the cerebellum is connected with the brain stem by three massive fiber bundles: the superior, middle, and inferior cerebellar peduncles. The superior peduncle extends to the mesencephalon, the middle peduncle to the pons, and the inferior peduncle to the medulla oblongata. The three peduncles con-

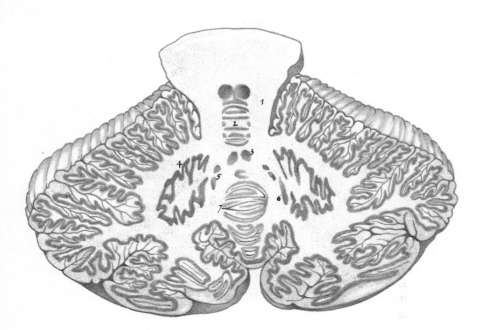

Figure 15–4 Cross-section of the central cerebellar nuclei.

1 superior cerebellar peduncle
2 lingula
3 fastigial nucleus
4 dentate nucleus
5 globose nucleus
6 emboliform nucleus
7 vermis

verge to the basal aspect of the cerebellum (see Fig. 14–2); at the level of the lateral recess of the fourth ventricle they unite to form a fibrous mass that enters the central white matter. The superior peduncles lie on either side of the superior medullary velum; the inferior peduncles are located caudal and medial to the large middle peduncle. Converging caudally, the inferior peduncles enclose the posterior medullary velum.

Through the superior peduncles pass mainly *efferent* fibers that originate from the dentate nucleus and nucleus interpositus. Many of these fibers cross the midline and end in the red nucleus of the mesencephalon; other fibers likewise cross and extend to the thalamus (Fig. 15–1). Through the middle cerebellar peduncle (brachium pontis) pass *afferent*, mostly decussating fibers arising from the pontine nuclei, which end in the hemispheres and in the central part of the vermis. The inferior cerebellar peduncle (restiform body) consists of *afferent* fibers from the spinal cord and the medulla oblongata. The medial part of the inferior peduncle is called the juxtarestiform body and contains *efferent* cerebellar projection systems to the vestibular nuclei and the reticular formation.

Chapter 16

The Spinal Cord

General Characteristics

The spinal cord is a slightly flattened cylindrical mass of nerve tissue, about 44 cm long, suspended freely in the vertebral canal. It is enveloped by three meninges: Between the outer membrane (dura mater) and the interior surface of the vertebral canal lies the epidural space, which is filled with adipose tissue and has a venous plexus (Fig. 16–1). The spinal cord weighs 35 to 38 gm. Its transverse diameter in the thoracic segment is 10 mm, and reaches 12 to 14 mm in the cervical and lumbar segments; its sagittal diameter is between 8 and 9 mm.

Its upper boundary is the exit of the first spinal nerve, located between the atlas and occipital bone. The structural transition to the medulla oblongata is fairly gradual. Caudally, the spinal cord extends as far as the upper margin of L2, but individual variations occur; in neonates, the spinal cord extends as far as L3. The caudal end (conus medullaris) continues caudally in a massive thread-like structure called the filum terminale. This structure, 1 mm thick and made up of pial tissue, continues free within the dural sac over a further distance of about 15 cm (internal filum terminale). The terminal part (external filum terminale) continues outside the dura and finally attaches to the periosteum of the dorsal aspect of the first coccygeal vertebra.

Gross Anatomy

The spinal cord shows two fusiform swellings: the cervical and the lumbosacral intumescences. The former extends between C5 and T1 and the latter, between L1 and S2. These swellings are caused by the large numbers of cells required for innervation of the extremities.

The surface of the spinal cord shows some grooves that divide it into funiculi. The anterior aspect shows the anterior median fissure, with a depth of about 3 mm. The posterior median sulcus is shallow; the dorsal median septum extends from the central canal to the posterior median sulcus.

The lateral aspect shows the exits of the ventral and dorsal roots. The dorsal roots emerge from a delicate groove called the dorsolateral sulcus. The ventral roots arise more irregularly from an area known as the ventrolateral sulcus. In the cervical cord, a posterior intermediate sulcus is found between the dorsolateral and the posterior median sulci. The sulci divide the white matter of the spinal cord into several funiculi. The posterior funiculus is located between the median septum and the dorsolateral sulcus; the lateral funiculus, between the dorsal and ventral roots; and the anterior funiculus, between the ventral median fissure and the anterior root.

THE GRAY MATTER

The gray matter occupies a central position in the spinal cord. It consists of nerve cells which, as viewed in three dimensions, are arranged in columns (Fig. 16–2). In a transverse section the gray matter assumes the shape of a letter H, in which a posterior, a lateral, and an anterior horn can be distinguished. The anterior horn is rather sturdy, whereas the posterior horn is slender and long, extending to quite near the dorsolateral sulcus. The transverse bar is known as central intermediate substance. In the center of this substance the central canal extends as a vestige of the lumen of the neural tube. In adults this canal shows interruptions caused by local accumulations of ependymal breakdown products. Both on the ventral and on the dorsal sides

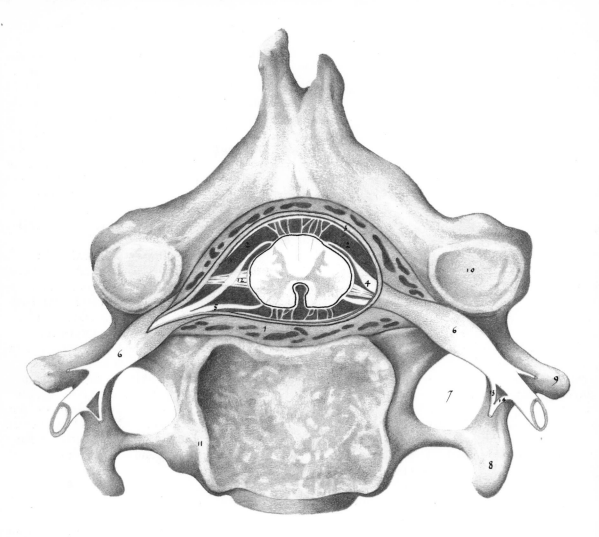

Figure 16–1 Horizontal section through cervical vertebral column and spinal cord. Note the subarachnoid and the epidural space (according to Sobotta).

1 epidural space with venous plexus
2 subarachnoid space
3 spinal dura mater
4 dorsal root
5 ventral root
6 spinal ganglion
7 transverse foramen
8 anterior tubercle
9 posterior tubercle
10 superior articular process
11 uncinate process
12 denticulate ligament
13 white communicating branch
14 gray communicating branch

of the central canal, numerous nerve fibers cross the midline (anterior and posterior gray commissure).

The ratio between gray matter and white matter is not the same at all levels. The gray matter is greatly increased at the sacral level, diminishes at the thoracic level, and increases again at the cervical level. The white matter gradually increases in volume in a caudocranial direction.

THE WHITE MATTER

The white matter consists of large numbers of myelinated or unmyelinated fibers, most of which take a longitudinal course (whereas the fibers in the gray matter take a more horizontal course). Fibers of four different types are found in the white matter: (a) fibers from the dorsal roots (exclusively in the posterior funiculus), (b) axons of the long ascending systems, (c) axons of the descending supraspinal systems, and (d) association fibers (propriospinal system). The association fibers are present in all three funiculi and lie against the gray matter; they connect the various spinal cord levels and integrate the activity of the spinal segments. More than two-thirds of the nerve fibers in the white matter of the spinal cord belong to the propriospinal system.

Apart from nerve cells and nerve fibers, the spinal cord contains neuroglia, ependymal cells, and blood vessels. The ependymal cells line the central canal (so far as it has a lumen); to the periphery they continue in long extensions that sometimes reach as far as the surface of the spinal cord.

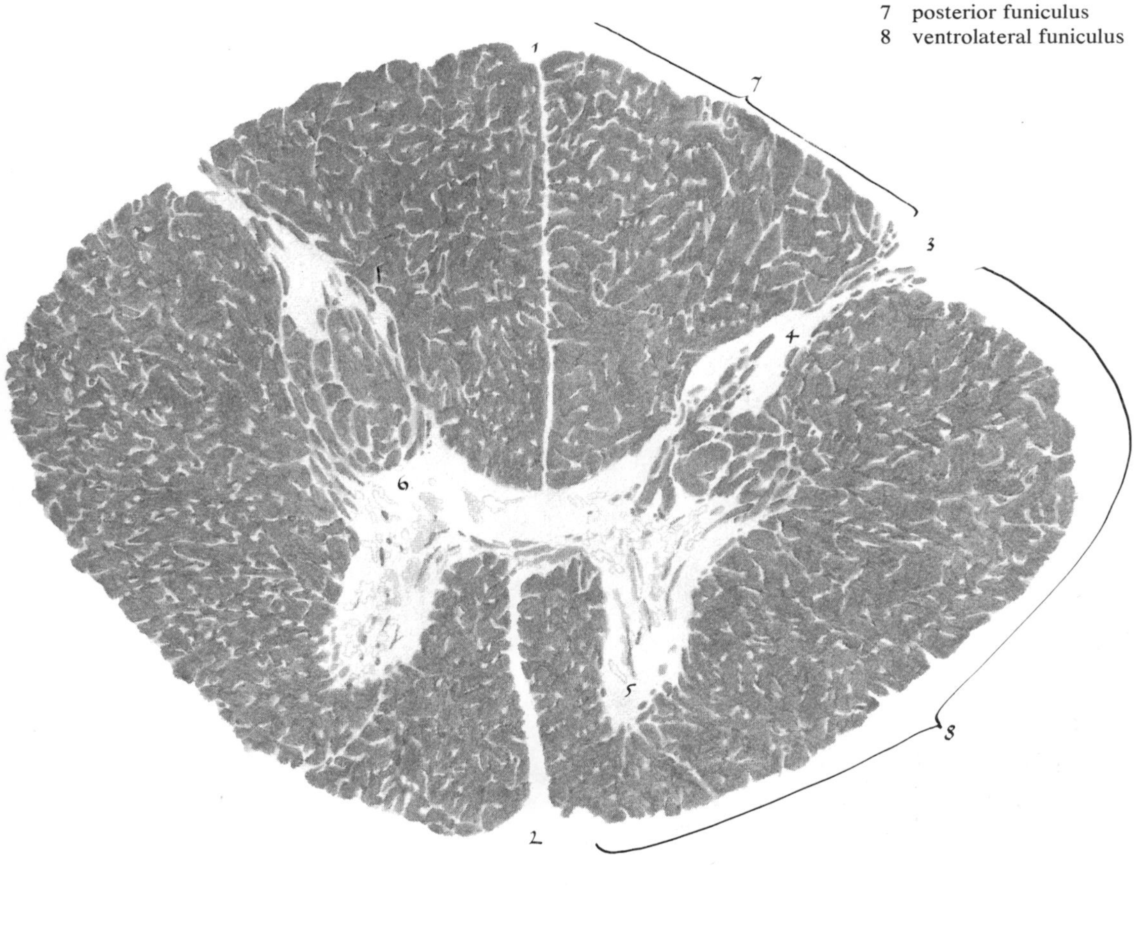

Figure 16–2 Horizontal section through the cervical region of the spinal cord (C1). The pyramidal fibers extend deep into the posterior horn of the spinal cord.

1 posterior median sulcus and septum
2 anterior median sulcus
3 dorsolateral sulcus
4 posterior horn
5 anterior horn
6 pyramidal fibers
7 posterior funiculus
8 ventrolateral funiculus

SPINAL CORD SEGMENTS

The regular succession of exiting roots seems to support the hypothesis that the spinal cord is organized in segments. Grossly a length of spinal cord that supplies dorsal and ventral roots for a pair of spinal nerves is interpreted as a spinal cord segment.

Structurally, however, there are no indications of segmentation because entering dorsal root fibers that have divided into an ascending and a descending branch (page 139) produce collaterals to the gray matter over a distance of a few "segments" above and below the level of entry. On the other hand, the ventral roots arise from the anterior horn cells localized in the same segment; these cells are not arranged in clusters within the segments but rather as "columns of cells," and extend far beyond the boundaries of the segments.

In spite of all these objections, the external segmentation caused by the roots is used to divide the spinal cord into eight cervical, twelve thoracic, five lumbar, five sacral, and one or two coccygeal segments. The localization of each segment can be determined with accuracy, and this has great clinical advantages.

Transverse sections through the various segments immediately reveal how much they differ in form. The cervical segments are broad (Fig. 16–3), with well developed white matter; the posterior funiculus is clearly divided into a medial gracile fasciculus and a lateral cuneate fasciculus. At the level of the cervical intumescence the anterior horn is very broad; a number of delicate extensions of gray matter are seen near the angle between anterior and posterior horns (reticular process).

The morphology of the thoracic segments varies with their level. In the lower segments the cuneate fasciculus disappears in the posterior funiculus. Lateral to the intermediate gray substance the lateral horn extends between T1 and L2; the lateral horn consists of a nucleus (intermediolateral nucleus), which gives rise to preganglionic myelinated fibers that exit via the ventral root. Medially on the base of the posterior horn, Clarke's nucleus dorsalis gives rise to the dorsal spinocerebellar tract. The thoracic segments are less broad than the cervical, partly as a result of a reduction in the gray matter but also because the number of ascending nerve fibers is diminished.

The lumbar segments (Fig. 16–4) are virtually circular. The gray matter is well developed; the posterior horn is short and wide, whereas the anterior horn is plump. Clarke's nucleus dorsalis is well defined, and in a caudal direction the white matter becomes a thinner and thinner layer of fibers.

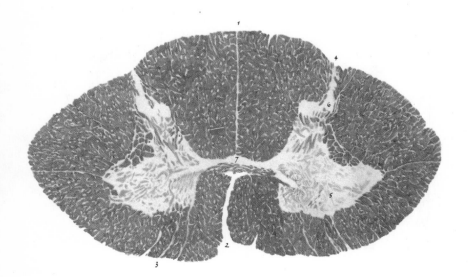

Figure 16–3 Horizontal section at the level of C7.

1 posterior median sulcus
2 anterior median sulcus
3 ventrolateral sulcus
4 dorsolateral sulcus
5 anterior horn
6 posterior horn
7 central gray substance

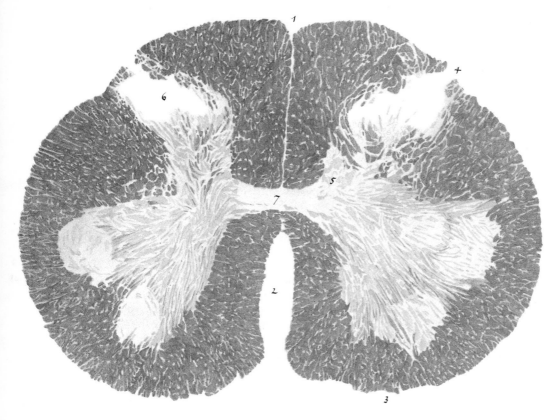

Figure 16–4 Horizontal section at the level of L4.

1 posterior median sulcus
2 anterior median fissure
3 ventrolateral sulcus
4 dorsolateral sulcus
5 Clarke's nucleus dorsalis
6 posterior horn (gelatinous substance)
7 central gray substance.

The sacral segments are smaller. The gray matter has a thick intermediate part and gradually loses its characteristic butterfly configuration.

VERTEBROSPINAL TOPOGRAPHY

The difference in length between the spinal cord and the vertebral column (as a result of the so-called ascent of the spinal cord) has its consequences for the course of the spinal roots on their way to the intervertebral foramina. In addition, of course, there is displacement of spinal cord segments in relation to the vertebrae of the same designation. The upper, cervical pairs of roots take a virtually horizontal course, perpendicular to the axis of the spinal cord. The lowest pairs of roots, however, are forced to take an ever longer, obliquely descending course on their way to the proper exits. The entire sheaf of obliquely descending roots is known as the cauda equina (horsetail).

The relations between spinal cord segments and vertebral bodies are variable. In most cases we find the following relative positions:

C1: opposite the occipital foramen magnum and the space between atlas and occipital bone,

C2: opposite the dens axis and atlas,

C3-C7: above the correspondingly numbered vertebrae,

C8: opposite the intervertebral disk between C6 and C7,

T1-T11: below the correspondingly numbered vertebrae,

T12: opposite the intervertebral disk between T10 and T11,

L1-L3-S1: opposite vertebral bodies T11, T12 and L1,

L2: opposite the disk between T11 and T12,

L4-L5: on either side of the disk between T12 and L1,

S2-S5: lower one-third of vertebral body L1,

Conus: opposite the disk between L1 and L2.

FIXATION OF THE SPINAL CORD IN THE VERTEBRAL CANAL

The outer surface of the spinal cord is separated from the dural sac by a CSF-filled space called the subarachnoid space. The CSF helps to "carry" the spinal cord, as it were. Untoward displacements of the spinal cord within the dural sac are prevented by: (a) the fusion of the dura with the perineurium of the emerging spinal nerves, (b) the denticulate ligament, and (c) the numerous arachnoidal trabeculae extending between dura mater and pia mater, especially on the ventral and dorsal side of the spinal cord (Fig. 16–1).

The frontally oriented denticulate ligament is a pia mater septum located between the ventral and dorsal roots, which connects the lateral aspect of the spinal cord with the dura mater. Its margin facing the dura is festooned between the attachment points (18 to 22), which alternate with the nerves passing through, attach to the dura mater, and thus cause partial separation of the subarachnoid space into anterior and posterior halves.

Mobility of the Spinal Cord

Flexion of the vertebral column extends the dorsal aspect of the intervertebral disks and thus causes elongation of the ligamentum flava. The walls of the vertebral canal increase in length. During extension of the vertebral column, the vertebral canal shortens. The difference in length between maximum flexion and maximum extension of the column ranges from 5 to 9 cm (Louis, Laffont et al., 1967). The lengthening (or shortening) of the vertebral canal is not evenly distributed over its total length but correlates with the flexibility of the vertebral column; the largest differences in length, therefore, occur in the cervical and lumbar regions.

During normal movements the spinal cord is not displaced relative to the vertebral column. In maximum flexion and extension, however, the spinal cord segments are displaced toward the vertebrae near the top of the curve of flexion (C6 in the cervical and L4 in the lumbar region, respectively). The segment opposite these two roots (C6 and L4), however, is not displaced. This means that tensile stress is exerted not on the entire length of the spinal cord but only on certain parts of it. During hyperflexion movements, overextended regions can be seen (C6-T2 and L4-S5) beside regions without increased tensile stress (T4-L2). The total lengthening of the spinal cord can be as much as about 43 mm (Louis, Laffont et al., 1967). Since the lengthening is to be provided largely by the regions exposed to tensile stress, it is understandable that these regions may be in jeopardy during hyperflexion. Certain neurologic disorders (paraplegia, quadriplegia) that develop after traumatic lesions of the vertebral column (without radiologic changes) might be attributable to a spinal cord lesion resulting from hyperextension.

Chapter 17

The Meninges

Between the CNS and the interior wall of the skull or vertebral canal, three membranes concentrically enclose the nervous system. From the outside in, these membranes are the dura mater (pachymeninx), the arachnoid, and the pia mater; the last two membranes together form the leptomeninx. The CSF-filled space between the pia mater and the arachnoid (the subarachnoid space) is of great importance for the adaptation of the cerebrum to the skull. Since the relations between dura mater and skull differ from those between dura mater and vertebral canal, they will be discussed separately.

Cerebral Meninges

DURA MATER

The dura mater is a strong membrane made up of numerous collagenous bundles; in maturity it is loosely attached to the interior surface of the skull. The dura is divided into an outer (periosteal) and an inner (meningeal) layer. With the exception of the so-called venous sinuses of the dura mater (see below), these two layers are firmly fused. In adults, the dura can be separated from the cranial bone with relative ease; only along the cranial sutures, on the petrosal bone, near the sella turcica, and on the lamina cribrosa of the ethmoid bone is the attachment firmer. The outer surface of the detached dura is rough, whereas the inner surface is perfectly smooth. In infants, the attachment is so firm that dura and skull cannot be dissected free. The venous sinuses of the dura mater are special blood vessels that drain the venous blood from the brain to the internal jugular vein. These sinuses are thin endothelial tubes which, so to speak, are "embedded" in the dura. Apart from the endothelium, these blood vessels have no proper wall.

Duplicatures

Arising from the dura mater, several septa extend between various parts of the brain and divide the cranial cavity into compartments. This ensures better fixation of the brain mass within the skull and prevents untoward movements of brain parts. The principal dural duplicatures are the falx cerebri, the tentorium cerebelli, the diaphragma sella, and the falx cerebelli.

The *falx cerebri* (Fig. 17–1) arises from the crista galli of the ethmoid bone, along the midline of the cranial roof, and extends to the internal occipital protuberance. The upper margin encompasses the superior sagittal sinus. The free lower margin of the falx encompasses the inferior sagittal sinus, which opens into the sinus rectus (see Fig. 18–13). The falx is a deep, sagittal dural septum that separates the hemispheres. The corpus callosum is located below the free margin of the falx.

The *tentorium cerebelli* forms a roof over the cerebellum located in the posterior cranial fossa. The occipital lobe of the cerebrum is located above the tentorium. The line of attachment follows a groove in the occipital bone in which the transverse sinus is located, and then a groove in the petrosal bone in which the superior petrosal sinus lies (Fig. 17–2); it ends near the posterior clinoid process. The falx cerebri is attached to the center of the tentorium; this attachment encompasses the sinus rectus, which collects the blood from the central gray substance and drains it to the confluence of sinuses (see below).

When we follow the lower margin of the falx cerebri in an occipital direction, the falx seems to divide itself into two leaves that form the tentorium or at least its superior layer. The free lower margin of the falx is continuous with the free margin of the tentorium; this margin extends rostrally and attaches to the anterior clinoid process (Fig. 17–1). Between the dorsum sellae

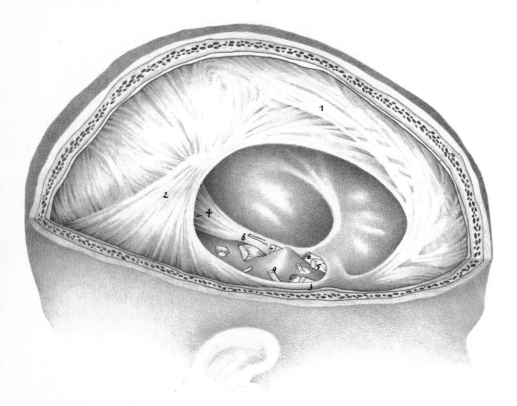

Figure 17–1 Cerebral dura mater and cerebellar tentorium (according to Rauber-Kopsch).

1 falx cerebri
2 cerebellar tentorium
3 anterior clinoid process
4 tentorial notch
5 optic nerve
6 internal carotid artery
7 oculomotor nerve
8 trochlear nerve
9 oculomotor nerve

Figure 17–2 Base of the brain, with dura mater in situ; entries of the cranial nerves. The sinus cavernosus and the trigeminal space are open on the right side.

1 anterior meningeal artery
2 lamina cribrosa
3 optic nerve
4 internal carotid artery
5 diaphragma sellae
6 infundibulum
7 oculomotor nerve
8 trochlear nerve
9 trigeminal nerve
10 abducens nerve
11 glossopharyngeal nerve, vagus nerve, accessory nerve
12 hypoglossal nerve
13 facial nerve, intermediate nerve, labyrinthine artery, vestibulocochlear nerve
14 greater petrosal nerve
15 middle meningeal artery
16 frontal branch of middle meningeal artery
17 meningeal branch of occipital artery
18 trigeminal ganglion
19 transverse sinus
20 cavernous sinus
21 superior petrosal sinus
22 sigmoid sinus

and the free margin of the tentorium lies a U-shaped opening (tentorial notch), which encompasses the brain stem and part of the cerebellar lingula (Fig. 17–2).

The anterior end of the tentorium is slightly twisted so that the insertion of the free margin and that of the tentorium proper decussate before attaching to the anterior and posterior clinoid processes, respectively; between the decussation and the attachment, the dura is perforated by the oculomotor (3rd cranial) nerve. The trochlear (4th cranial) nerve perforates the dura behind the oculomotor nerve. The two nerves then pass through the wall of the sinus cavernosus to the superior orbital fissure and the orbit. The anterior attachment of the tentorium also forms the roof and the medial wall of the sinus cavernosus.

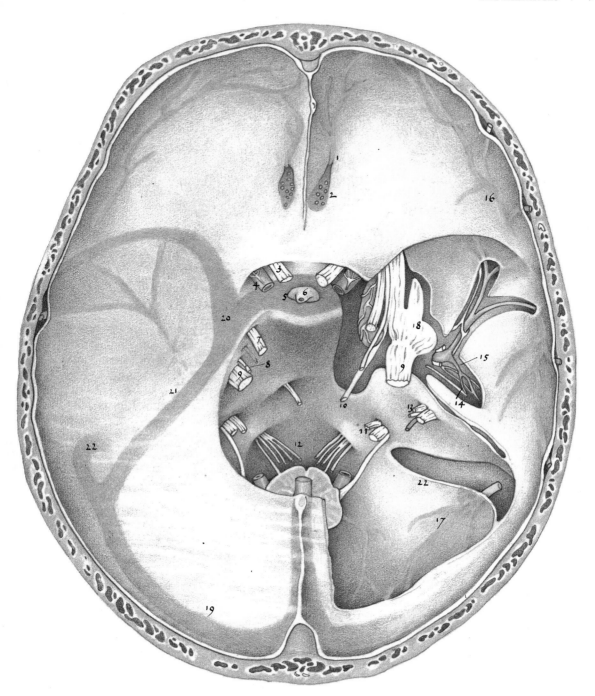

Falx cerebri and tentorium cerebelli together form what could be described as an interior "overpass" in both the sagittal and the horizontal planes. In neonates, this overpass is of great importance because it prevents cranial deformations.

The *diaphragma sellae* is a small dural fold that closes the entrance to the sella turcica. In this way the hypophysis is enclosed in an osteofibrous chamber. The diaphragm has a small circular aperture through which the infundibulum passes.

The *falx cerebelli* arises from the undersurface of the tentorium near the internal occipital protuberance. The free margin of the falx extends between the cerebellar hemispheres.

Innervation

The dura mater of the cranial roof is hardly sensitive to pain, but the basal part of the dura and the large blood vessels do have pain perception. The anterior cranial fossa and the tentorium cerebelli are innervated by branches of the ophthalmic division and meningeal branches of the maxillary division of the trigeminal (5th cranial) nerve. The middle cranial fossa is innervated by branches of the maxillary and the mandibular division of the trigeminal nerve. The subtentorial part of the dura is innervated mainly by ascending branches of the 2nd and 3rd cervical nerves, which enter the cranial cavity via the foramen magnum. Participation of the glossopharyngeal and vagus nerves in the sensory innervation of the dura mater is uncertain.

Postganglionic fibers from the superior cervical ganglion reach the dura along the adventitia of the large arteries (internal carotid and middle meningeal arteries). These are probably vasomotor fibers.

Vascularization

The vascularization of the dura mater is totally independent of that of the brain. The arteries extend in the periosteal layer of the dura and leave deep grooves in the cranial bones. Despite their name (meningeal arteries), these blood vessels vascularize mainly the skull (Fig. 17–2).

The anterior cranial fossa is vascularized by branches of the anterior and posterior ethmoid arteries. The middle cranial fossa is vascularized by the middle meningeal and the accessory meningeal arteries and by a branch of the ascending pharyngeal artery that enters via the foramen lacerum. The posterior cranial fossa is vascularized by branches of the occipital artery, which have entered the skull via the jugular and the mastoid foramen.

The Middle Meningeal Artery and Extradural Hemorrhages. The middle meningeal artery is the principal dural artery; it is a branch of the maxillary artery and enters the cranial cavity through the spinous foramen (Fig. 17–2). Within the skull it divides into an anterior and a posterior branch. The former extends anteriorly to the anterior cranial fossa, while the latter takes an arching course in a superoposterior direction and vascularizes the occipital bone, the parietal bone, and part of the cerebellar tentorium.

Lesions of the middle meningeal artery often result from head injuries (fracture of the skull). In many of these cases, a convexity fracture arises from the parietal region and extends perpendicular to the middle meningeal artery. Because the artery is attached to the cranial bone, shearing forces involved in the fracture can cause vascular rupture. The high blood pressure produces an increasing extradural (epidural) hematoma; the dura is loosened from the interior surface of the skull, and the resulting rapid increase in intracranial pressure necessitates acute surgical intervention (decompression via trephination).

THE LEPTOMENINX (PIA AND ARACHNOID)

The arachnoid ("spider's web") consists of a thin layer of flat cells immediately next to the dura. Dura and arachnoid are connected by a neurothelial layer and by the so-called anchor veins, the traversing veins originating from the cortex and on their way to the venous sinuses. The arachnoid is not of the same thickness throughout and, unlike the pia mater, does not enter the grooves of the brain surface; the subarachnoid space is, therefore, of very variable

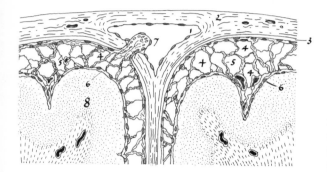

Figure 17–3 Transverse section through the superior sagittal sinus; meninges and subarachnoid space (according to Weed).

1 superior sagittal sinus
2 dura mater
3 subdural space (potential)
4 subarachnoid space
5 arachnoid trabecula
6 pia mater
7 arachnoid granulation (pacchionian granulation)
8 cerebral cortex

size. Most of the more marked dilatations of this space (cisterns) are localized on the basal side of the brain.

Numerous trabeculae arise from the interior surface of the arachnoid and bridge the subarachnoid space to connect the arachnoid with the pia (Fig. 17–3). Near the cisterns, these trabeculae are underdeveloped or absent.

The surface of fixed brain specimens is covered by pia and arachnoid, while the dura and the corresponding outer layer of the arachnoid have usually remained on the interior surface of the skull.

Subarachnoid Space

The subarachnoid space contains CSF and the larger blood vessels that vascularize the brain. In some areas of the base of the brain there are considerable dilatations of this space (cisterns). The capacity of the subarachnoid spaces of the brain is about 25 ml.

The principal *cisterns* are the cisterna magna, pontine cistern, and interpeduncular cistern. The cisterna magna is located in the angle between cerebellum and medulla oblongata and communicates with the fourth ventricle via the

median aperture (foramen of Magendie). Caudally, the cisterna magna communicates with the subarachnoid space around the spinal cord. The dorsocaudal wall of the cisterna magna is adjacent to the posterior atlantooccipital membrane. The pontine and the interpeduncular cisterns are dilatations on the ventral side of the pons and the mesencephalon. They contain the basilar artery and the circle of Willis, respectively. The (superior) cisterna ambiens is located between the splenium and the upper surface of the cerebellum and contains the pineal body.

Arachnoidal (Pacchionian) Granulations

These are sacs of arachnoidal tissue that protrude into the cavity of the superior sagittal sinus and other venous canals of the skull (Fig. 17–3). Macroscopically they look like villus-shaped buds that are connected with the subarachnoid space by a slender stalk, surrounded by the dura (Fig. 17–3). These buds increase in size and number with increasing age.

The subarachnoidal sacs are lined with a delicate layer of mesothelium. Each sac contains a reticulum of collagenous fibers with fibrocytes and macrophages. Venous blood and CSF are separated only by the mesothelium with its basement membrane and the endothelium of the sinus. Jayatilaka (1965) and Gomez and Potts (1974) described in these sacs tangles of tubules connecting the subarachnoid space with the venous space. The CSF, they maintained, reached the blood via these tubules, which were kept open by the colloid osmotic pressure of the blood and the hydrostatic pressure of the CSF. However, other authors have refuted the existence of these tubules.

CSF Circulation

Once the CSF reaches the subarachnoid space via the apertures in the roof of the fourth ventricle (Fig. 17–4), it disperses around the brain and spinal cord, and forms a "water cushion" that suspends these structures. The CSF ascends through the tentorial incisure and along the undersurface and the convexity of the hemispheres as far as the vertex, where the arachnoidal granulations ensure its absorption into the

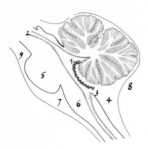

Figure 17–4 Midline section through cerebellum and brain stem, communication between fourth ventricle and cisterna magna (from Benninghoff).

1 fourth ventricle
2 cerebral aqueduct
3 median aperture of fourth ventricle (foramen of Magendie)
4 cisterna magna
5 pons
6 medulla oblongata
7 pontine cistern
8 arachnoid
9 interpeduncular cistern

venous blood of the superior sagittal sinus and other veins. A proportion of the CSF is absorbed along the roots of the spinal and cranial nerves, or directly from the veins in the subarachnoid space. About 250 ml of CSF is produced per day; the ventricles and aqueduct contain about 35 ml, while about 100 ml is contained in the total subarachnoid space.

Microscopic Structure of the Leptomeninx

The arachnoid consists of a delicate network of low-density connective tissue and is lined by a few layers of flat (mesothelial) cells. Numerous delicate trabeculae arise from the arachnoid and continue in the upper layer of the pia mater (Fig. 17–3). Although the arachnoid is usually described as avascular, this membrane supplies the anatomic substrate (trabeculae) for the course of many small blood vessels to the brain surface (Fig. 17–3). All blood vessels and nerves within the subarachnoid space are therefore lined with arachnoid tissue. The subarachnoid space is effectively sealed off from the dura by many tight junctions between the cells of the arachnoid.

Subdural Space. The boundary between dura and arachnoid is often regarded as a potential crevice in which both the interior aspect of the dura and the exterior aspect of the arachnoid are lined with mesothelial cells. This crevice does not communicate with the subarachnoid space but, via the perineurium of the nerves, is in communication with the cervical lymph nodes. Electron microscopic studies of the borderline

area between the two meninges (Andres, 1967; Nabeshima et al., 1975), however, revealed no crevice but an area in which numerous cell extensions are entangled. Between the extensions there are fairly wide intercellular spaces in which a filamentous substance is contained. The extensions are kept together by desmosomes; this layer of cells is called a ''neurothelium.'' The so-called subdural space probably results from postmortem vacuolation of the neurothelium.

Structure of the Pia Mater. Two layers can be distinguished in the pia mater: the epipia and the intima-pia. The epipia is continuous with the arachnoid and is sometimes regarded as arachnoid proper; the intima-pia is a leaf of low-density connective tissue localized against the glial membrane that bounds the brain surface. A distinctly plicated basement membrane separates the intima-pia from the glial membrane. The pia follows all the configurations of the brain surface, but the arachnoid does not. The pia is highly vascular, the blood vessels being embedded in some connective tissue of the pia mater proper. As they enter the brain and spinal cord, blood vessels are enveloped over some distance by a perivascular sheath of pia and arachnoid (perivascular space of Virchow-Robin). The two layers ultimately fuse with the adventitia of the arterioles, so that the capillaries are not separated from the nerve tissue by extravascular connective tissue structures. The CSF in the perivascular space is believed to receive and neutralize the shock effect of the pulse wave.

Blood-Brain Barrier. As the perivascular spaces of Virchow-Robin disappear, the small arterioles and capillaries within the brain are enveloped solely by glia extensions. Only the capillary endothelium with its basement membrane and the pericapillary glia extensions separate the blood plasma from the intercellular space; the pericapillary glia extensions form a sheath. The functional characteristics of the endothelium or of the glia sheath ensure selective passage of substances from the blood to the nerve cells. The CNS is inaccessible to many substances that circulate in the blood (pigments, drugs, antibodies, etc.). After being injected into the blood stream, these substances do not reach the neurons of the CNS, hence the term blood-brain barrier.

Spinal Meninges

Around the foramen magnum, the dura mater divides into an outer leaf (vertebral periosteum) and an inner leaf (spinal dura mater in the proper sense). Between these two leaves there remains a space that contains fat and a venous plexus (epidural space).

Where the roots of the spinal nerves perforate the dura, they are provided with a dural sheath as far as the intervertebral foramen. As the nerves reach the intervertebral foramen, the dural sheath fuses with the periosteum. The ventral and dorsal roots of C1 to T8 pass through the dura mater separately, for the most part; the dural sac becomes singular only at the site of union of the two roots (see Fig. 16–1). Singular dural portals are found below T8. The nerves of the cauda equina are likewise enclosed by a long dural sheath.

EPIDURAL SPACE

The outer leaf of the dura already merges into the periosteum of the vertebral arches and ligamenta flava in 18-month-old infants. The two dural leaves fuse at the foramen magnum and mark the cranial boundary of the epidural space. Its caudal boundary is determined by the caudal end of the sacral canal (sacral hiatus), which is closed by a layer of connective tissue. The dural sac terminates at the approximate level of the first sacral vertebra.

The epidural space encompasses veins, arteries, and nerve roots. The veins form the internal vertebral plexus, which drains the blood from the spinal cord and the wall of the vertebral canal. This plexus is localized in the ventrolateral part of the epidural space; right/left connections are found, and it is noticed that the internal diameter of the ventrally located veins is considerable. This causes the venous plexus to resemble a kind of rope ladder (Luyendijk, 1962). The internal vertebral plexus has no valves; consequently, carcinoma metastases located in the lower half of the body can reach the brain via this plexus in response to acute abdominal straining (such as occurs with coughing and sneezing).

LUMBAR PUNCTURE

Samples of CSF can be obtained by lumbar puncture, a widely used technique that is usually not dangerous. The needle is inserted between L4 and L5 or between L5 and S1 and introduced into the dural sac. At this level there is no risk of inadvertent puncture of the spinal cord. The needle is inserted exactly in the median plane, from a caudal direction at an angle of 70° with the surface of the back. Having passed the ligamentum flavum (indicated by a somewhat resilient resistance), the needle is advanced a few millimeters until CSF is seen to escape. Lumbar puncture can be dangerous in patients with increased intracranial pressure.

Chapter 18

Vascularization of the Central Nervous System

The arterial vascularization of the CNS shows various morphologic characteristics that are explained, in part, by embryonic development and by special demands made on the blood circulation in connection with metabolism. Nerve tissue is exceedingly sensitive to reduction of the blood supply because the metabolism is aerobic and the oxygen consumption virtually constant. A diminished oxygen supply, therefore, immediately reduces the metabolism. Within five seconds of interruption of the cerebral circulation, loss of consciousness ensues. After an interruption lasting about four minutes, certain areas of the cerebral cortex are irreversibly damaged. This is why the vascular system of the brain should ensure fairly constant perfusion.

The vascularization of the brain is anatomically and functionally different from that of other organs. The regulation of the cerebral circulation is largely "autonomic": For example, the vasoconstriction that generally follows a significant decrease in blood pressure does not occur in the brain. The blood supply to the CNS is regulated by three major arterial systems: (a) the system of the carotid artery, (b) the system of the vertebral artery, and (c) the vertebroaortomedullary system, which comprises the anterior and posterior radicular arteries that supply the spinal cord with blood via the so-called corona vasorum.

The following sections separately discuss the vascularization of the brain and that of the spinal cord.

Cerebral Vascularization

The rapid growth of the brain during the fetal and postnatal periods is supported by the vascular system in that it receives preferential treatment, as indicated by the fact that the oxygenated blood supplied is free from any admixture of venous blood. This is ensured by the fact that the great aortic branches destined for the head arise from the aortic arch proximal to the site of origin of the ductus arteriosus. Moreover, the oxygenated blood is transported to the brain by the shortest route, through blood vessels without ramifications. In this respect the two major supply systems — the carotid and the vertebral systems — are comparable (Fig. 18–1).

CHARACTERISTICS OF THE CEREBRAL ARTERIES

The Superficial Vascular Network

The cerebrum differs from other organs in the unusual arrangement of its vascular pattern. The cerebrum is an organ without a hilus, and its main supplying branches are located basally and therefore eccentrically. From this basal origin, the cerebral arteries are distributed over the brain surface, from which they ramify perpendicularly into the brain tissue so that the intracerebral circulation flows from the inside out (*centripetal circulation*). The supplying arteries can be compared with an annular network from which branches extend from the periphery to the center (Van den Bergh, 1960). This is in marked contrast to the arrangement of the vascular pattern of other organs, in which the main arterial branches first reach a more or less central position in the organ (kidney, spleen), and then supply the organ with blood via terminal branches that extend from the center to the periphery (*centrifugal circulation*).

Although the intracerebral vascular network is of the centripetal type, it includes a few

Figure 18–1 Schematic representation of the vascularization of the brain from the aortic arch and the subclavian artery (according to Chusid).

1 carotid sinus
2 external carotid artery
3 internal carotid artery
4 vertebral artery
5 subclavian artery
6 basilar artery
7 ophthalmic artery
8 posterior cerebral artery
9 eyeball
10 aortic arch

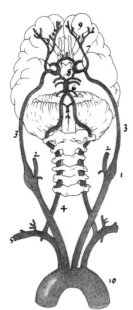

smaller centrifugal arteries, the choroid arteries, which occupy a special position in the vascularization of the brain.

Cortical and Central Branches

The arterial vascular network of the CNS can be divided into a central and a peripheral system. The central system originates from the cerebral arterial circle and from the proximal segments of the three principal cerebral arteries. The central arteries reach their territories from the base of the brain; they enter the brain via the anterior perforated substance and the posterior perforated substance. The main branches are the striate branches, which supply a large part of the basal ganglia and the internal capsule.

The peripheral system comprises the arteries of the cortex and of the white matter, which originate from the distal segments of the three principal cerebral arteries. The peripheral branches form a superficial plexus in the pia mater, from which smaller "terminal" branches enter the brain tissue and end in the cerebral cortex (the cortical branches). Other branches (medullary branches) pass through the cortex and end in the white matter.

Anastomoses between the Cerebral Arteries

The anastomoses between the supplying arterial systems can be divided into three levels: (a) anastomoses between the intracranial and the extracranial circulations, which in the normal situation are inactive (see below); (b) anastomoses between the carotid and the vertebral system on the base of the brain (arterial circle of Willis); and (c) anastomoses between the leptomeningeal arteries on the exterior surface of the brain.

The existence and functional significance of leptomeningeal anastomoses have been widely debated. According to Cohnheim (1872), all cerebral arteries are terminal vessels; Beevor (1909), however, postulated that the anastomoses between the various principal arteries are more important than those between branches of the same artery. Others (van den Eecken and Adams, 1953; van den Eecken, 1959) demonstrated that the largest anastomoses are always found along the borderline regions of the three major cerebral arteries and have their origin in two different arteries.

Histologic Characteristics

The histologic structure of the cerebral arteries differs substantially from that of other arteries of comparable size; their walls are less thick due to the much thinner muscular layer in the tunica media and the underdeveloped tunica adventitia. They have no external elastic membrane, but the internal elastic membrane is extremely thick. The collagenous and elastic fibers of the adventitia show an annular arrangement. The wall of the cerebral arteries comprises about 22 per cent collagenous fibers, 2 per cent elastic fibers, and about 74 per cent muscular tissue. Some authors (Goerttler, 1953) have postulated that the reduced thickness of the wall results from the fact that the cerebral arteries are located in a CSF-filled space (the subarachnoid space). Because in maturity the skull has become a well closed unit, the CSF cannot be compressed; consequently it "supports" the vascular wall and bears part of the mural tension.

In this context it may be mentioned that the typical difference in mural structure between

Figure 18–2 Schematic representation of the normal course of the cerebral arteries at carotid arteriography. The middle cerebral artery is shown in black, while the anterior cerebral artery is in white (according to Krayenbuhl and Yasargil).

1   internal carotid artery
2   ophthalmic artery
3   petrosal bone
4   dorsum sellae
5   anterior cerebral artery
6   pericallosal artery
7   frontopolar artery
8   callosomarginal artery
9   anterior choroidal artery
10 orbitofrontal artery
11 prerolandic artery
12 temporal arteries
13 posterior parietal artery

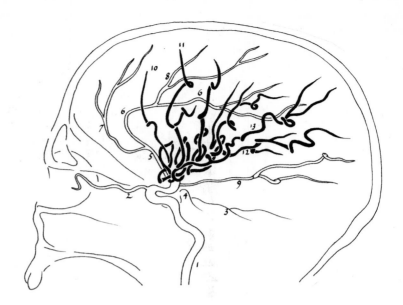

cerebral and extracerebral arteries does not become apparent until the fontanelles have disappeared and the skull has become a rigid enclosing structure. Prior to the disappearance of the fontanelles, there is no structural difference between intracranial and extracranial arteries.

THE SYSTEM OF THE CAROTID ARTERY

The carotid system is the largest system supplying the brain and comprises the common carotid artery and the internal carotid artery with its terminal branches. In anatomic specimens it can be seen that the internal carotid could be regarded as the direct continuation of the common carotid. The two arteries are in line and both are without complex ramifications. The external carotid, however, should be viewed as a large lateral branch of the carotid system (Fig. 18–1), for its diameter is smaller and it has a characteristic, rich pattern of ramification. Arteriography reveals that the internal carotid first fills with contrast medium, and only subsequently the external carotid.

The internal carotid ascends almost perpendicularly in the cervical region, passes behind the stylohyoid muscles and reaches the entry of the carotid canal of the cerebral base. Through this canal it extends to the interior surface of the skull; in the bony canal, the artery is surrounded by a plexus of small veins and sympathetic nerve branches that originate from the sympathetic trunk. The artery enters the carotid sulcus of the sphenoid bone through the foramen lacerum. In the sulcus, the artery lies in the space of the sinus cavernosus and has close relations with the third, fourth, and sixth cranial nerves and the ophthalmic nerve. This part of the course of the internal carotid (see Fig. 17–2) is called C4 by radiologists.

In the immediate vicinity of the anterior clinoid process, the artery abruptly turns in a superoposterior direction (Fig. 18–2) and produces the ophthalmic artery (carotid siphon, area C3). The artery then perforates the dura mater (see Fig. 17–2) and enters the subarachnoid space, passing alongside the hypophysis (C2). The terminal segment (C1) of the carotid produces several terminal and lateral branches (posterior communicating, anterior choroid, and anterior cerebral arteries). The trunk of the artery continues laterally as the middle cerebral artery. The terminal branches of the internal carotid already form part of that remarkable arterial ring of the cerebral base, the circle of Willis.

The internal carotid artery can be regarded as a kind of "short circuit" (Fig. 18–1) in the vascular system of the head, through which blood can pass directly from the aorta to the cerebrum without any deviation through the facial, mandibular, or oral vascular regions. The internal carotid exclusively supplies the cerebrum and the eyeball with the eye muscles and other tissues of the orbital region. The external carotid, however, vascularizes the face and the cranial wall with its dural lining and part of the cervical region. In the head there are two, functionally almost independent circulations: the intracranial (internal carotid) and the extracranial (external carotid). Anatomically there are anastomoses between these two circulations (see below); these anastomoses can play an important role in developmental disorders, for example, with anomalies of the cerebral circulation.

Branches of the Internal Carotid Artery

Collateral Branches. In its course through the carotid canal and sinus cavernosus, the internal carotid artery gives rise to small branches extending to the tympanic cavity (caroticotympanic branch) and to the trigeminal ganglion and the hypophysis. The principal side branch of the internal carotid is the ophthalmic artery.

OPHTHALMIC ARTERY. This artery arises from the convexity of the carotid knee, medial to the anterior clinoid process, and along with the optic nerve enters the orbit through the optic canal. It vascularizes the eye (central retinal artery, posterior and anterior ciliary arteries), the lacrimal gland (lacrimal artery), and the extrinsic eye muscles (muscular branches). Other branches are the supraorbital artery, the dorsal artery of the nose, and the frontal artery. These three branches anastomose with arteries of the extracranial circulation (superficial temporal and angular arteries). In the event of obstruction of the internal carotid, these collateral anastomoses can develop into new supply routes along which the blood of the external carotid artery can reach the intracranial vascular system.

Terminal Branches

ANTERIOR CEREBRAL ARTERY. This artery, about 3 mm in diameter, arises from the terminal ramification of the internal carotid and extends between the optic nerve and the cerebral base to the longitudinal cerebral fissure, where the two vessels communicate via a transverse anastomosis (anterior communicating artery) and follows the upper margin of the corpus callosum on the medial aspect of the hemisphere. The terminal branch of the anterior cerebral artery (the pericallosal artery) leaves the corpus callosum near the splenium and ascends to the area of the precuneus, as far as the parietooccipital fissure.

From its origin to the level of the rostrum, this artery gives rise to two or three side branches (frontobasal, frontopolar, and callosomarginal arteries). From the initial segment of the anterior cerebral and anterior communicating arteries, numerous small branches arise to supply the corpus callosum, the septum pellucidum, and part of the caudate nucleus and hypothalamus. Known as anteromedial arteries (Fig. 18–3), these enter the brain through the medial part of the anterior perforated substance. Proximal to the anterior communicating artery arises the last central branch, the recurrent artery (Heubner), which supplies the head of the caudate nucleus, the anterior limb of the internal capsule, and parts of the septum.

ANTERIOR COMMUNICATING ARTERY. This is a transverse anastomosis between the two anterior cerebral arteries at the level of the optic chiasm. Its diameter varies from 1 to 3 mm, and its length also varies but rarely exceeds 3 mm. In a study of 2359 cases (Piganiol et al., 1960) the communicating artery was found lacking in 0.5 per cent; in 3.8 per cent it was filiform and nonfunctional.

MIDDLE CEREBRAL ARTERY. This artery (Fig. 18–2) can be regarded as the direct continuation of the internal carotid. It curves around the temporal pole of the hemisphere and reaches the lateral cerebral fissure; near the limen insulae it curves dorsally again and divides into several cortical branches (sylvian arteries) that extend along the surface of the insula. Many of these branches are located in the depth of the sulci and are hidden from direct view. They vascularize most of the convexity of the hemispheres. From the initial segment of the middle cerebral artery

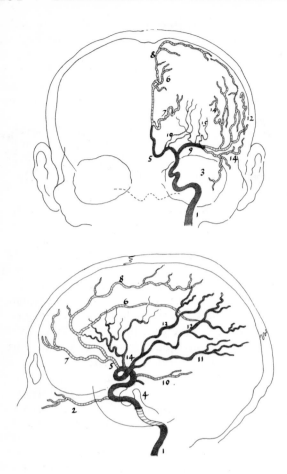

Figure 18–3 Schematic representation of normal carotid arteriograms. A, Anteroposterior projection; B, lateral projection (according to List, Barge and Hodges).

1	internal carotid artery
2	ophthalmic artery
3	orbit
4	dorsum sellae
5	anterior cerebral artery
6	pericallosal artery
7	frontopolar artery
8	callosomarginal artery
9	middle cerebral artery
10	anteromedial arteries and anterior choroidal artery
11	temporal arteries
12	posterior parietal artery
13	anterior parietal artery
14	lateral frontobasal arteries
15	central branches of middle cerebral artery

arises the anterior choroidal artery; this enters the sulcus between the temporal lobe and the brain stem, there to reach the choroid fissure, and then extends to the choroid plexus of the lateral ventricle.

The principal cortical branches of the middle cerebral artery extend in a fan-shaped pattern. They are (Fig. 18–2) (a) the lateral frontobasal artery, which supplies the orbital region, (b) the triangular artery, which vascularizes the motor area of speech, (c) the prerolandic artery, which supplies the central sulcus and adjacent areas, (d) the anterior and posterior parietal arteries, which vascularize the parietal lobe, and (e) the temporal arteries, which supply the temporal lobe.

The small central branches arise from the proximal segment of the middle cerebral artery and extend to the deep structures of the hemispheres. They enter the brain through the anterior perforated substance. Two groups can be distinguished: the medial striate branches, which vascularize the caudate nucleus and the internal capsule, and the lateral striate branches, which pass through the internal capsule and vascularize parts of the caudate nucleus (Fig. 18–3A). Intracranial hemorrhages are often due to rupture of one of these branches.

POSTERIOR COMMUNICATING ARTERY. This artery anastomoses the internal carotid artery with the posterior cerebral artery, a branch of the basilar artery (Fig. 18–4). Its diameter is 1 to 2 mm. Bilateral absence of this artery is found in 0.4 per cent of cases (Laveille, 1966); unilateral absence in 3.6 per cent. Instances of hypoplasia, however, are far more numerous. The posterior communicating artery gives rise to the posteromedial branches, which enter the brain through the tuber cinereum and the interpeduncular fossa. The rostral group of branches vascularizes the hypophysis and tuber cinereum; some extend further into the brain and vascularize large parts of the thalamus. The caudal group vascularizes the mamillary bodies, the subthalamus, and parts of the mesencephalon (tegmentum, pes pedunculi).

THE SYSTEM OF THE VERTEBRAL ARTERY

The vertebral artery is the first branch to arise from the subclavian artery; it extends in a superior direction along the posterior aspect of the anterior scalenus muscle and enters the transverse foramen of the sixth (sometimes the fifth) cervical vertebra. It continues through the transverse foramina of the vertebrae above this level and is located ventral to the exiting spinal cord nerves. The artery curves laterally and reaches the transverse foramen of the atlas, whereupon it curves medially again, perforates the posterior atlantooccipital membrane and foramen magnum, passes through the dura, and finally enters the posterior cranial fossa. The curvatures of the vertebral artery shortly before it enters the cranial cavity are "spare" loops, which prevent traction on the artery during movements of the head (Fig. 18–1).

At the level of the lower margin of the pons, the two vertebral arteries fuse to constitute a single vessel, the basilar artery. At the level of the mamillary bodies the basilar artery divides into its terminal branches, the posterior cerebral arteries.

On morphologic grounds, the vertebral artery can be compared with the carotid system. Both arteries ascend perpendicularly (see Fig. 18–8) without important ramifications (apart from the external carotid artery). Both perforate the cerebral base via a peculiarly tortuous route ("carotid siphon," "vertebral siphon"). The major difference is that the two vertebral arteries fuse to become a single vessel (basilar artery), whereas the internal carotid arteries continue individually. Hemodynamically, however, there is a permanent separation of the two flows within the basilar artery: The blood from the left vertebral artery flows through the left side of the brain stem, and that from the right vertebral artery flows through the right side of the brain stem.

Branches of the Vertebral Artery

The system of the vertebral artery vascularizes the brain stem and the cerebellum as well as a considerable part of the basal aspect of the

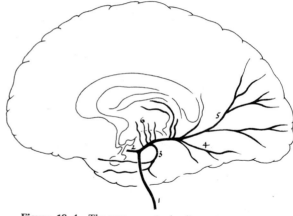

Figure 18–4 The posterior cerebral artery at vertebral arteriography (according to Krayenbuhl and Yasargil).

1 basilar artery
2 posterior communicating artery
3 anterior temporal artery
4 lateral branch of posterior cerebral artery
5 medial branch of posterior cerebral artery
6 interpeduncular arteries

hemispheres, including the occipital lobe. The pattern of ramification is characterized by trunks that extend on the basal surface of the brain stem, from where they give rise to side branches that form an annular pattern around the brain stem. In principle, three groups of branches can be distinguished: the paramedian arteries (short, slender branches that enter the tissues on either side of the midline), the short circumferential arteries, and the long circumferential arteries.

The vertebral artery produces two important branches destined for the medulla and the superior part of the spinal cord: the anterior and the posterior spinal arteries. The former arises at the level of the pyramid (see Fig. 11–3). The artery descends to the midline and unites with its contralateral counterpart to form the anterior spinal artery. This artery, which extends in the midline over the spinal cord, anastomoses with the ventral radicular arteries from C4 on. The posterior spinal artery descends on each side along the dorsal aspect of the spinal cord. This artery is often a side branch of the posterior inferior cerebellar artery.

The Basilar Artery

The two vertebral arteries unite on the ventral side of the medulla to form the basilar artery. The left vertebral artery is usually more developed than the right; this may have important consequences in the event of occlusion of the larger artery. The basilar artery extends in a superior direction along the median pontine sulcus and, at the level of the dorsum sellae, divides into its two terminal branches, the posterior cerebral arteries. The anastomoses between these arteries and the posterior communicating arteries close the arterial circle of Willis.

Branches of the Basilar Artery

POSTERIOR CEREBRAL ARTERY. The proximal part of the artery is separated from the superior cerebellar artery by the oculomotor nerve; at this level its diameter is about 3 mm. The artery curves around the cerebral peduncle as far as the lateral geniculate body, where it divides into its two large terminal branches, the medial and the lateral branches. The posterior cerebral artery vascularizes the basal part of the temporal lobe, the occipital lobe, the tectum, the pineal body, and parts of the thalamus (pulvinar), the dorsal part of the internal capsule, and the lateral geniculate body (see Figs. 11–3 and 18–4).

Cortical branches of the posterior cerebral artery are the quadrigeminal artery (for the tectum), the posterior choroidal arteries (for the plexus of the third and the lateral ventricles), the medial branch (for the occipital lobe), and the lateral branch (for the temporal lobe). Central branches are the interpeduncular arteries, which perforate the posterior perforated substance and vascularize the posterior part of the thalamus, the internal capsule, and the subthalamus.

CEREBELLAR ARTERIES. The cerebellum is vascularized by three arteries: the superior cerebellar artery and the anterior inferior cerebellar artery, which arise from the basilar artery, and the posterior inferior cerebellar artery, which originates from the vertebral artery (see Fig. 18–6). The superior cerebellar artery arises from the basilar artery proximal to its terminal bifurcation. It extends in the sulcus between peduncle and pons and vascularizes the superior aspect of

the cerebellum and the superior cerebellar peduncle. The anterior inferior cerebellar artery is quite variable. It arises from the middle part of the basilar artery, extends in a laterodorsal direction, produces small branches to the brain stem, and ends on the basal side of the cerebellum in the area of the flocculus. It vascularizes the pyramis, the flocculus, and the tuber. The posterior inferior cerebellar artery arises from the vertebral artery. First it extends on the lateral surface of the medulla, and then reaches the undersurface of the cerebellum. It vascularizes the uvula, nodulus, tonsil, and parts of the cerebellar hemispheres.

VASCULAR COMPARTMENTS IN THE BRAIN STEM

The vascular areas of the brain stem are shown in Figure 18–5. The ventral part of the pons is vascularized by the paramedian and the short circumferential arteries. The tegmentum (reticular formation, facial nucleus, abducens nucleus, and trapezoid body) is vascularized by

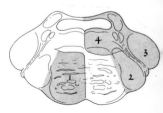
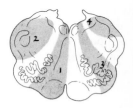
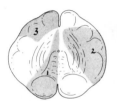

Figure 18–5 Vascular areas of the arteries of the brain stem. A, Pons; B, cranial part and C, caudal part of medulla oblongata (according to Carpenter).

A
1 paramedian arteries
2 short circumferential arteries
3 anterior inferior cerebral artery
4 long circumferential arteries
B
1 anterior spinal artery
2 posterior inferior cerebral artery
3 vertebral artery
4 posterior spinal artery
C
1 anterior spinal artery
2 vertebral artery
3 posterior spinal artery

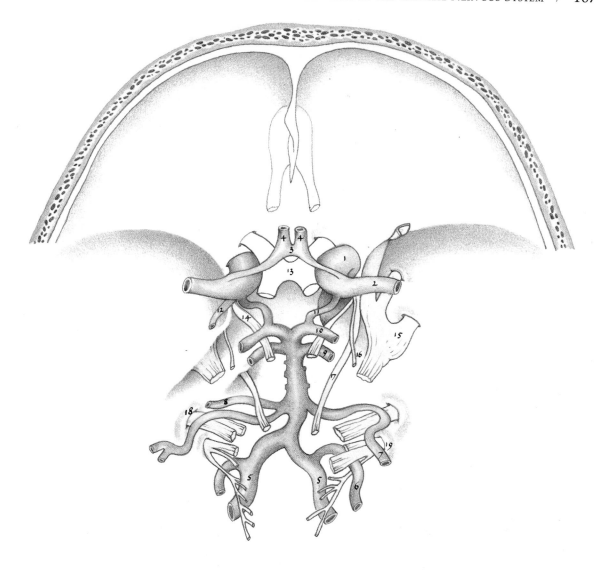

Figure 18–6 Base of cerebrum, circle of Willis, and cranial nerves (according to Walsh).

1 internal carotid artery
2 middle cerebral artery
3 anterior communicating artery
4 anterior cerebral artery
5 vertebral artery
6 posterior inferior cerebellar artery
7 anterior inferior cerebellar artery
8 labyrinthine artery
9 superior cerebellar artery
10 posterior cerebral artery
11 posterior communicating artery
12 anterior choroidal artery
13 optic chiasm
14 oculomotor nerve
15 trigeminal nerve
16 trochlear nerve
17 abducens nerve
18 facial nerve, intermediate nerve, vestibulocochlear nerve
19 glossopharyngeal nerve, vagus nerve, accessory nerve

the long circumferential arteries. The most lateral part of the pons (brachium conjunctivum, brachium pontis) lies within the territory of the superior and anterior inferior cerebellar arteries.

In the medulla oblongata, at the level of the olive, a wedge-shaped zone on either side of the midline is vascularized by the anterior spinal arteries. Lateral to each zone lies an area vascularized by direct branches from the vertebral artery. The posterior inferior cerebellar artery and posterior spinal artery vascularize the dorsolateral part of the medulla oblongata. At the level of the nuclei of the posterior funiculus there are three vascular areas: a ventral area (anterior spinal artery), a lateral area (vertebral artery), and a dorsal area (posterior spinal artery).

THE ARTERIAL CIRCLE OF WILLIS

The circle of Willis (circulus arteriosus) is a virtually annular double anastomosis between the two carotid arteries on the one hand and the carotid artery and basilar artery on the other hand, localized at the base of the brain. In this ring an anterior and a posterior segment can be distinguished. The anterior segment comprises the distal part of the internal carotid artery (C1), the proximal part of the anterior cerebral artery, and the anterior communicating artery (Fig. 18–6); the posterior segment comprises the posterior communicating arteries (right and left) and the initial part of the posterior cerebral arteries. This vascular ring gives rise to all arterial branches that extend to the cerebral hemispheres.

The circle of Willis shows many variations. The "normal" vascular pattern described in manuals and atlases is actually found in less than 40 per cent of cases. These "perfect" circles, with well developed component parts and anastomoses (anterior communicating artery, posterior communicating arteries) with a diameter of at least 2 mm, provide optimal conditions for an effective collateral circulation. An occlusion of one of the large supplying arteries can be compensated by the well developed communicating arteries (Fig. 18–6). However, when one or several communicating arteries are underdeveloped or even rudimentary, the anastomosis between the large supplying arteries is not available; these arteries function independently, and consequently the vascular continuum, which ensures the vascularization of the brain, is affected.

Lazorthes et al. (1968) distinguished between circles with "autonomic supplying arteries" and circles with mutually "dependent supplying arteries," according to the level of development of the communicating arteries. The communicating arteries are ill developed in the former type of circle and well developed in the latter. The situation confronted in other cases is that the area of one main artery is markedly expanded at the expense of the other (for example, the posterior cerebral artery, branch of the internal carotid artery). In this context Lazorthes (1968) used the designations "piliers dominants" (dominant columns) and "piliers dominés" (dominated columns).

An analysis of the anatomic data that characterize a well developed circle of Willis indicates the following characteristic features:

(a) The components of the circle are direct branches from the supplying arteries: topographically, the circle constitutes the *"portal" of the cerebral circulation* and is therefore localized proximal to the entire arterial system of the brain.

(b) The anastomoses in the circle (communicating arteries) should be well developed to provide a kind of arterial "traffic circle" with various possibilities of circulation.

(c) The circle is localized in the subarachnoid space. This localization permits a particular histologic structure of the arterial wall (thin, muscular wall), with its functional implications.

(d) Branches from the extracranial arterial system do not reach the circle of Willis. The extracranial and intracranial circulations function largely independently.

Functionally, the circle of Willis plays an important role as the route via which collateral circulation can be quickly established. With well developed communicating arteries, even occlusion of the internal carotid artery can be overcome. Particularly in the case of gradual occlusion, such as in atheromatous lesions, these anastomoses are very valuable. Even in normal situations, the circle of Willis is of great importance, for example, in order to overcome the temporary interruption of flow in the vertebral artery that occurs when the head is thrown back

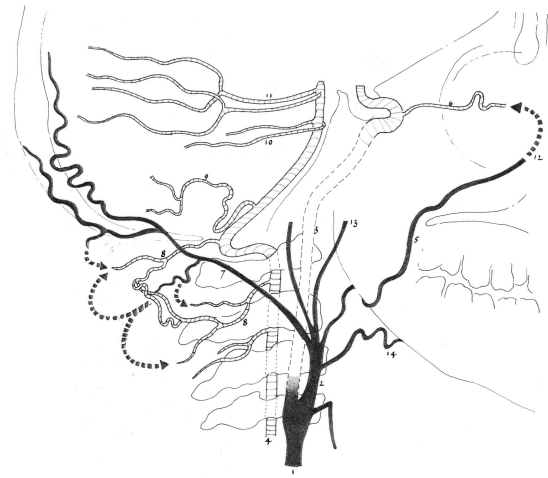

and at the same time turned. Several investigators (Toole and Tucker, 1960) have, in fact, demonstrated that forced head movements can cause simultaneous compression of the carotid and the vertebral arteries. According to these and other authors, the circle of Willis functions not only in vascular diseases but also in normal situations by virtue of variations in the direction of flow in accordance with the localization of the diminished blood flow.

ANASTOMOSES BETWEEN INTRACRANIAL AND EXTRACRANIAL CIRCULATION

These anastomoses are fairly extensive, but their functional value as a collateral route is small. A distinction is made between normal and abnormal anastomoses.

Figure 18–7 Normal anastomoses between extra-cranial and intracranial circulation (arteriogram); the anastomosing arteries are indicated by dark dashed lines (according to Krayenbuhl and Yasargil).

1 common carotid artery
2 external carotid artery
3 internal carotid artery
4 vertebral artery
5 facial artery
6 ophthalmic artery
7 occipital artery
8 muscular branches of vertebral artery
9 posterior inferior cerebellar artery
10 superior cerebellar artery
11 posterior cerebral arteries
12 angular artery
13 maxillary artery
14 lingual artery

Normal anastomoses link the external carotid artery to the ophthalmic artery and, via this artery, to the circle of Willis. A second group connects the vertebral artery with the occipital artery, a branch of the external carotid (Fig. 18–7). The principal anastomoses between the external carotid and the ophthalmic artery are the following:

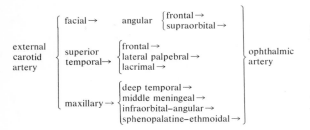

The second group of normal anastomoses is localized in the occipital region and ensures communication between the muscular branches of the vertebral artery and the branches of the occipital artery. Through these branches the blood can reach the distal segment of the vertebral artery if its proximal segment is obstructed.

The functional value of these anastomoses depends mostly on the speed with which the main artery is occluded; rapid obstructions cannot be effectively compensated by these anastomoses, but gradual obstructions could be, in favorable cases.

Abnormal anastomoses are vestiges of vessels that normally disappear in the course of embryonic development (Fig. 18–8). They can be found between the carotid and basilar arteries (trigeminal, auditory, and hypoglossal arteries) and between the internal carotid and middle meningeal arteries (stapedial artery). The presence of these abnormal anastomoses is usually associated with other anomalies of the circle of Willis.

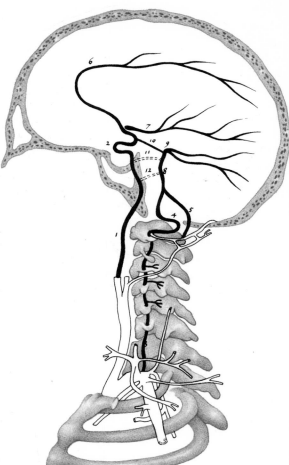

Figure 18–8 Abnormal anastomoses (dotted) between the carotid and the vertebral system (according to Krayenbuhl, modified).

1 internal carotid artery
2 carotid siphon
3,5 vertebral artery
4 vertebral siphon
6 anterior cerebral artery
7 middle cerebral artery
8 basilar artery
9 posterior cerebral artery
10 posterior communicating artery
11 trigeminal artery
12 auditory artery

INNERVATION OF THE CEREBRAL ARTERIES

Carotid System

One or two fairly thick nerve branches arise from the superior cervical ganglion and, together with the internal carotid artery, enter the cranial cavity through the carotid canal. Within the sinus cavernosus these nerves divide into several branches (carotid branches) that gradually form a periarterial sympathetic plexus. The terminal branches of the internal carotid artery are accompanied by branches from this plexus. According to Chorobski and Penfield (1932), the periarterial sympathetic plexus receives parasympathetic fibers originating from the intermediate nucleus (7th cranial nerve) via the greater petrosal nerve (Fig. 18–9). Chorobski and Penfield maintained that the parasympathetic fibers can cause vasodilation of the intracerebral and pia mater arteries. Lazorthes (1965), however, believed that the greater petrosal nerve receives sympathetic branches from the carotid plexus because the distal segment of the petrosal nerve contains numerous unmyelinated fibers after crossing the carotid (Fig. 18–9).

the fibers around the posterior cerebral artery is uncertain; according to Lazorthes, this artery is innervated by branches that have entered the skull along with the vertebral artery.

Vertebral Artery

The vertebral artery is innervated by the anterior and posterior vertebral branches. These nerves are branches of the cervical sympathetic trunk (middle cervical ganglion and stellate ganglion, respectively). Above C5 the two nerves divide into several branches that form a periarterial plexus. The vertebral plexus is reinforced by afferent (sensory) fibers from the first and second cervical nerves and by sympathetic fibers from the superior cervical ganglion. The vertebral plexus enters the cranial cavity and innervates the basilar artery and its branches. Scattered nerve cells are found in the meshes of the plexus.

Vascularization of the Spinal Cord

The spinal cord is vascularized by arteries that belong to several areas: the cervical segment by branches of the subclavian artery, the thoracic segment by the intercostal arteries, and the lumbosacral segment by a direct branch from the aorta (great radicular artery).

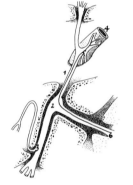
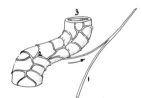

Figure 18–9 Parasympathetic innervation of the cerebral arteries according to Chorobski and Penfield (A) and according to Lazorthes (B).

A
1   greater petrosal nerve
2   geniculate ganglion
3   facial nerve
4   internal carotid artery
5   periarterial plexus
6   parasympathetic fibers
    of facial nerve
B
1   greater petrosal nerve
2   periarterial sympathetic
    plexus
3   internal carotid artery

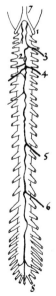

Figure 18–10 Arteries supplying the anterior spinal artery.

1   vertebral artery
2   anterior spinal artery
3   cervical radicular branches
4,5 anterior radicular artery
6   great radicular artery
7   basilar artery
8   crossing branches

Circle of Willis

The various links of the circle of Willis are surrounded by periarterial networks of myelinated and unmyelinated fibers. The large arteries of the cerebral base seem to be better innervated than the smaller cortical branches. The origin of

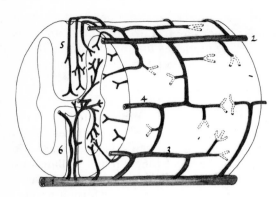

Figure 18-11 Vascularization of the spinal cord (according to Benninghoff).

1 anterior spinal artery
2 posterolateral spinal artery
3 anterolateral spinal artery
4 lateral spinal artery
5 fissural artery
6 sulcus artery

GENERAL VASCULAR PATTERN

The spinal branches enter the vertebral canal through the intervertebral foramina, whereupon each branch divides into several branches for vascularization of the vertebrae. The anterior and posterior radicular arteries are destined for the spinal cord (Fig. 18-10). The anterior radicular arteries supply the anterior spinal artery. The posterior radicular arteries are variable and little known.

The anterior spinal artery extends along the anterior median fissure over the entire length of the spinal cord. This artery vascularizes the anterior two-thirds of the cord, the posterior one-third being vascularized by the posterolateral spinal arteries. The latter begin cranially as branches of the vertebral artery and descend along the dorsal aspect of the cord, medial to the dorsal roots. The smaller branches of these arteries form the corona vasorum, an annular system from which small branches enter the spinal cord proper.

Channels of Supply

Cervical Region. Beside two or three radicular arteries that arise from the vertebral artery, there is a fairly large branch from the highest intercostal artery, which enters the vertebral canal through C6 or C7. Other radicular arteries originate from the deep cervical artery (C3 or C4).

Thoracic Region. The vascularization of the thoracic region is less abundant. The only channel of supply is one anterior radicular artery, which usually originates from the sixth intercostal artery.

Lumbosacral Region. This region is richly vascularized by the great radicular artery (Adamkievicz, 1882), which reaches the spinal cord above the lumbar intumescence. According to Lazorthes (1968), this artery accompanies one of the three last thoracic nerves in 75 per cent of cases, while in the remaining 25 per cent it accompanies the nerve of L1 or L2. This is the most important artery for the spinal cord, usually localized on the left. The conus medullaris is vascularized by an anastomosis between the great radicular artery and two posterior radicular arteries (Fig. 18-10).

Venous Circulation

The veins of the brain do not accompany the arteries but form a separate plexus, which drains mainly into the venous sinuses of the dura mater. The venous plexus is divided into a superficial and a deep system. The superficial vessels drain the cortex and the underlying white matter; the deep vessels drain the basal ganglia, the thalamus, the hypothalamus, etc.

DURA MATER SINUSES

The venous sinuses of the dura mater are endothelium-lined venous channels localized between the meningeal and the periosteal layers of the dura. Since the wall of these channels consists of stiff dural tissue, they are unable to change their diameter (due to lack of muscle cells) as other veins do. This is why the dural sinuses do not collapse when severed. Such special vessels are not found anywhere outside the brain. The sinuses and other cerebral veins have no valves. The largest dural sinuses meet in the *confluence of sinuses,* the venous space on the boundary between falx cerebri and cerebellar

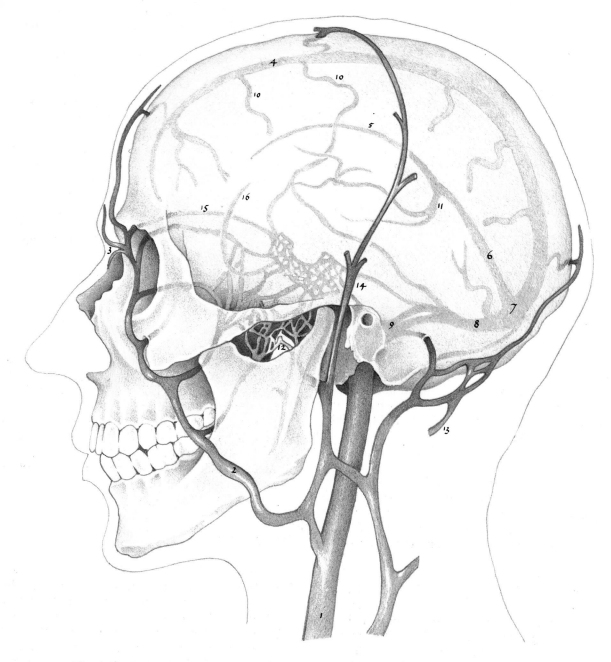

Figure 18–12 Anastomoses between the sinuses of the dura mater and the large veins of the head (according to Ferner and Kautzky).

1 internal jugular vein
2 facial vein
3 angular vein
4 superior sagittal sinus
5 inferior sagittal sinus
6 straight sinus
7 confluence of sinuses
8 transverse sinus
9 sigmoid sinus
10 anterior cerebral veins
11 great cerebral vein
12 pterygoid plexus
13 occipital vein
14 superficial temporal vein
15 superior ophthalmic vein
16 sphenoparietal sinus

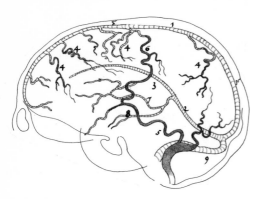

Figure 18–13 Superficial veins of the convex surface of the brain (phlebogram).

1 superior sagittal sinus
2 straight sinus
3 inferior sagittal sinus
4 ascending cerebral veins
5 temporooccipital vein (Labbé)
6 superior anastomotic vein (Trolard)
7 great cerebral vein
8 basal vein (Rosenthal)
9 transverse sinus

tentorium, opposite the internal occipital protuberance. From the confluence of sinuses arise the transverse sinuses (left and right) which, as the sigmoid sinus, continue as far as the jugular foramen, where they continue in the internal jugular veins (Fig. 18–12).

There are many variations of the confluence of sinuses: The superior sagittal sinus is often continuous with the right transverse sinus, in which case the straight sinus communicates with the left transverse sinus and there is no confluence of sinuses.

The superior sagittal sinus is located in the upper margin of the falx cerebri. On either side of the sinus there are dilatations of the lumen (lacunae), where the pacchionian granulations are invaginated. The inferior sagittal sinus extends in the free lower margin of the falx cerebri and joins the great cerebral vein to end in the straight sinus. This extends in an occipital direction, embedded in the cerebellar tentorium, and opens up into the confluence of sinuses.

The transverse sinus extends laterally in a broad, well defined groove in the occipital bone.

At the level of the base of the petrosal bone it curves down (sigmoid sinus) and reaches the jugular foramen (Fig. 18–12).

The sinus cavernosus is an irregular venous space beside the sella turcica. The lumen of this sinus is bridged by numerous dural trabeculae along which vessels and nerves extend. The two cavernous sinuses communicate via venous channels in front of and behind the hypophysis.

The superior and inferior ophthalmic veins and the sphenoparietal sinus drain into the sinus cavernosus; the blood is further drained off through the superior and inferior petrosal sinuses. The former connects the sinus cavernosus with the sigmoid sinus (Fig. 18–12) and extends along the line of attachment of the cerebellar tentorium; the latter connects the sinus cavernosus with the bulb of the jugular vein.

CORTICAL VEINS

The cortical veins comprise a superior and an inferior system. The superior system drains the blood to the superior sagittal sinus via 10 to 15 large veins. The inferior system drains into the cavernous sinus, transverse sinus, and great cerebral vein via Rosenthal's basal vein (Fig. 18–13). The two systems communicate via superficial anastomoses like the superior anastomotic vein (Trolard).

DEEP VEINS

Parts of the basal ganglia, choroid plexus, thalamus, and hypothalamus are drained by the thalamostriate vein, which extends in the terminal sulcus. At the level of the interventricular foramen the vein curves dorsally and enters the velum interpositum, where it continues as an internal cerebral vein. The two internal cerebral veins unite to form the great cerebral vein which in addition to the internal cerebral veins, receives the basal veins (Rosenthal) and the occipital veins. The great cerebral vein drains into the straight sinus.

Part III

Microscopic Anatomy of the
Central Nervous System

Chapter 19

Nerve Cells, Nerve Fibers and Synapses

The nervous system comprises nerve cells, nerve fibers, glia cells, and blood vessels. The nerve cells (neurons) differ from other cells in that they have extensions. In some neurons with long extensions the amount of cytoplasm in the extensions is sometimes much larger than that around the nucleus (perikaryon). The glia cells are far more numerous than the neurons. Electron microscope studies have shown that neurons are insulated from their environment by thin layers of glial cytoplasm. Only the sites of synapses are free from this glial lining. Besides neurons and glia cells there are numerous fibers, which are the main component of the white matter. The fibers, however, are not independent structures: Each fiber corresponds with a nerve cell. Blood vessels with accompanying connective tissue enter the CNS, but this connective tissue is always separated from the actual nerve tissue by a membrane of glial cytoplasm and a basement membrane.

Neurons are functionally involved in the generation and transmission of impulses. Moreover, they synthesize chemical substances (neurohormones, chemotransmitters) that are transported by the axons and released at specific sites. Neuroglia cells play a role in the transport of nutrients, oxygen, and carbon dioxide between nerve cells and capillaries. Moreover, they form myelin sheaths around the central axons.

Patterns of Organization

The neuron is the building block of the CNS. A chain of neurons is formed by several neurons linked in succession. The pattern of linkage of a collection of neurons determines their functional properties and spatial arrangement.

The neurons are topographically arranged in accordance with one of the following patterns: *a* as "cortex," *b* as "nucleus," or *c* as "reticular formation." Nuclei are accumulations of cells of a homogeneous neuron population from which one or several fiber bundle(s) extend(s) to its (their) proper destination. A reticular formation is a pattern of organization characterized by a rather diffuse cell matrix in which many myelinated fibers extend. The efferent fibers of the reticular neurons are not arranged in well defined bundles.

General Characteristics of Nerve Cells

A neuron consists of a cell body (perikaryon) and processes: the dendrites and the axon. The dendrites are usually markedly ramified, fairly thick, and relatively short. In many neurons the dendrites have small, bud-like excrescences (gemmules) that give them a thorny appearance. Axons synapse on the gemmules (Fig. 19–1). Since the gemmules can be very numerous, they greatly enlarge the available surface area for synaptic contacts between nerve cells. The axon can be very long (up to about 100 cm) and is slender and smooth. Its ramifications (collaterals) extend more or less at right angles. At its end, the axon divides into several delicate terminal branches (telodendrons), which end freely in a small bud.

The dendrites and the cell body receive impulses, while the axon conducts them. The site of contact between an axon and a dendrite or perikaryon of another neuron is called synaptic junction or synapse. It is at the synapse that impulse transmission takes place.

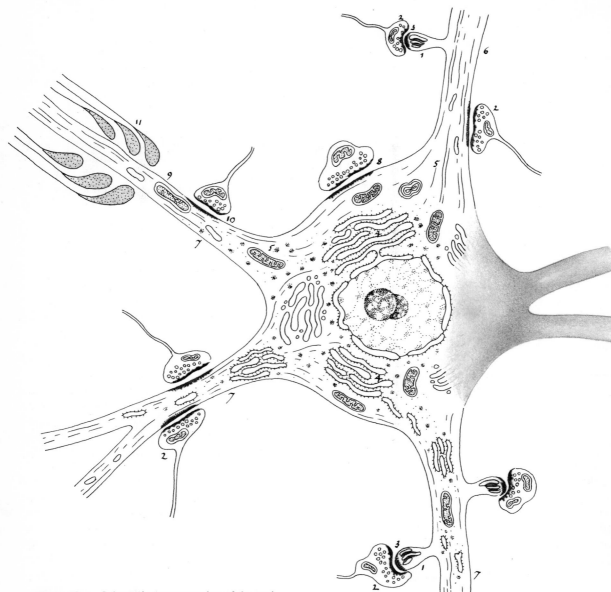

Figure 19–1 Schematic representation of the perikaryon of a nerve cell.

1 gemmule (spine)
2 end-feet ("boutons terminaux")
3 axodendritic synapse
4 Nissl bodies
5 microtubules and neurofilaments
6 apical dendrite
7 basal dendrites
8 axosomatic synapse
9 axon (initial segment)
10 axoaxonal synapse
11 beginning of the myelin sheath

TYPES OF NERVE CELLS

On the basis of the morphology of the extensions (processes), nerve cells are divided into multipolar, bipolar, and unipolar neurons. The multipolar nerve cells have several dendrites and a single axon; the bipolar nerve cells have one dendrite and one axon; the unipolar nerve cells have only one process, which divides into a peripheral branch (dendrite) and a central branch (axon). Unipolar nerve cells are found mainly in the spinal ganglia.

In modern classifications of neurons, the following criteria are applied: axon length, presence or absence of gemmules ("spines") on the dendrites, and morphology of the pattern of ramification of the dendrites. On the basis of these criteria, two neuron types are distinguished: class I neurons (Golgi cells of type I) with a long axon, many spines on the dendrites, and a virtually conical dendritic zone (see Fig. 35–1), like the large pyramidal cells of the cortex; class II neurons with a shorter axon and no or only a few spines on the dendrites and a variable "dendritic zone" (this type includes many "linking" or "intercalated" neurons).

ULTRASTRUCTURAL CHARACTERISTICS

Cell Membrane

The cell membrane of the neuron is visible only with electron microscopy. In thin sections, three layers can be distinguished in the cell membrane: two dark layers (about 25 Å thick) on either side of a lighter central layer (about 30 Å thick). The outer layer of the membrane is slightly thinner than the inner layer. The molecular structure of the cell membrane is still debated. On the basis of the difference in electrical properties between dendrites and axons, it is assumed that the structure of the membrane cannot be the same throughout.

Perikaryon

The perikaryon or cell body is the mass of cytoplasm that surrounds the nucleus of the cell.

The nucleus is rounded and usually has a central position, but in some cells (Clarke's dorsal nucleus) its position is eccentric. An eccentric position in other neurons would signify that the cell is damaged (as, for example, by severance of the axon). Characteristic features of the perikaryon are the Nissl bodies and the filamentous structures.

Nissl Bodies. The Nissl bodies present themselves in specimens as flakes that stain readily with basic dyes (methylene blue, cresyl violet). The Nissl bodies penetrate the proximal part of the dendrites but not the axon hillock or the axon proper. The Nissl bodies degenerate when the neuron is damaged (chromatolysis) and, of course, also when the axon is severed. On the basis of chromatolysis it is possible to determine which perikaryons belong to a given group of (experimentally) severed axons.

With the electron microscope the Nissl bodies are seen to consist of local accumulations of cisterns arranged in parallel; some of these cisterns belong to the agranular, while others belong to the granular endoplasmic reticulum (Fig. 19–2). Numerous free ribosomes are localized between the cisterns. The Nissl bodies are the principal protein-synthesizing organelles. In about three days, they synthesize as much protein as is contained in the neuron. These cytoplasmic proteins are in part drained off via the axon.

Filamentous Structures. The cytoplasm of both the perikaryon and the processes contains networks of delicate elements that can be stained microscopically with the aid of silver staining techniques. These filaments (neurofibrils) have long been (but no longer are) regarded as the conducting elements of the nervous system. Two types are distinguishable with electron microscopy: microtubules and neurofilaments. Microtubules are long tubular structures with a diameter of about 200 Å; they are found anywhere within the neuron. Neurofilaments are thinner structures (about 100 Å in diameter) that form networks in the cytoplasm.

Dendrites

Dendrites are neuron processes which, in principle, have the same structure as the cy-

Figure 19–2 Electron microscope view of a nerve cell. Note the Nissl bodies (magnification 6500 ×).

1 Nissl body

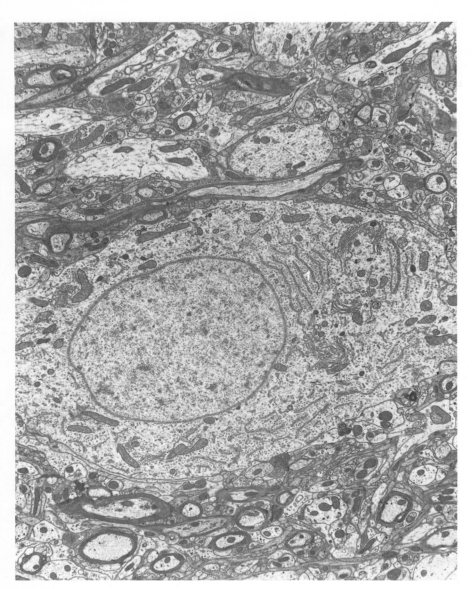

toplasm. Electron microscopy reveals that in the dendrites there are Nissl bodies, the Golgi apparatus, mitochondria, and many free ribosomes (Fig. 19–1). In somewhat longitudinally cut sections of dendrites, the numerous irregular evaginations and the irregular configuration of the circumference of the dendrites are conspicuous features.

The peripheral part of the dendrites is less rich in organelles than is the proximal part. Both parts are characterized by many microtubules, a few neurofilaments, and oblong mitochondria with longitudinal crista. The agranular endoplasmic reticulum consists of only a few flattened canaliculi localized immediately below the plasmalemma.

Gemmules. Gemmules are excrescences with a length of about 1 to 2 μm, with slightly swollen ends. They are clearly visible in Golgi preparations but can also be demonstrated by

Ehrlich-Dogiel's methylene blue method. They are very numerous in the large class I neurons, with estimates ranging from about 6000 to about 40,000 per neuron. The gemmules have a dual significance. To begin with, they enlarge the cell surface area for synaptic contacts; secondly, they are "plastic," that is, they can appear as required with a view to the necessary adaptation of the synaptic circuits (learning processes).

Axons

All neurons except a few have one axon (some, the so-called "amacrine cells" of the retina, have no axon), which arises from the axon hillock. This conical area of the perikaryon is characterized by the absence of Nissl bodies. The membrane of the axon is called axolemma. The axoplasm differs from the cytoplasm of the dendrites in that it has no Golgi apparatus or ergastoplasm, nor any free ribosomes. Moreover, most axons are enveloped by a sheath of a special fat-like substance, the myelin sheath. Thin axons have no sheath. Components of the axoplasm are cisterns of the agranular endoplasmic reticulum, mitochondria, microtubules, and neurofilaments. The terminal segment of the axon comprises numerous synaptic vesicles (see page 122).

The axon is divided into several parts. The most proximal part is called the initial segment and is located between the axon hillock and the beginning of the myelin sheath. Beneath the axolemma, this part contains an electron-dense layer of about 150 Å thickness (Palay et al., 1968). The initial segment is of central importance in generating the action potential. The second, longest part of the axon is the so-called conductive segment, with or without a myelin sheath that is interrupted at regular intervals by constrictions known as nodes of Ranvier (see Fig. 19–4). When the myelin sheath is absent, the fibers are described as unmyelinated. The end of the axon is the transmissive segment. In this segment the axon loses its myelin sheath and either terminates immediately or divides into several thin branches that end in swollen buttons (end-feet, or "boutons terminaux;" Fig. 19–1).

Nerve Fibers

A nerve fiber is the totality of an axon with its envelopes (myelin sheath, cytoplasm of Schwann cell, endoneurium); a bundle of nerve fibers constitutes a peripheral nerve. Groups of fibers are encased in a perineurium, and the entire nerve is enclosed by an epineurium. Unmyelinated and myelinated fibers are distinguished: The former are up to about 1 μm in diameter, while the latter range from 1 to about 20 μm in diameter.

PERIPHERAL AXON ENVELOPES

The conductive segment of the axon is usually enveloped by a fat-like sheath called a myelin sheath. In the peripheral nervous system this sheath is made up of lemmoblasts (Schwann cells), but in the CNS it consists of oligodendroglia cells. Numerous peripheral axons of the autonomic nervous system (ANS) are unmyelinated. These fibers are embedded in the cytoplasm of the lemmoblasts.

Axons without sheath ("naked axons") are found exclusively in the CNS (hypothalamus, Lissauer's marginal zone). Although they have no sheath, these axons are to some extent insulated from their environment by thin layers of glial cytoplasm.

THE MYELIN SHEATH

The myelin sheath consists of layers of double lemmoblast membranes wrapped around the axon. Each of these double membranes consists of two bimolecular lipid layers sandwiched between protein layers with a thickness of 30 Å. The myelin sheath as such is interrupted by the nodes of Ranvier (see below). Within a given axon, the length of the segments thus formed is constant. Thick axons have longer segments and conduct more rapidly than thin ones. A mesaxon is formed by invagination and fusion of the exterior surfaces of the cell membranes of the lemmoblast (Fig. 19–3). The peripheral axon lies embedded in the mesaxon, which is wrapped

Figure 19–3 Four successive stages of the spiralization of a Schwann cell. The black line in the myelin sheath (6) marks the fusion of the inner layers of the cell membrane.

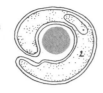

1 axon
2 cytoplasm of the Schwann cell
3 nucleus of the Schwann cell
4 outer layer of the cell membrane
5 mesaxon
6 fusion of the inner layers (thick line)

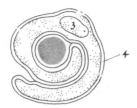

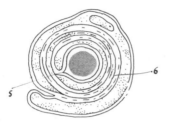

around the axon (Geren, 1954; Robertson, 1958). The cytoplasm of the lemmoblast is "squeezed out" as the interior surfaces of the membrane come together, whereupon these surfaces fuse. In this way the dark lines of the myelin layers are produced.

The boundary between two successive myelin segments (Fig. 19–4) is marked by an area without myelin sheath. These areas are called *nodes of Ranvier*. In peripheral nerves (Fig. 19–4) the axon is insulated from the extracellular space by a layer of lemmoblast cytoplasm at each area; central axons, however, are in direct contact with the extracellular space at these sites. If the axon of a myelinated fiber produces a side branch, the ramification always lies at a node of Ranvier; the side branch also has a myelin sheath.

UNMYELINATED FIBERS

These fibers consist of axons that are embedded in the cytoplasm of a chain of lemmoblasts but remain enveloped by the cellular liminal plane of the lemmoblast — an "envelope" which via a mesaxon is connected with the outer liminal plane of the lemmoblast. In this way, several axons can be accommodated in the cytoplasm of a single lemmoblast (Fig. 19–5).

Synapses

The synapse is a morphologic specialized site of contact between two neurons, where impulse transmission and integration of information take place. The term synapse was introduced by Sherrington in 1897. The structure of the synapse, however, can be visualized only by electron microscope methods and was not revealed until the 1950s (Palade and Palay, 1954; De Robertis, 1954).

The synapse can be divided into the presynaptic membrane, the postsynaptic membrane, and the synaptic cleft in between. The width of

around it several times. The nucleus of the lemmoblast lies on the outer aspect of the myelin sheath, against the outer liminal plane. Electron microscope studies of the myelin sheath reveal a constellation of alternating thick and thin lines (Fig. 19–4). The thick lines indicate the fusion of the interior surfaces of the cytoplasm membranes, while the thin lines in between ("intraperiod lines") are caused by the contact planes of the exterior surfaces. The interior cell membrane of the lemmoblast (Fig. 19–3) is connected with the first myelin layer by the inner mesaxon. The more peripheral layer is connected with the cell membrane by the outer mesaxon.

The myelin sheath is believed to develop as a result of rotation of the original mesaxon

Figure 19–4 Electron microscope view of a node of Ranvier in a peripheral nerve (magnification 32,000×).

1   node of Ranvier
2   myelin sheath
3   end of myelin segment
4   outer part of the cytoplasm of the Schwann cell
5   myelin loops indicating the end of the myelin segment
6   inner part of the cytoplasm of the Schwann cell
7   axon

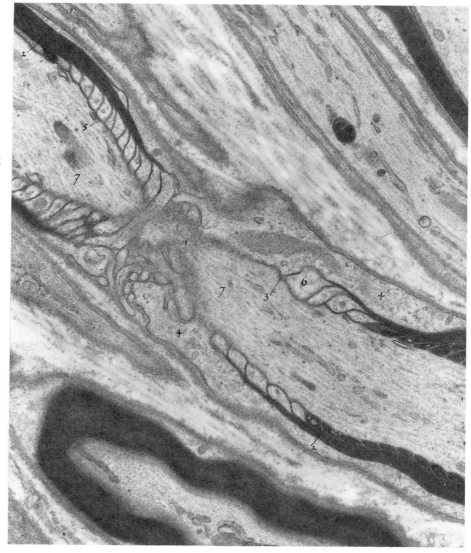

the synaptic cleft is 200 to 300 Å. The plasma membranes on either side of the cleft are of different structure; this asymmetry expresses the functional polarity of the synapse.

Most synapses are located between the end-foot ("bouton terminal") of an axon and a dendrite or perikaryon (axodendritic or axosomatic synapses). In some instances, synapses have been demonstrated also between two axons (axo-axonal synapses), or between two dendrites (dendrodendritic), or between a dendrite and a soma (dendrosomatic). Morphologically, synapses can be divided into terminal and collateral synapses.

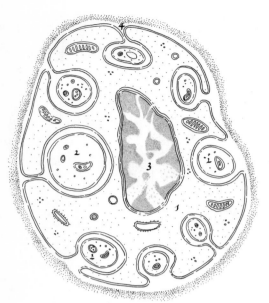

Figure 19–5 A Schwann cell with unmyelinated axons.

1 cytoplasm of the lemmoblast
2 unmyelinated axons
3 nucleus of the lemmoblast
4 mesaxon

TERMINAL SYNAPSES

Axodendritic: This is the most common type. The axon synapses with one or several dendrites, mainly on the gemmules (Figs. 19–6 and 19–7).

Axosomatic: The synapse lies between the axon and the membrane of the perikaryon.

Axo-axonal: The presynaptic axon can terminate on the initial segment of another axon or on its terminal segment (telodendrion).

Dendrodendritic: These synapses have so far been found only in certain areas of the CNS (olfactory bulb, thalamus). Characteristically, they are often found as pairs of "opposite-poled" (reciprocal) synapses.

Synaptic Glomeruli: These structures consist of an accumulation of many synapses (axodendritic, axo-axonal, etc.), separated from the environment by a glia capsule. Typical examples are the glomeruli of the olfactory bulb and those of the granular layer of the cerebellum.

COLLATERAL SYNAPSES

Collateral synapses are sites of contact between a point somewhere along the course of an axon and a postsynaptic element ("boutons en passant"); the axon then continues its course and terminates on another dendrite or another perikaryon.

CHEMICAL AND ELECTRICAL SYNAPSES

When impulse transmission involves the release of chemical substances (transmitters) in the synaptic cleft, the synapse is described as a chemical synapse. This is the most common type of synapse in higher mammals.

In invertebrates, a second type of synapse is found, the so-called electrical synapse. Recent research, however, has revealed electrical synapses also in higher vertebrates and they probably occur in humans as well. In these synapses, no transmitters are used. Instead, they have a virtually obliterated synaptic cleft (about 20 Å wide), in which direct electrical transmission is possible. Morphologically, the electrical synapses are symmetric, that is, the structures of the presynaptic and postsynaptic membranes are identical. Impulse transmission is (usually) possible in both directions.

Structure of Chemical Synapses

The boutons contain many mitochondria, synaptic vesicles, and small cisterns of the endoplasmic reticulum. The synaptic vesicles (Fig. 19–8) are rounded structures with a diameter of 200 to 700 Å. They are for the most part accumulated against the presynaptic membrane and contain high concentrations of transmitter substance. Of the various morphologic types, the following are the most widely known:

(a) round, electron-lucent vesicles about 400 Å in diameter, usually found in asymmetric synapses and probably excitatory; they contain acetylcholine, among other substances;

(b) oval, electron-lucent vesicles with a

Figure 19–6 Group of end-feet around a central dendrite; axodendritic synapses (magnification 25,000 ×).

1 dendrite
2 axons
3 axodendritic synapses

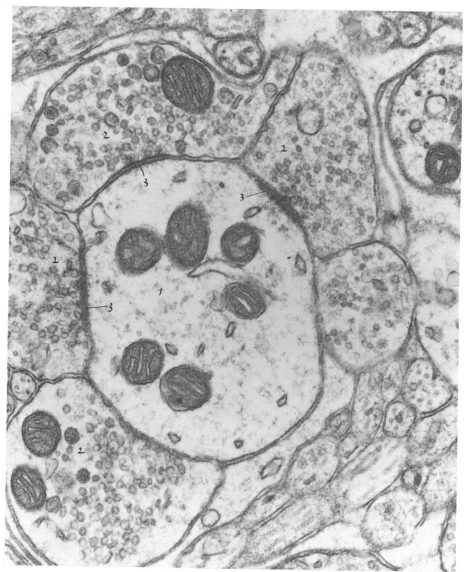

maximal diameter of about 500 Å, found mainly in symmetric synapses and containing the inhibitory transmitter glycine, among other substances;

(c) electron-dense vesicles with a diameter of 400 to 600 Å, which contain catecholamines (e.g., norepinephrine, which is the transmitter in postganglionic orthosympathetic neurons).

The presence of synaptic vesicles in the presynaptic element is an important argument in favor of the postulate that the synapse permits only one-way transmission.

The presynaptic membrane shows a few electron-dense swellings separated by thin membrane segments. In frozen corrosion preparations one sees a characteristic reticular image of dark and light spots ("presynaptic grid"), with meshes that are about 200 Å wide (Fig. 19–8). It

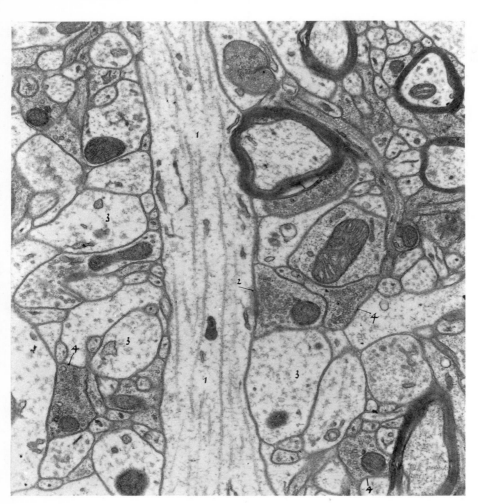

Figure 19–7 Axodendritic synapse on an apical dendrite of a pyramidal cell in the cerebral cortex of a c[a]t (magnification 16,000 ×).

1 apical dendrite of the pyramidal cell
2 axodendritic synapse
3 dendrites
4 axons with synaptic vesicles

is probably through these meshes that the transmitters are released into the synaptic cleft. The synaptic cleft is a space about 200 Å wide, filled with a substance that contains carbohydrate.

The structure of the postsynaptic membrane varies. A layer of an electron-dense substance is often found lying against this membrane (Figs. 19–6 and 19–7). On the basis of electron microscopic findings, Gray (1959) distinguished two synapse types: Type I is characterized by a thick continuous subsynaptic membrane and a synaptic cleft with a width of 300 Å, filled with dense extracellular substance; type II is characterized by local swellings in the presynaptic and postsynaptic membranes. Type I synapses (asymmetric synapses) are mainly localized on the gemmules of the dendrites, whereas type II synapses (symmetric synapses) are for the most part axosomatic. Gray's two types, however, are the extremes of a whole range of intermediate forms.

Impulse Transmission in the Synapse

As an action potential arrives in the presynaptic ending, the permeability of the membrane to Ca^{++} ions is increased. Many synaptic vesicles fuse with the presynaptic membrane and release their contents into the synaptic cleft. The released transmitter diffuses within about 1 milli-second to the postsynaptic membrane and combines with specific receptor proteins. Consequently the permeability of the postsynaptic membrane changes slightly (see page 129). This change of permeability, however, is determined by the transmitter-receptor combination, not by the transmitter only. The transmitter released into the synaptic cleft is rapidly broken down by the enzymes present in the cleft.

TRANSMITTERS

The following transmitters have so far been identified:

Acetylcholine (ACh). The cholinergic synapses contain acetylcholine in the synaptic vesicles. As an impulse arrives in the presynaptic element, acetylcholine is released into the synaptic cleft. Ca^{++} ions seem to be required in order to cause the vesicles to "rupture." The excess of acetylcholine in the synaptic cleft is broken down by the enzyme acetylcholinesterase into choline and acetic acid. This breakdown is very important. When the transmitter continues to act too long, the postsynaptic neuron is unable to repolarize and finally becomes unable to fire an impulse.

Cholinergic transmission occurs in many parts of the peripheral nervous system (motor end-plate, autonomic ganglia, and between parasympathetic postganglionic endings and effector cells). Most cholinergic synapses are excitatory with the exception of the inhibitory action of the vagus nerve (parasympathetic) on the heart.

Monoamines. Monoamines result from decarboxylation of amino acids. In terms of their activity as transmitters, two groups are distinguished: catecholamines (dopamine, norepinephrine, epinephrine) and indolamines (serotonin). The catecholamines are derived from tyrosine (or phenylalanine) and are found in the so-called electron-dense granules of certain nerve endings.

Centrally, high concentrations of catecholamine are found in the brain stem (e.g., in the locus ceruleus). Extensions from here have been demonstrated in the hypothalamus and the limbic system; other (descending) fibers reach the spinal cord. The substantia nigra and the nigrostriatal fibers are rich in dopamine (see stratum). The cerebellum and the cerebral cortex, on the other hand, show very low concentrations of catecholamine.

The indolamines are derived from tryptophan. The best known indolamine is serotonin (5-hydroxytryptamine; 5-HT). From the raphe nuclei in the brain stem, serotonergic fibers ascend to the diencephalon; these fibers play an important role in the regulation of the sleep-wake rhythm.

Other Transmitters. The amino acids glycine and gamma-aminobutyric acid (GABA) are believed to act as inhibitory neurotransmitters. Additional neurotransmitters will undoubtedly be identified in future studies.

Figure 19–8 Schematic representation of the structure of a presynaptic terminal bouton. The presynaptic membrane shows the so-called presynaptic grid. Note the synaptic vesicle shortly before release of its contents into the synaptic cleft (according to Akert).

1 microtubules
2 mitochondrion
3 synaptic vesicles
4 presynaptic grid
5 release of neurotransmitter into the synaptic cleft

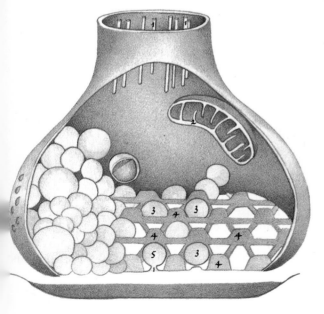

Chapter 20

Action Potentials and Synaptic Potentials; Neuronal Circuits

Nerve Signals

The CNS can be regarded as an information-processing apparatus. Data on the environment or on the organism itself reach the CNS via certain channels (afferent nerves). These data are analyzed and processed in the appropriate centers, whereupon signals are sent back via the efferent nerves to the executive organs (muscles and glands). These signals activate the muscles by which the individual responds to certain changes in the environment or in his own body. The numerous vital data (changes in temperature, sound, light, physical injury) cannot be processed as such by the nervous system; these data first must be "translated" into a language the nervous system understands. The translating is done in the receptors (sensors), which in many instances consist of sensory nerve endings distributed over the entire body. In other instances (internal ear, retina) the receptors are specialized cells with which an afferent nerve fiber synapses.

The receptors are sensitive to a particular form of energy (adequate stimulus), which they convert to a change in electric potential (receptor potential). The amplitude of the receptor potential varies with the stimulus intensity and can therefore be regarded as an analogous signal. When the receptor potential is strong enough to depolarize the first node of Ranvier, an action potential develops in the afferent nerve. Light, pain, and pressure stimuli are all converted to action potentials (digital signal), which are conducted at different speeds through the afferent nerves to specific areas of the CNS.

The entire activity of the nervous system is based on the transport and transmission of nerve signals. The transport is effected by the action potentials in the axons; these fibers are specialized in the transport of signals over long distances without addition or loss of information on the way. The transmission and assimilation of the nerve signals is effected by the synaptic potentials (see below). Action potentials and synaptic potentials are of an entirely different nature.

TOPOGRAPHY OF SIGNAL TRANSMISSION

The transmission of signals is of great importance in processing information. This transmission takes place (Fig. 20–1):

(a) in the receptors, in which external or internal stimuli are converted to receptor potentials; when the receptor potential attains its liminal value, an action potential is fired off;

(b) between neurons (synapses), action potentials are converted to synaptic potentials;

(c) between efferent neurons and the executive organs (e.g. muscles), action potentials are converted to end-plate potentials.

ACTION POTENTIALS

The impulse conduction in the axon is associated with electric phenomena that can be registered with the aid of derivation electrodes and electronic gear. The term action potential is therefore used as a synonym for nerve impulse, although strictly speaking it covers only one aspect of a nerve impulse.

Impulse conduction in nerve fibers has several important characteristics:

(a) The impulse obeys the all-or-nothing law, which is to say that intensification of the stimulus

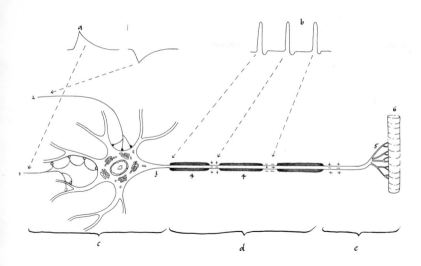

Figure 20–1 The functional components of a nerve cell. When the sum of the (excitatory and inhibitory) synaptic potentials attains the threshold value in the area of the initial segment, an action potential is fired off.

a synaptic potentials
b action potentials
c receptive part
d conductive part
e transmissive part
1 excitatory ending
2 inhibitory ending
3 initial segment of the axon
4 myelin segments
5 telodendrion
6 muscle

in excess of the threshold value does not increase the impulse amplitude.

(b) The impulse amplitude remains constant, regardless of the length of the axon.

(c) Having conducted an impulse, the fiber is absolutely refractory (not at all excitable) for a brief time (0.4 to 2 msec), and subsequently remains relatively refractory (excitable only to a limited extent) until it recovers full excitability.

(d) The action potential leaps, so to speak, from one node of Ranvier to the next (saltatory pulse conduction). Of course this applies only to myelinated fibers, for the nodes of Ranvier are the only sites at which ions can pass through the membrane and cause its depolarization. This is why impulse conduction in myelinated fibers is a generative process, which is renewed at each next node of Ranvier.

CODE OF THE NERVOUS SYSTEM

Action potentials traveling through a given nerve fiber are always constant in amplitude. This is why the amplitude cannot be used to transmit information. However, the information can be coded by modulating the frequency of the action potentials fired off, that is, by changing the number of action potentials conducted via a

nerve fiber per unit of time. The frequency of the action potentials is proportionate to the logarithm of the stimulus intensity. Other factors that play a role in the coding of information are (a) the length of the intervals between successive action potentials and (b) the fact that the information is always conducted through several channels, each with its own frequency.

SYNAPTIC POTENTIALS

Excitation of the perikaryon or of a dendrite of a nerve cell produces no all-or-nothing signal but local polarization (depolarization or hyperpolarization) of the postsynaptic membrane. The excitatory change of potential (EPSP) results from the fact that the released transmitter combines with "receptors" in the subsynaptic membrane. Consequently the permeability of this membrane to various ions changes. The ion migrations (influx of Na^+ and efflux of K^+) are responsible for the small circular currents that cause the local depolarization of the postsynaptic membrane. The depolarization effected by a single EPSP is usually unable to generate an action potential (subliminal stimulus). A second subliminal stimulus, at least if it follows the first quickly enough, further depolarizes the postsynaptic

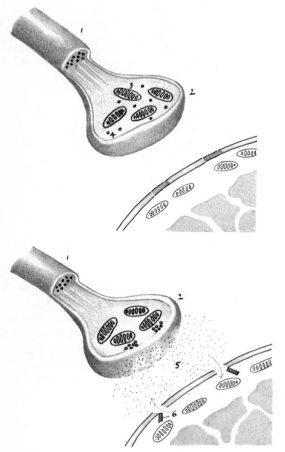

Figure 20–2 Release of transmitter into the synaptic cleft. The combination of transmitter and receptor proteins in the subsynaptic membrane causes a change in permeability.

1. axon
2. axon ending
3. mitochondrion
4. synaptic vesicle
5. transmitter released into the synaptic cleft
6. receptor proteins in the plasma membrane

neuron is increased (hyperpolarization). The inhibitory phenomena are in many ways similar to excitatory phenomena. The released transmitter changes the permeability of the postsynaptic membrane in such a way that K^+ and Cl^- ions migrate to the extracellular space. The cell becomes less excitable (increased threshold value) and more EPSPs are required to generate an action potential. Inhibition means that the normal excitability of the neuron is diminished, but not that the neuron becomes absolutely refractory.

Localization of the Inhibitory Mechanisms

In vertebrates, all inhibitions take place exclusively in *central* structures (spinal cord or brain). Afferent signals always give rise to excitatory phenomena; inhibition occurs only if an inhibitory link cell is included in the neuron chain.

Disinhibition

When an inhibitory link cell is inhibited by another inhibitory cell, the result is "facilitation;" double inhibition leads to facilitation. This phenomenon is known as disinhibition — the inhibition of an inhibitory effect.

Presynaptic Inhibition

Inhibition of a neuron can either be achieved by hyperpolarization of the entire postsynaptic membrane (postsynaptic inhibition) or result from preceding partial depolarization of the presynaptic endings. In the latter case, the action potentials that arrive in the presynaptic ending find an already partly depolarized membrane, which reduces the amount of excitatory transmitter released. Reduction of released transmitter means diminution of the excitatory effect on the postsynaptic membrane (smaller EPSPs) and less chance for the postsynaptic neuron to attain the threshold value. This reduction results from the activity of a special synapse at the presynaptic nerve ending, an axo-axonal synapse (Fig. 19–1).

membrane (summation effect). Several EPSPs generated in rapid succession are summated until the threshold value (about −55 mV) is attained. At that moment an action potential is generated in the axon hillock (Fig. 20–2).

Inhibitory Postsynaptic Potentials

The term inhibitory postsynaptic potential (IPSP) applies when the membrane potential of a

Presynaptic inhibition is based on preceding excitation of the presynaptic membrane. No inhibitory transmitter is then released. An important difference between presynaptic and postsynaptic inhibition is that in the former the cell membrane of the postsynaptic element fully retains its excitability in response to impulses that reach the cell via other synapses, whereas postsynaptic inhibition reduces the excitability of the entire neuron. Presynaptic inhibition makes it possible to suppress certain channels that transport less relevant information.

THE CELL MEMBRANE AS AN APPARATUS OF INTEGRATION

The surface of the neurons is strewn with thousands of synapses (excitatory and inhibitory), which cover an important part (15 to 29 per cent) of the available surface area. Many neurons can therefore be influenced by stimuli from widely diverse sources (Fig. 20–3).

The balance between excitatory and inhibitory influences determines whether a neuron does or does not generate an action potential or whether its firing rate decreases or increases. The receptor part of the membrane can therefore be regarded as a kind of mosaic of activating and inhibiting contact sites. The following aspects are of importance in this context:

(a) The topographic distribution of the synapses follows a fixed pattern. This means that a given group of afferent fibers always synapses with a characteristic part of the postsynaptic neuron (the parallel fibers of the cerebellum, for example, synapse exclusively on the gemmules of the dendrites of the Purkinje cell).

(b) The localization of the synapses on the perikaryon or on the dendrite tree is of great importance. Since the synaptic potentials travel passively (decremental conduction), the synapses on the body or trunk of the dendrites can more readily cause the cell to fire than those on the peripheral part of the dendrites, which are further away from the axon hillock. A synapse is generally as much more effective as its distance from the axon hillock is shorter. This also applies to inhibitory synapses.

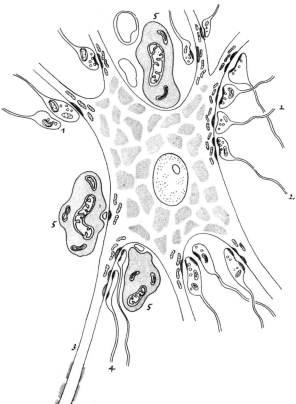

Figure 20–3 The surface of the perikaryon and dendrites is partly covered with synapses. Glial extensions line the remainder.

1	axoaxonal synapse
2	axosomatic synapse
3	axon
4	axoaxonal synapse
5	glial cytoplasm

(c) Recent research has led to the suspicion that synapses are not rigid but plastic structures. In the course of life, many new synapses probably develop as a result of frequently recurring stimuli, such as increased reflex activities, new modes of behavior, and training of intellectual functions.

Neuronal Circuits

The neurons are linked in circuits. Some of these circuits consist of no more than two neurons with a synapse in between; others com-

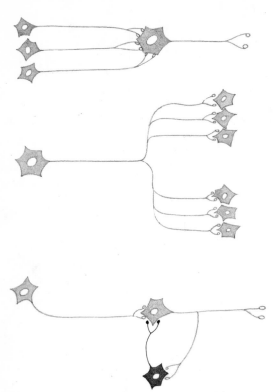

Figure 20–4 Examples of neuronal connections. *A*, Convergence: several presynaptic nerve cells synapse with the same postsynaptic neuron. *B*, Divergence: the axon of a neuron repeatedly ramifies and synapses with several other neurons. *C*, Recurrent inhibition: the axon of neuron colored light gray (at night) produces a recurrent branch that synapses with the inhibitory neuron colored dark gray, the axon of which synapses with the perikaryon of the original neuron.

prise hundreds or even thousands of synapsing neurons.

Open and closed circuits are distinguished. An open circuit consists of a chain of neurons in which impulses travel in one direction (Fig. 20–4). In a closed circuit, impulses can travel in both directions because one or several neurons are interposed between the recurrent axon collateral or a nerve cell and the perikaryon of this nerve cell.

More complex structures are the so-called closed multicatenary circuits, in which many neurons are interposed between the recurrent axon collateral of a neuron and its perikaryon. In view of the enormous number of neurons and the even larger number of synapses, it is not surprising that neuronal circuitry can be complicated beyond imagination.

The importance of a study of the architecture of a circuit lies in the fact that the connection diagram of the neurons within a circuit is closely related to the function of that circuit.

REGULATORY CIRCUITS

Some nuclei in the diencephalon and telencephalon are characterized by the fact that their efferent fibers for the most part project back (via the thalamus or otherwise) to the cerebral cortical areas from which their afferent fibers originate. These nuclei are thus part of a circuit: cerebral cortex–nucleus I–nucleus II, etc.–cerebral cortex. This is evident especially in the basal ganglia, the neocerebellum, and certain parts of the limbic system. Such circuits are known as cortical regulatory circuits.

It is of essential importance for the function of a regulatory circuit that information from elsewhere can come in at each connection, and that there are also collaterals that leave the circuit. The nuclei of a regulatory circuit probably function as comparators, that is, as components of a servo-mechanism based on the feedback principle.

Many neuronal connections involve combinations of the two basic principles of convergence and divergence.

CONVERGENCE AND DIVERGENCE

The axon of a neuron divides into many branches that synapse with different other

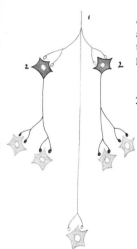

Figure 20-5 Inhibitory cells can also suppress the "noise" around a "main line" of information transfer by inhibiting traffic in parallel pathways.

1 main line
2 inhibitory cells

FACILITATION

The arriving subliminal stimuli, which partly depolarize the postsynaptic neuron, "prime" the neuron; that is to say, they facilitate attainment of the threshold value by newly arriving stimuli which, of their own accord, would be unable to cause the neuron to fire. This phenomenon is called facilitation. There are two possibilities: The subliminal stimuli (EPSPs) arrive simultaneously via different synapses (spatial facilitation), or many subliminal stimuli arrive via the same synapses in rapid succession (temporal facilitation).

OCCLUSION

neurons (Fig. 20–4). In this case the impulses that originate from this cell are dispersed *(divergence)*. On the other hand, a neuron can be influenced by impulses that come from many different other neurons *(convergence)*. Convergence and divergence are the morphologic substrate of certain physiologic properties of the neuronal circuits (such as facilitation and occlusion).

When there is partial overlap at the synapses of two or more axons, the response after simultaneous excitation of these axons can be less than the sum of the separate excitations of the same axons. This phenomenon is described as occlusion; it is based on the same process as facilitation, the difference being that in occlusion each stimulus is assumed to be sufficiently strong to cause the postsynaptic neurons to fire.

Chapter 21

Flows of Axoplasm; Degeneration and Regeneration of Nerve Fibers

The perikaryon plays the role of a trophic center of the neuron. The principal components of the cell are synthesized very near the nucleus and then transported to dendrites and axon. Since no significant protein synthesis occurs in the axon the enzymes, lysosomes, mitochondria, etc. have to be transported to the axon endings over long distances.

The studies of Weiss and Hiscoe (1948) revealed that the axoplasm is constantly moving from proximal to distal levels, at a speed of about 2 mm per day. Mitochondria, lysosomes, and formed elements are taken along with this flow. Autoradiographic studies have shown that certain substances (protein molecules, neurosecretions) move to the axon endings at a much higher speed (up to 2500 mm per day). Two different proximodistal flows have since been distinguished in the axoplasm: a slow flow that transports organelles and other formed elements, and a rapid flow that transports protein molecules. The latter flow can be stopped by local application of colchicine to the axon. Microtubules seem to be important for the rapid transport of proteins.

Some of the materials that arrive in the axon ending are used for transmission in the synapse; some of the remaining materials return to the perikaryon in a distoproximal flow of axoplasm.

Lesions of Nerve Cells and Nerve Fibers

With regard to the effect of a lesion, the neuron can be divided into a perikaryon and an axon. The perikaryon is, among other things, the trophic center of the cell. Destruction or a serious lesion of the perikaryon leads to destruction of the neuron with all its processes.

Severance of the axon has consequences for the distal fragment as well as for the proximal fragment and the perikaryon. The consequences for the neuron are much more serious as the distance between severance and the perikaryon is decreased.

CHANGES OF THE DISTAL SEGMENT OF THE AXON

These changes are known as anterograde degeneration (wallerian degeneration) and are very pronounced. Both the axon and the myelin sheath (if present) are destroyed over their entire length, including the terminal axon branches (telodendrion; Fig. 21–1). The axon first starts to swell and then fragments. The myelin sheath fragments within the cytoplasm of the Schwann cells; numerous lipid droplets form simultaneously. The Schwann cells become hypertrophic and divide. Two weeks after the lesion the degenerated myelin fragments are subject to chemical changes that make it possible to stain them with osmic acid (the principle of the Marchi technique). Myelin of intact axons cannot be stained by the Marchi technique. This difference in stainability makes it possible to stain degenerating axons in test animals and to follow them after an experimental lesion.

The Schwann cells (or the oligodendrocytes) detach themselves from the sheath and scavenge the degenerated myelin and axon fragments.

CHANGES OF THE PROXIMAL SEGMENT OF THE AXON

These changes are known as retrograde degeneration and involve not only the axon (retrograde fiber degeneration) but the perikaryon as well. Severances very near the perikaryon can lead to destruction of the neuron.

In the case of less severe lesions we find a characteristic reaction in the perikaryon, known as chromatolysis. The cell nucleus assumes an eccentric position, and the Nissl bodies shrink

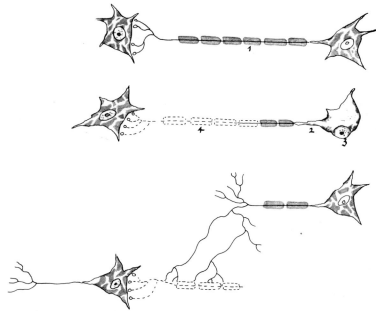

Figure 21–1 Anterograde and retrograde degeneration. After severance of an axon, the distal fragment degenerates (anterograde or wallerian degeneration). At the same time, retrograde degenerative changes occur (retrograde fiber degeneration, chromatolysis). In *C*, the regenerating nerve fibers seek to establish contact with the peripheral, partly degenerated myelin sheath. *A*, Normal neuron. *B*, Neuron after severance. *C*, Regenerating nerve fibers.

1 myelinated axon
2 retrograde degeneration
3 chromatolysis
4 anterograde (wallerian) degeneration

and fragment against the cell membrane. At the same time there is an increase in the number of mitochondria and lysosomes. The glia cells in the vicinity of the damaged perikaryons divide and encircle the nerve cells, probably preparatory to phagocytosis.

Regeneration

Regeneration of the peripheral axons often starts before the degenerative phenomena (particularly chromatolysis) reach a culmination. Successful regenerative processes call for the formation of a guiding tissue along which the regenerating axons can grow. The so-called Büngner bands provide this guidance.

The Büngner bands are chains of cells that fill the now hollow nerve fiber sheaths; the cells are formed by proliferation of Schwann cells. From the proximal end of the severed nerve, filaments grow toward the Büngner bands; once arrived, the growth buds of the regenerating axons enter these bands. They initially lie at the periphery of these bands, but subsequently one of the nerve fibers assumes a central position in the band. The central fiber develops a new myelin sheath and replaces the original axon, whereas the peripheral fibers gradually disappear. The optimal growth rate of a central growth bud in a Büngner band is about 4 mm per day.

The space between the two cut surfaces of the nerve is filled by cicatricial tissue. When this tissue is too hard and too fibrous, or when the nerve stumps are too far apart, the regenerating nerve fibers degenerate and no restoration of continuity is achieved. In these cases a so-called amputation neuroma develops in the proximal stump.

Regeneration in the CNS is less effective because the growing growth buds are rarely able to pass the glial cicatrices; and central regeneration is further impeded by the absence of Büngner bands.

Chapter 22

Transmission of Information to the Central Nervous System

Impulses from the periphery (skin and specialized senses) and from the interior of the body reach the CNS as electric signals via the peripheral nerves. The incoming information initiates processes that lead to a perception (processing and assimilation of information).

This information is supplemented and compared with similar information stored in the memory; the result is a motor response or a mental phenomenon.

Afferent impulses to the CNS (specialized senses excepted) pass through the processes of the peripheral sensory neurons. The perikaryons of these neurons are located outside the CNS in the spinal ganglia and in the ganglia of the cranial nerves. The peripheral processes of the sensory neurons accompany the nerves as afferent nerve fibers. They are part of mixed nerves (comprising both motor and sensory fibers) and of predominantly sensory nerves (skin). The latter also contain efferent autonomic fibers for innervation of blood vessels, glands, and smooth muscles in the skin. Afferent and efferent fibers cannot be separated histologically.

Receptor Types

Receptors can be classified on the basis of structure, nature of the adequate stimulus, functional properties, etc. Morphologically they can be divided into free and encapsulated receptors. A *free receptor* is a plexus of unmyelinated fibers in direct contact with tissue components; an *encapsulated receptor* is characterized by an enveloping capsule of connective tissue that separates it from adjacent tissues. In both types, the nerve endings are unmyelinated.

Receptors can also be classified on the basis of the type of information received and passed on. For example:

exteroceptors are localized in the skin and subcutaneous tissue and receive information from the environment; they include mechanoreceptors (pressure, traction), thermoreceptors (cold, heat), and nociceptors (pain);

proprioceptors are localized in the locomotor apparatus (muscles, tendons, joints), of which muscle spindles and tendon corpuscles are the best-known representatives; they register changes of movement and posture;

visceroceptors are localized in the visceral walls, which provide information on, for example, the tension in the walls of bowels and blood vessels.

Structure of the Receptors

The structure of the receptors is highly variable, and consequently numerous structural types are distinguished (corpuscles of Pacini, Meissner, Merkel, Golgi-Mazzoni, Ruffini, etc.). It was formerly believed that for each modality of perception a separate receptor existed (Müller's theory of specific nervous energy): The Meissner corpuscles were believed to be involved in tactile perception, the Ruffini corpuscles in heat perception, the Krause corpuscles in cold perception, and the free receptors in pain perception.

It is now understood that no type of receptor is specific for a particular sensory modality. The cornea, for example, possesses only free nerve endings but is nevertheless sensitive to both pain and pressure. The external ear is sensitive to heat, cold, pain, and touch but possesses only two receptor types: free receptors and nerve endings on hair follicles.

Encapsulated receptors are found only in hairless skin. The physical properties of the capsules determine which quality of the mechanical stimulus can depolarize the receptive membrane.

mammals. The nerve fibers enter the external epithelial layer and form two concentric spirals. The outer spiral lies in the connective tissue capsule, while the inner spiral is localized in the external epithelial layer. Larger hair follicles are innervated by several nerve fibers.

Encapsulated Nerve Endings (Mechanoreceptors)

The best known mechanoreceptors are the corpuscles of Pacini and of Meissner. The former are elliptical structures with a length of 3 to 4 mm, in which a thick myelinated nerve fiber terminates. These corpuscles are located in the subcutaneous tissues of the hand and foot, but also in deep structures like mesentery, pleura and pancreas. The corpuscles consist of several concentric layers of flat cells (lamellae), which can shift their relative positions in response to pressure. Each lamella is separated from the next

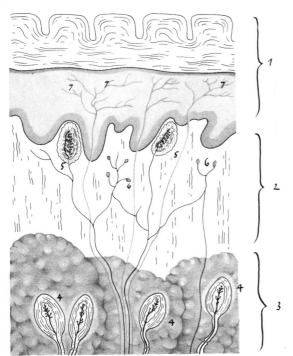

Figure 22–1 Schematic representation of some free and encapsulated skin receptors.

1. epidermis
2. dermis
3. subcutaneous adipose tissue
4. Pacini corpuscles
5. Meissner corpuscles
6. free nerve endings
7. C-fibers ("pain fibers")

Figure 22–2 Microscopic structure of a Meissner corpuscle (touch and pressure).

1. connective tissue capsule
2. nerve fiber
3. supporting cells

Figure 22–3 Structure of a Pacini corpuscle (pressure and vibration).

1. fibrous lamellae
2. central mass
3. nerve fiber
4. blood capillary

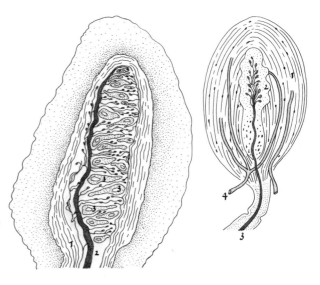

Free receptors result from ramification of thin sensory nerve fibers. Immediately beneath the dermis these fibers lose their myelin sheath and form dense networks immediately beneath the epidermis, where they end in small button-like swellings (Fig. 22–1). The free nerve branches are very numerous. They are localized mainly beneath the epidermis but can be found also in the connective tissue between the intestines, around muscles, and in the walls of viscera.

Nerve Endings on the Hair Follicles

These structures reach the highest degree of development in the tactile vibrissae of many by a space that contains a network of delicate collagenous fibers and a few isolated cells. Capillaries enter the capsule. The central nucleus of a Pacini corpuscle consists of the unmyelinated ending of the nerve fiber, which is enclosed in a separate internal capsule (Fig. 22–3).

Meissner corpuscles are found in the so-called nervous papillae of the palmar and plantar skin. They possess a thin envelope in which delicate connective tissue ramifications lie perpendicular to the longitudinal axis of the corpuscle. In the interior, flat epithelioid cells are found around which the naked ending of a sensory nerve is wrapped. Each corpuscle is innervated by one to four afferent fibers (Fig. 22–2).

Functional Aspects

The adequate stimulus for mechanoreceptors is deformation of the tissue surrounding them. They can be functionally divided into rapidly and slowly adapting mechanoreceptors. The former include Pacini bodies and tactile vibrissae; the latter include the Merkel corpuscles and Ruffini corpuscles.

Adaptation is defined as the diminishing excitability of a receptor with increasing time. Constant stimulation as a rule leads to reduced receptor activity. Rapidly adapting receptors are involved especially in the registration of abrupt changes in stimulus intensity; receptor activity disappears completely after a while. Slowly adapting receptors constantly provide information on a particular condition (for example, body posture). The proprioceptors (muscle spindles, tendon corpuscles) are slowly adapting receptors; so are pain receptors.

Proprioceptors, Muscle Spindles, and Tendon Corpuscles

Proprioception is the processing of sensory information from the locomotor apparatus (muscles, tendons, joints). Part of this information is used for the unconscious control of muscles

during a wide variety of movements; another part serves to give conscious awareness of body posture and motor activity.

MUSCLE SPINDLES

Scattered through the muscles are numerous small (about 7 mm long) structures that consist of special muscle fibers with a highly differentiated innervation (muscle spindles; Fig. 22–4). These structures are enclosed by a fusiform capsule that contains a lymph-like fluid. A muscle spindle comprises six to eight striated muscle fibers (intrafusal muscle fibers). *Long* fibers running through the total length of the muscle spindle and connected with the endomysium of ordinary (extrafusal) muscle fibers are distinguished from *short* fibers, which number four to five per spindle and in turn are connected with the long fibers.

Afferent Innervation. The middle part of the long and short intrafusal fibers differs from the more polar parts in that it is slightly thickened and contains many nuclei. This middle (equatorial) part is not contractile but is abundantly provided with sensory endings. The ends of the intrafusal fibers are striated and contractile. Since the muscle spindle is in parallel connection with the extrafusal muscle fibers, the middle part of the muscle spindle is pulled out when the muscle stretches. This also happens when the ends of the muscle spindle contract. The middle part of the long fibers functions as a sensor. The afferent nerve branches (*primary sensory nerve branches*) are wrapped spirally around the equatorial part of the long and short intrafusal fibers. These primary sensory branches unite to form a nerve fiber with a thickness of about 12 μm, so that each muscle spindle has only one primary afferent fiber (I_a-fiber). These fibers conduct at a speed of about 80 m/sec. Around the short intrafusal fibers one also finds the terminations of secondary afferent fibers (*secondary sensory nerve branches*). These branches continue in a thinner (about 6 μm) afferent nerve fiber (group II). They conduct at a speed of about 50 m/sec.

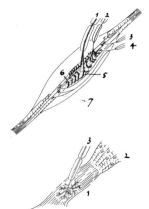

A
1   I_a-fiber
2   II-fiber
3,4 γ-fibers
5   annulospiral nerve ending (yellow)
6   short intrafusal fiber
7   long intrafusal fiber (contractile part)
B
1   tendon
2   muscle
3   I_b-fiber

Figure 22–4   Innervation of proprioceptors. *A*, Muscle spindle. *B*, Golgi (tendon) corpuscle (according to Bernards and Bouman).

Efferent Innervation.   The muscle spindle is a complicated complex of sense organs. Apart from the primary and secondary sensory nerve branches, the muscle spindle also has an efferent innervation. The polar, contractile parts of the intrafusal fibers are efferently innervated by thin motor nerve fibers (γ-fibers). They are divided into γ_1-fibers (which innervate the long intrafusal muscle fibers) and γ_2-fibers (which innervate the short intrafusal fibers). The γ_1-fibers are 3 to 5 μm thick and conduct at a speed of about 20 m/sec; the γ_2-fibers have a diameter of 1 to 2 μm and conduct at a speed of 10–15 m/sec.

Function.   The muscle spindles are sensitive to stretch. When the equatorial (sensor) part of the long and short fibers is stretched in a longitudinal direction, the I_a-fibers and the group II fibers fire action potentials. The equatorial part can be stretched when the entire muscle is stretched or when the striated ends of the intrafusal fibers contract as a result of activity in the γ-system. When the entire muscle is stretched, the afferent I_a-fiber ends give information on the *speed of the change,* while the secondary afferent nerve branches give information on the *change in length* of the muscle. The short intrafusal fibers thus function as "length detec-

tors" and provide the spinal cord with static information; the long intrafusal fibers on the other hand provide phasic information on the speed of muscle stretching and function as "change detectors."

Stimuli that enter via the γ-fibers shorten the intrafusal muscle fibers and keep the muscle spindles slightly stretched. In this way, minor differences in muscle length can be registered. A decrease in muscle length, too, is registered by a reduction of the firing rate of the muscle spindle. The γ-activity serves the purpose of "standardization," which enables the muscle spindle to adapt itself to the change in the length of the muscle fibers.

When a striated muscle relaxes, a certain "baseline activity" of the muscle spindles remains intact by virtue of the constant discharge of the γ-neurons. This activity increases the firing rate of the I_a-fibers and ensures that both the muscle itself and the muscle spindles remain "primed."

TENDON CORPUSCLES

These receptors are structurally less complicated and have no efferent innervation. The receptor has a capsule that encloses the transition from muscle to tendon (Fig. 22–4). Tendon corpuscles are connected in series between bone and muscle, and are therefore activated both at passive stretching and at active contraction of the muscle. They provide information on the tension in the tendon and function as "tension detectors."

Classification of the Sensory Nerve Fibers

The sensory nerve fibers vary in diameter. The diameter correlates with the speed of conduction: the thicker the fiber, the higher the speed of conduction. The afferent fibers of the dorsal root are classified as shown in Table 22–1.

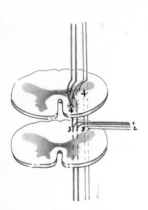

Figure 22–5 Division of dorsal root fibers.

1 dorsal root fibers (thick)
2 dorsal root fibers (thin)
3 division of dorsal root fibers
4 collaterals of the ascending dorsal root fibers

Dorsal Roots

The axons of the spinal ganglion cells enter the spinal cord via the dorsolateral sulcus. Each dorsal root comprises a large number of fibers (about 20,000) with widely diverse diameters. Distinction is made between a medial bundle (with thick fibers) and a lateral bundle (with thinner axons). The thick fibers arise from large, encapsulated receptors (touch, pressure and fibration receptors, proprioceptors). The thin fibers conduct stimuli from temperature, pressure, and pain receptors. Immediately after entering the spinal cord, the thick fibers divide into an ascending and a descending branch, with many collaterals to the gray matter of the cord (Fig. 22–5). The thin, lateral root fibers likewise divide into an ascending and a descending branch (T-shaped division); the former extends over one to two segments through Lissauer's marginal zone (see page 144).

Table 22–1 THE AFFERENT FIBERS OF THE DORSAL ROOTS

Group	Diameter (μm)	Conduction Speed (m/sec)	Stimulus	Receptor
I_a	12–20	70–120	stretch	muscle spindle
I_b	12–20	70–120	stretch	tendon corpuscles
II	6–12	36–75	stretch, pressure movement	muscle spindle joint receptor
III	2–5	12–30	deep pressure	Pacini corpuscles
IV	0.5–2	1.5–2	pain fibers, C-mechanoreceptors	free nerve branches

Chapter 23

Microscopic Structure of the Spinal Cord

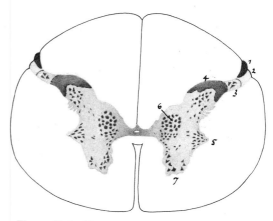

Figure 23–1 Topography of the principal cell groups in a horizontal section through T10.

1 dorsal root fibers
2 Lissauer's marginal zone
3 posteromarginal nucleus
4 substantia gelatinosa
5 intermediolateral nucleus
6 Clarke's dorsal nucleus
7 motoneurons of the anterior horn

Transverse sections of the spinal cord that are stained by the Nissl method or one of its variants provide a relatively simple (if incomplete) impression of the gray matter. These sections are therefore suitable for a first discussion of the structure of the spinal cord.

Cytoarchitectonic Data

Anterior Horn. The anterior horn contains the large perikaryons of the motor anterior horn cells (α-motoneurons), whose fibers ensure the innervation of the extrafusal muscle fibers of the skeletal muscles. In addition to these cells, there are smaller γ-neurons for innervation of the muscle spindles.

Results of physiologic experiments indicate the existence of a third cell type, the so-called Renshaw cell, which morphologically has not yet been demonstrated with certainty. Recurrent axon collaterals of an α-motoneuron synapse on the Renshaw cells; the axon of the Renshaw cell synapses with the same cell body from which the axon collaterals arise (see Fig. 24–4).

Interneurons. Interneurons exceed other nerve cell types in number, and are particularly numerous in laminae VII, VIII, and IX. Against expectations, studies by the Golgi method have revealed that these cells are "class-I cells;" cells with short axons (class II) are believed to occur only in lamina II (substantia gelatinosa). The axon of an interneuron extends over one or several segments either homolaterally or contralaterally, via the gray commissures. The spi-

nal segments are thus connected with each other. The dendrites of the interneurons are long and often exceed the boundaries of the laminae in which their perikaryon is located.

Lateral Horn. A group of visceral efferent cells is located in the lateral horn of the thoracic and the proximal part of the lumbar spinal cord (intermediolateral nucleus, C8–L3). Their cell body is oval or fusiform, with thin dendrites and a pale cytoplasm. The axons leave the spinal cord with the ventral roots; beyond the intervertebral foramen, they leave the spinal nerve and extend as preganglionic fibers to the sympathetic trunk or the prevertebral ganglia.

A second group of visceral efferent fibers is located in the sacral segment of the spinal cord (S1, S2, S3). Their axons accompany the corresponding ventral roots as preganglionic fibers and extend to the (parasympathetic) intramural ganglia.

Posterior Horn. These cells are morphologically very different. Characteristic are the large cells of Clarke's dorsal nucleus (C8–L4), with thick myelinated axons (dorsal spinocerebellar tract) and an eccentric nucleus (Fig. 23–1). The mid-region of the posterior horn contains the so-called nucleus proprius, which consists of

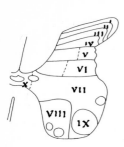

Figure 23–2 General diagram of Rexed's layers in the spinal cord of a cat (according to Rexed).

Figure 23–3 Boundaries of Rexed's layers in the human spinal cord. Lamina IX consists of several cell islets (according to Carpenter).

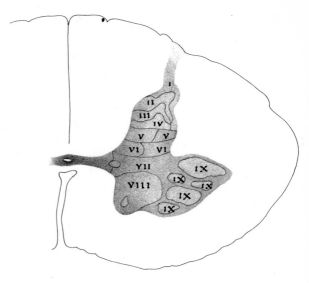

large cells with numerous long dendrites. Many interneurons, too, are found scattered in the posterior horn.

Rexed's Layers

Modern research using sophisticated fiber degeneration techniques calls for a division of the gray matter in which the synaptic junctions of the arriving fibers are taken into account. For this purpose Rexed (1954) prepared a cytoarchitectonic "atlas" in which nine layers (laminae) are distinguished. Although this atlas is based on the cat, a similar division seems to apply to humans.

A lamina in Rexed's atlas is an area with certain characteristics, but the boundaries from other laminae are not always well defined. Some laminae are identical with long-known nuclei, but others are less clearly defined areas (Figs. 23–2 and 23–3).

Lamina I comprises large and medium-size cells, lying fairly far apart (posteromarginal nucleus). The dorsal root fibers pass through this layer but hardly synapse with the cells in it.

Lamina II used to be known as the substantia gelatinosa. It comprises many small cells (class-II neurons) whose axons extend through Lissauer's marginal zone over two to three segments and then return to the substantia gelatinosa. Afferents to these neurons are axons of the fairly large pyramidal cells of lamina IV (see below). Lamina II is perforated by many thick fibers from the dorsal root on their way to their respective destinations. These thick fibers, however, do not synapse here.

Laminae III and IV consist of morphologically different, generally larger cells, with characteristic large pyramidal cells in lamina IV, in which many fibers from the skin receptors (exteroceptive stimuli) synapse. This area serves as center for many exteroceptive reflexes. Laminae I through IV together constitute the apex of the posterior horn.

Laminae V and VI can be divided into a lateral and a medial area. Many proprioceptive fibers from muscles and joints and corticospinal fibers from the cerebral cortex synapse here. These laminae can be regarded as a center of integration of reflex activities, because proprioceptive as well as corticospinal impulses converge on the same neurons.

Lamina VII is a very extensive area that comprises well known nuclei like Clarke's dorsal nucleus. Lamina VII enters the anterior horn in the cervical and lumbar tumescences of the spinal cord. Important spinocerebellar tracts arise from this lamina, which is likewise an important center of integration for many reflexes.

Lamina VIII is variable; it is sometimes confined to the medial part of the anterior horn. Some axons of the cells of lamina VIII are believed to cross the midline in the anterior white commissure.

Lamina IX comprises many groups of motor anterior horn cells and both large and small neurons (α-neurons and γ-neurons). It can be regarded as the primary motor area in the spinal cord.

FUNCTION OF REXED'S LAYERS

The morphologic features of the various laminae in the spinal cord are associated with certain functional activities. In this respect, laminae I through IV can be regarded as the areas on which exteroceptive signals synapse. Most proprioceptive signals go to laminae V and VI. Lamina VIII is required for postural and other reflexes.

The neurons in lamina IV respond mainly to mechanical stimuli that originate from small receptor areas. The receptor area of a neuron is defined as that area in the periphery from which the neuron can be activated.

Signals from the skin and viscera (exteroceptive and interoceptive stimuli) converge on the cells of lamina V. Physiologically, many other (lamina IV) cells prove to also converge on each cell.

The cells of lamina VI are activated by (active and passive) movement, in accordance with the terminations of many fibers from receptors in the locomotor apparatus. Synaptic transmission in laminae IV through VI can be influenced by impulses from supraspinal centers (cerebral cortex, reticular formation) and by impulses from lamina II (substantia gelatinosa). Many spinal neurons are sensitive to stimuli from various sources; this is due to the convergence of the arriving stimuli on these cells.

Excitation of the corticospinal tract and a few supraspinal centers exerts a marked influence on synaptic transmission in laminae IV, V, and VI; transmission can be either facilitated or inhibited (see page 158). Synaptic transmission in laminae I through III is probably subject to the modulating influence of the substantia gelatinosa.

On the basis of these and other observations, the transmission and assimilation of signals in the spinal cord is currently considered to be a flexible process. Despite the close agreement between the localizations of the terminations of the afferent fibers and the functions of the laminae, the spinal cord is not a rigid complex of separate channels through which information from various receptors is conducted. The processing of information for spinal reflexes and the selection and transmission of information to higher nerve centers are dependent, to a considerable degree, on the supraspinal control of sensory transmission and the activity of the substantia gelatinosa, among other things.

Termination of the Root Fibers

THICK ROOT FIBERS

Some 65 per cent of the thick fibers traverse a small part of the posterior funiculus, enter the gray matter of the posterior horn (Fig. 23–4), and then synapse. Other fibers accompany the posterior funiculus over three to four segments above the level of entry before they enter the posterior horn. Some 25 per cent of the thick fibers of the

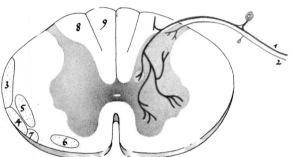

Figure 23–4 Terminal ramification of the dorsal root fibers. The thin fibers do not extend beyond lamina IV; the thick fibers synapse in laminae IV to IX.

1	thick dorsal root fibers
2	thin dorsal root fibers
3	posterior spinocerebellar tract
4	anterior spinocerebellar tract
5	lateral spinothalamic tract
6	anterior spinothalamic tract
7	spinoolivary tract
8	fasciculus cuneatus
9	fasciculus gracilis

dorsal root ascend in the funiculus to the posterior column nuclei of the medulla oblongata, where they finally synapse. As a result, fibers from caudal roots are pushed more and more medially by fibers from cranial roots; this causes the typical lamination of the posterior funiculus (page 150 and Fig. 25–1). The thick root fibers that have entered the posterior horn terminate with axodendritic or axosomatic synapses on the cells of the gray matter. The synapse can lie between laminae IV and IX, with a certain predilection for laminae IV, VI, and VII.

Lissauer's marginal zone (dorsolateral tract) consists of a small light-colored area localized lateral to the incoming dorsal root fibers. The zone is usually found between the surface of the spinal cord and the most peripheral cells of lamina I (posteromarginal nucleus). The shape of the zone is variable: Sometimes it is a thin but fairly broad layer (Fig. 23–1), but in other cases it is a narrow but deep wedge between the dorsal root fibers and the lateral funiculus of the white matter of the cord.

The marginal zone comprises a population of thin myelinated and unmyelinated fibers, about half of which are dorsal root fibers on the way to their terminations in the posterior horn. The other half are propriospinal fibers (axons of the small neurons of the substantia gelatinosa), which ascend or descend over two or three segments and reenter the substantia gelatinosa.

THIN ROOT FIBERS

The thinner, lateral fibers of the dorsal root (pain, temperature, deep pressure, visceroceptive stimuli) likewise divide into a T and run in Lissauer's marginal zone over one or two segments. Little is known about the further course of these fibers and their terminal synapses because thin fibers do not readily stain. Some of these fibers synapse with the large cells of lamina I, while others terminate with synapses on the dendrites of the small neurons of the substantia gelatinosa (lamina II and the dorsal part of lamina III). Fibers of a third group penetrate deeper and synapse with the medial neurons of lamina IV.

Structure of the Substantia Gelatinosa

This area differs markedly from the other layers of the spinal cord in that it contains many small neurons with short axons (class-II neurons). A highly characteristic feature of the substantia gelatinosa is the absence of an exit channel. The axons of the small cells remain close to their cells or reenter the substantia gelatinosa after ascending or descending in Lissauer's marginal zone.

Entry channels to the substantia gelatinosa are (a) thin lateral fibers of the dorsal root and (b) axon collaterals of fairly thick dorsal root fibers that have their terminal synapses in the deeper layers of the posterior horn (Fig. 23–5). The thick fibers enter on the inferior side of the substantia gelatinosa, while the thin fibers enter on the superior side.

The substantia gelatinosa also contains the so-called P-cells. The perikaryon of these cells is usually located in lamina III, whence the axon ascends to the substantia gelatinosa. The ends of the axons of these cells are essential components of the synaptic glomeruli that characterize this substance (Fig. 23–5). The P-cells are thought to be under direct control of the supraspinal systems.

The exit channel of the substantia gelatinosa is probably formed by large neurons (T-cells)

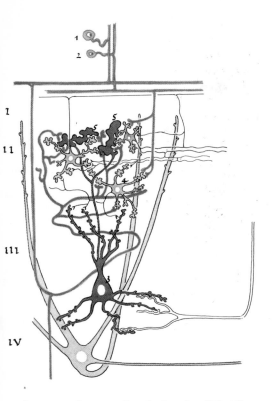

Figure 23–5 Structure of the substantia gelatinosa. The collaterals of the thick dorsal root fibers synapse with the thickened ends of the pyramidal cells of lamina IV and with dendrites of the cells of the substantia gelatinosa (synaptic glomeruli). The axons of the latter cells return from Lissauer's marginal zone to the substantia gelatinosa (according to Szentágothai, slightly simplified).

1 spinal ganglion cell with thick fiber
2 spinal ganglion cell with thin fiber
3 pyramidal cell of lamina IV
4 small neurons of the substantia gelatinosa
5 synaptic glomeruli

whose perikaryon lies in lamina IV. These cells have long radial dendrites that enter the substantia gelatinosa on the inferior side and synapse with the thin axons of the cells of this substance.

The substantia gelatinosa seems to function as a kind of filter for incoming sensory stimuli. According to Voorhoeve, the entire substantia gelatinosa system clearly impresses one as being capable of exerting a modulating influence on the synaptic transmission from the primary afferents to the posterior horn cells.

Chapter 24

Motoneurons, Motor Units, and Reflexes

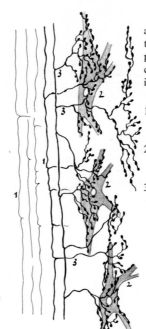

Figure 24–1 Axodendritic and axosomatic synapses between the collateral branches of posterior funiculus fibers and the cells of the anterior horn (according to Cajal).

1 ascending thick and thin fibers of the posterior funiculus
2 cells of the posterior horn with vertically arranged dendrites
3 collateral axon branches that synapse with the cells

Morphology of the Motoneurons

The α-motoneurons are localized in lamina IX. They are among the largest nerve cells (30 to 70 μm in diameter) and have a large, round central nucleus. The Nissl bodies are coarsely granular and the cells are multipolar, with numerous dendrites in mainly vertical arrangement (Fig. 24–1). Horizontal sections show only a small part of the dendritic tree, that is, the processes that lie perpendicular to the longitudinal axis of the spinal cord. These horizontal dendrites extend into lamina VIII. The dendrites that parallel the longitudinal axis of the spinal cord sometimes exceed the boundaries of the segment in which their perikaryon is located.

Organization of the α-Neurons

The large motoneurons of the anterior horn are arranged in oblong nuclei that parallel the longitudinal axis of the spinal cord. The localization of these nuclei depends on the topographic localization of the innervated muscles; generally, the medial (erector) muscles of the trunk are innervated by the most medial neurons. The lateral muscles of the trunk and those of the humeroscapular and pelvic zones are innervated by the intermediate nucleus. Finally, the most lateral neurons innervate the distal muscles of the extremities. For this purpose the cervical and lumbar spinal cord tumescences with a number of nuclei (anterolateral, posterolateral, and retroposterolateral nuclei) develop (Fig. 24–2). Neurons that innervate extensors are localized

ventrally in the anterior horn; the opposite applies to neurons that innervate flexors.

Ventral Roots

The ventral root consists of axons of the motoneurons of the anterior horn. The ventral roots between T1 and L2 also contain axons of the cells of the intermediolateral nucleus (preganglionic sympathetic fibers), which originate from lamina VII. The numbers of axons of ventral roots vary widely and depend on the musculature to be innervated.

The diameter of the ventral root axons ranges from 3 to 14 μm. The thickest axons (10 to 14 μm) belong to the α-motoneurons; other fibers with a diameter of 3 to 6 μm are the γ-efferent fibers. The preganglionic fibers have a diameter of 3 to 10 μm (B-fibers).

MOTOR UNIT

The term "motor unit" applies to the totality of an α-motoneuron, including its axon and all muscle fibers innervated by this axon. A distinction is made between a small and large motor

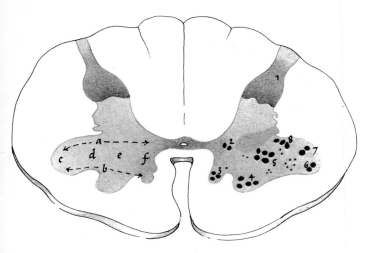

Figure 24-2 Topography of the motoneurons in the anterior horn of the spinal cord.

a   flexors
b   extensors
c   hand
d   arm
e   shoulder
f   trunk
1   substantia gelatinosa
2   posteromedial nucleus
3   anteromedial nucleus
4   anterior nucleus
5   central nucleus
6   anterolateral nucleus
7   posterolateral nucleus
8   retroposterolateral nucleus

unit: Muscles involved in delicate movements have small motor units, whereas those involved in the performance of crude, vigorous movements can do with large motor units. The smallest units have fewer than ten muscle fibers per axon.

The muscle fibers of a motor unit are usually scattered over a given part of the muscle; a transverse section reveals many fibers corresponding with different units.

SLOW AND FAST MUSCLES

A distinction is made between slow ("red") and fast ("white") muscles. The former have many mitochondria and oxidative enzymes in the cytoplasm, whereas the latter possess fewer mitochondria but have an abundance of glycogen. The red muscles are important for body posture and are virtually indefatigable (antigravitational muscles). The white muscles are muscles of movement; they can develop considerable force but tire easily. Red muscles have small and white muscles have larger motor units.

TROPHIC FUNCTION OF THE MOTONEURONS

The muscle fibers are subject to the metabolic influence of the innervating nerve fibers. Denervated muscle fibers degenerate. If the nerve fails to regenerate, then the muscle may be completely destroyed. Muscle degeneration is partly dependent on lack of activity, but this is probably not the only cause of degeneration. Nothing is yet known with certainty about the existence of trophic substances that could affect the motor end-plate.

Peripheral Motor Paralysis.   Damage to motoneurons of the anterior horn, the ventral root, or the peripheral nerve causes flaccid paralysis of the muscle, associated with atonia (lack of muscular tone) and areflexia (absence of reflexes). Denervated muscles show spontaneous contractions of isolated muscle fibers (fibrillations). Electrical stimulation of the muscle via the nerve has no effect. Only direct galvanic stimulation proves able to cause contraction of the muscle fibers.

Reflexes

The anatomic substrate of a reflex is the route followed by the stimulus from the peripheral receptor to the effector organ (muscle). This route is known as a reflex arc and can be summarized as follows:

receptor → afferent nerve → reflex center →
                     efferent nerve → effector.

Evidently the term "reflex center" refers to the spinal cord or brain stem. The reflex arc is

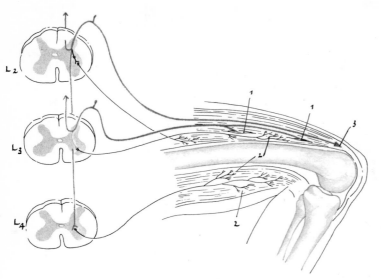

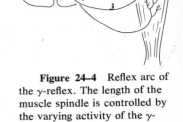

Figure 24–4 Reflex arc of the γ-reflex. The length of the muscle spindle is controlled by the varying activity of the γ-neurons (according to Carpenter).

1   muscle spindle
2   motor end-plate
3   γ-efferent fiber

Figure 24–3   Reflex arc of the knee tendon reflex (according to Carpenter).

1   muscle spindle
2   motor end-plate
3   Golgi's tendon corpuscle

interrupted once or several times in the reflex center (synapses); via the synapses the reflex activity can be enhanced or suppressed in response to the influence of certain spinal or supraspinal centers.

STRUCTURAL CHARACTERISTICS OF THE REFLEX ARC

The following are the structural characteristics of the reflex arc:

(a) the length of the arc and the thickness of the afferent and the efferent segment of the arc;

(b) the number of synapses of the neuronal circuit in the reflex center; the simplest reflex minimally involves two neurons with an intermediate synapse (monosynaptic reflex), but many reflexes involve several interneurons between the afferent and the efferent neuron (multisynaptic reflexes);

(c) the localization of the synapses involved in the reflex arc (ipsilateral, heterolateral, etc.);

(d) the connection pattern of the interneurons in the reflex center, which can cause different mechanisms such as facilitation, reciprocal inhibition, disinhibition, and modulation of the reflex activity by higher centers.

In terms of the morphology of the reflex arc, a distinction is made between monosynaptic and multisynaptic, unilateral and bilateral, and monosegmental and polysegmental reflexes.

STRETCH REFLEX

The stretch reflex (myotatic reflex) is the basic element of many servo-mechanisms that are of fundamental significance for postural motor activity. A muscle attuned to a certain length tends to maintain this length and resists any "imposed" increase in length with increased tone. The stretch reflex is the muscle's reaction to forces that want to cause an abrupt elongation of its fibers.

Stretching of the muscle fibers causes the primary sensory endings of the muscle spindles to fire off impulses. These impulses travel through the I_a-fibers to the spinal cord, where they monosynaptically cause the α-motoneurons to discharge. As a result the muscle is shortened and the original situation restored. This can be viewed as a feedback mechanism in which the increase in muscle fiber length acts as an anomaly; the change in tone is then centrally controlled (Fig. 24-3). The stretch reflex is monosynaptic, ipsilateral, and monosegmental. In some cases (such as knee tendon reflex) the change is phasic; in other instances it can be gradual and tonic.

GAMMA REFLEX

The parallel-connected muscle spindle has the special advantage of its ability to continue firing during active shortening of the muscle. In principle, a shortening of this kind causes relaxation of the intrafusal fibers with the associated decrease in the firing rate of the I_a-fibers. However, such an effect is undesirable because the activity of the α-motoneurons diminishes and the muscle relaxes as the result of the diminished input of impulses. This untoward effect is abolished by virtue of a shortening of the intrafusal fibers as a result of increased activity of the γ-neurons, which keeps the impulse frequency in the I_a-afferents constant. In this way the muscle spindle is again "standardized" for a new length; this calls for a synaptic junction between the α- and the γ-neurons (α-γ linking).

During voluntary movements or postural changes the activity of the γ-fibers changes so that the length of the intrafusal muscle fibers increases or decreases in order to ensure an equal stretching of the equatorial primary sensory ending. The discharge activity of the muscle spindle consequently shows the necessary adaptations during the movement so that the α-motoneurons receive sufficient afferent impulses for persistent discharge.

The γ-reflex plays an important role in the control of voluntary and involuntary movements, particularly in slow postural changes. According to the "gamma-loop" theory (Merton, 1953), each movement could be produced via preceding excitation of the γ-neurons (Fig. 24-4). This results in an increased impulse frequency in the I_a-afferents, which in a reflex causes the corresponding α-neurons to discharge. It is therefore possible to induce a movement from the γ-system (contraction via the gamma-loop). The gamma-loop can be schematically represented as follows:

γ-neuron $\rightarrow$ muscle spindle $\rightarrow$ afferent I_a-fiber $\rightarrow$ α-motoneuron $\rightarrow$ skeletal muscle.

The α-γ linking is disregarded in this representation.

The theory of the gamma-loop "promotes" the γ-system to a leading factor in the induction of movement. It is therefore very important to know from which areas of the CNS excitation of the γ-system can be achieved: from the I_a-afferents, from various skin receptors, via interneurons, or from supraspinal neurons (reticular formation, cerebral cortex, lateral vestibular nucleus). From these areas, a strong modulating influence can be exerted on the γ-system.

AUTOGENOUS INHIBITION

The "serially" connected tendon corpuscles can be regarded as tension detectors. An increase of the tension in a tendon above a certain value activates these corpuscles, which fire off action potentials via the I_b-afferent fibers. Impulses through these fibers inhibit the muscle via interneurons and facilitate the antagonists. In this way, muscles are protected from excessively strong contractions (Fig. 24-3).

Chapter 25

The Long Ascending Systems

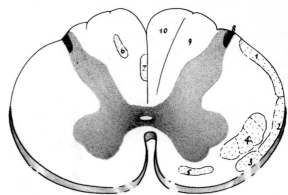

Figure 25–1 Schematic representation of the ascending fiber systems of the spinal cord.

1 posterior spinocerebellar tract
2 anterior spinocerebellar tract
3 spinoolivary and spinotectal tract
4 lateral spinothalamic tract
5 anterior spinothalamic tract
6 interfascicular fasciculus (descending)
7 septomarginal fasciculus (descending)
8 Lissauer's marginal zone
9 fasciculus cuneatus
10 fasciculus gracilis

Of the extensive flow of information constantly supplied to the CNS, one part remains in the spinal cord to be processed to unconscious reflex activity, while another part reaches the cerebellum or the thalamocortical system to lay the foundation for the conscious perception of the various sensory qualities. The latter information travels via the so-called ascending oligosynaptic systems. These nerve pathways consist of parallel chains of three neurons, counting from the spinal ganglion cell to the thalamus. The three successive neurons are (a) spinal ganglion cell, (b) neuron in the spinal cord or brain stem (second order neuron), and (c) neuron in the thalamus (third order neuron). The oligosynaptic systems are, therefore, interrupted at least twice by synapses. Other systems are interrupted more frequently by synapses (multisynaptic systems) and form rather diffuse fiber bundles that ascend to the brain stem through the lateral funiculus.

The oligosynaptic systems show a well defined somatotopic arrangement. The peripheral receptive areas are localized in the nerve tract in accordance with a fixed pattern. In the more diffuse multisynaptic systems, however, no somatotopia is found.

Oligosynaptic Systems

The oligosynaptic systems can be divided into three systems: the dorsal, the spinothalamic, and the spinocerebellar systems.

DORSAL SYSTEM

This system is localized in the posterior funiculus and has two parts: the fasciculus gracilis and the fasciculus cuneatus. These bundles are made up of thick dorsal root fibers that ascend uninterrupted to the posterior funiculus nuclei of the medulla oblongata (Fig. 25–1), where they synapse. The dorsal system is phylogenetically young and most developed in humans; it comprises mainly fibers that originate from the extremities. In humans, this means fibers with a length of about 150 cm.

Topography

Some of the thick axons of the dorsal root remain in the posterior funiculus, where they arrange themselves in closely packed longitudinal fiber bundles. The ascending fibers join the fibers from lower segments and arrange themselves lateral to these fibers, thus producing a layered organization. The fibers from the sacral, lumbar, and lower thoracic levels are localized medially and constitute the fasciculus gracilis. The other fibers (from thoracic and cervical segments) are localized laterally and constitute the fasciculus cuneatus (Fig. 25–2).

The fibers of these two fasciculi synapse in two nuclei in the caudal part of the medulla oblongata: the nucleus gracilis and the nucleus cuneatus. The axons of the cells of the nuclei of the posterior funiculus (second neuron) cross the midline and extend cranially as the medial lemniscus as far as the ventral posterolateral nucleus of the thalamus, where they synapse. The lemniscus fibers produce few, if any, collaterals to the reticular formation (see below).

Descending Fibers

Because all incoming dorsal root fibers divide in a T-shaped bifurcation, there are also descending fibers, which generally are shorter than the ascending fibers. The descending bundles are localized in the so-called interfascicular fasciculus and the septomarginal fasciculus. These fibers synapse in the gray matter of the spinal cord, a few segments below the level of their entry.

Morphology and Functional Aspects of the Nuclei of the Posterior Funiculus

Histologically, the nucleus gracilis can be divided into three areas: a rostral area with a reticular structure, a midportion with numerous "cell nests," and a rather inconspicuous inferior area with more scattered cells. The nucleus cuneatus likewise shows local differences.

The termination of the fibers is not yet completely known. Research findings indicate that the distribution of the nerve endings has a fixed, clearly somatotopic pattern. Moreover, there seems to be a correlation between the topography of the nerve endings and the nature of the information transmitted: Proprioceptive fibers synapse with the rostral area of the gracile nucleus, and exteroceptive fibers with the "cell nest" zone. The nucleus gracilis and the nucleus cuneatus are synaptic nuclei where the impulse transmission between the first and the second neurons of the dorsal system takes place.

The functional role of the nuclei of the posterior funiculus can be envisaged more easily when we compare them with a preamplifier with circuitry for noise suppression and channel separation. Trains of information-rich impulses are identified and amplified. At the same time, the less differentiated activity in adjacent fibers ("noise") is suppressed, which benefits the so-called "marginal contrast." The suppression of the "noise" ensures that only sharply focused, information-rich firing patterns have access to the thalamus. In view of the convergence of several axon endings on a synaptic cell, it is likely that even in these nuclei a degree of integration of the information takes place, with the corresponding transformation of the impulse code.

An additional factor of great importance is that the impulse transmission in the nuclei of the posterior funiculus is subject to the direct influence of the cortex via the collaterals of the corticospinal fibers. Via these fibers, the cortex controls the amount of information admitted to the higher centers of the nervous system. It is a remarkable fact that a typical motor system like the corticospinal tract (pyramidal tract) can regulate the impulse transmission in a sensory system.

Sensory Modalities in the Dorsal System

The thick fibers of the dorsal system originate from exteroceptors (touch and pressure receptors like the hair follicles and the Meissner corpuscles, deep pressure and vibration receptors like the Pacini corpuscles) and from proprioceptors (I_a-fibers and receptors in tendons and joints). The I_a-fibers arise mainly from C2–T6 and end in the so-called external cuneate nucleus.

The sensory modalities transmitted through the fibers of the dorsal system are delicate touch and pressure, along with proprioceptive perceptions like angle accelerations in movements of the extremities, and registration of the spatial

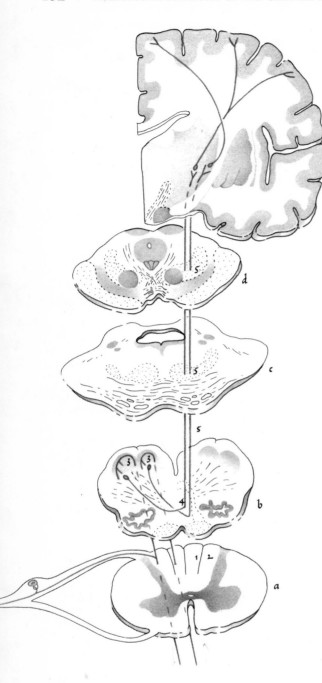

Figure 25–2 Schematic representation of the course of the fibers of the dorsal system. This oligosynaptic system consists of a chain of three neurons with two synapses (partly according to Rasmussen).

a spinal cord
b medulla oblongata
c pons
d mesencephalon
e thalamus and cortex
1 fasciculus gracilis
2 fasciculus cuneatus
3 nuclei of the posterior funiculus
4 decussation of the medial lemniscus
5 medial lemniscus
6 thalamus (ventral posterolateral and mediolateral nucleus)

position of the extremity. The dorsal fibers are modality-specific, and this specificity is maintained throughout the tract as far as the thalamus.

SPINOTHALAMIC SYSTEM

The spinothalamic fibers arise from a diffuse, fairly extensive area of the posterior horn, which has not yet been defined with certainty. They probably originate from laminae I, VI, and VII. Most of these fibers cross the midline in the anterior white commissure, one or more segments above the level of origin, and ascend in the contralateral lateral funiculus as the lateral spinothalamic tract (pain and temperature sense) and as an anterior spinothalamic tract (touch). Both tracts show a somatotopic arrangement. Some of the fibers of the anterior spinothalamic tract end in the reticular formation of the medulla oblongata or in the lateral reticular nucleus. The other fibers join the lateral spinothalamic tract at the approximate level of the lower margin of the olive. The lateral spinothalamic tract is involved in pain perception. This tract extends in the lateral funiculus, dorsal to the anterior spinocerebellar tract (Fig. 25–1).

Many fibers of the spinothalamic tract terminate in the reticular formation of the brain stem. At the level of the boundary between pons and mesencephalon, the remaining spinothalamic fibers join the medial lemniscus. This is why

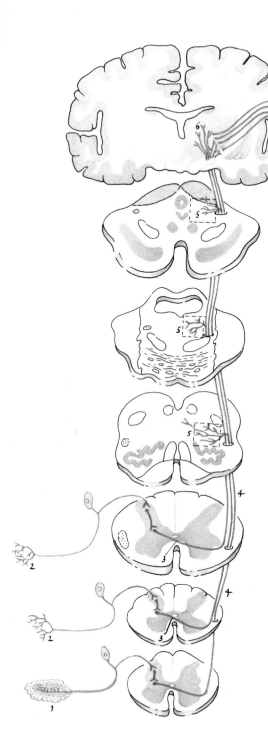

Figure 25–3 Schematic representation of the course of the lateral spinothalamic tract (pain and temperature sense). Some of the ascending spinothalamic fibers terminate in the reticular formation.

1 Meissner corpuscle
2 free nerve endings (pain receptors)
3 anterior white commissure
4 lateral spinothalamic tract
5 synapsing spinothalamic fibers in the reticular formation
6 thalamus (ventral posterolateral nucleus, posterior nucleus, and intralaminar nuclei)
7 cortex (areas 40 and 43)

the dorsal system, medial lemniscus, and spinothalamic tract are collectively known as the "lemniscal system."

The second neuron of the spinothalamic tract terminates partly in the ventral posterolateral nucleus of the thalamus; other fibers, however, synapse in the intralaminar nuclei, the posterior nucleus, and the magnocellular part of the medial geniculate body.

Unilateral severance of the lateral spinothalamic tract causes analgesia (absence of pain sense) and thermoanesthesia (absence of cold and heat sense) in the contralateral side of the body; the loss of sensibility applies to the body surface but not to the viscera. The loss begins about one segment below the level of the spinal cord lesion, owing to the oblique course of the decussating fibers in the white anterior commissure (Fig. 25–3).

Vital and Gnostic Sensibility

The above has shown that some sensory modalities (touch pressure) are transmitted through two separate fiber systems. This corresponds with the difference between "vital" (protopathic) and "gnostic" (epicritic) sensibility. Vital sensibility supplies information on a given change in progress but gives little information on the intensity, localization, and cause of the change. On the other hand, vital perceptions are associated with a distinct affective component (pleasant, unpleasant). Gnostic sensibility is mainly involved in the registration of quantitative aspects of perception, like the exact localiza-

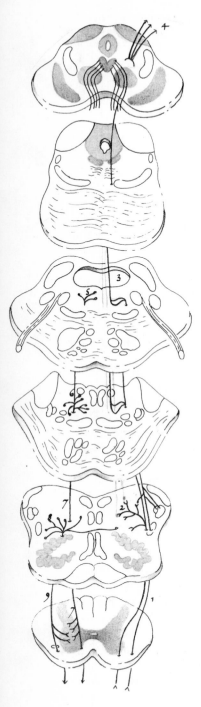

Figure 25–4 Schematic representation of the connections between the spinal cord and the reticular formation. On the right, the spinoreticular tract. On the left, the reticulospinal systems (according to Carpenter).

1 spinoreticular tract
2 synapsing fibers in the reticular formation
3 central tegmental fasciculus
4 reticulothalamic fibers
5 oral pontine reticular nucleus
6 caudal pontine reticular nucleus
7 anterior reticulospinal tract
8 gigantocellular reticular nucleus
9 lateral reticulospinal tract

tion of the source of stimulation, delicate gradations in the intensity of stimulation, and stereognostic aspects (the ability to recognize an object with the eyes closed).

Spinothalamic fibers transmit mostly vital sensory modalities, while the delicately discriminative modalities travel through the dorsal system. Disorders of the latter system lead to deficiencies such as diminished stereognosis, two-point discrimination at greater distances, and difficulties in determining the spatial position of the extremities.

Multisynaptic Spinothalamic Systems

These systems consist of thin fibers, probably originating from laminae V and VII. The fibers pass to the lateral funiculus and terminate in the reticular formation of the brain stem (Fig. 25–4). Some of these fibers synapse in the gigantocellular reticular nucleus, while others continue to the pons and terminate in the caudal pontine reticular nucleus. Both reticular nuclei largely project to the intralaminar nuclei of the thalamus. These fibers belong to the extralemniscal system, which is the phylogenetically oldest connection between spinal cord and thalamus. The system is multisynaptic, not somatotopic, and is highly sensitive to anesthetics.

OLIGOSYNAPTIC VERSUS MULTISYNAPTIC SYSTEMS

A comparison of the most striking characteristics of the oligosynaptic and multisynaptic systems casts some light on the remarkable differences between and even contradictory characteristics of the two systems, which are listed in Table 25–1. The anatomic and functional contrast between these systems is not a source of conflict but a necessity for cooperation; the transmission of information to the thalamocortical area demands a high degree of cooperation between the lemniscal and the extralemniscal system. The efferent impulses that travel through the extralemniscal system play an exceedingly important role: regulation of the level of activity of the cerebral cortex (see page 200). The "attention state" is controlled by the reticular formation (via the ARAS system), which in turn receives impulses through the spinoreticular fibers, etc. This means that the attention state depends largely on the magnitude of the sensory input. The reticular formation ensures a sufficient degree of cortical activity so that sensory stimuli arriving through the lemniscal system remain clear and sharp until they are perceived. Dysfunction of the extralemniscal system causes such a degree of reduction of cortical activity that the sensory stimuli that normally arrive through the lemniscal system remain unperceived.

Spinocerebellar Tracts

POSTERIOR SPINOCEREBELLAR TRACT

This tract is localized superficially in the lateral funiculus, near the posterior horn. The fibers arise from the homolateral lamina VII (Clarke's nucleus dorsalis), whence they curve to reach the lateral funiculus (Fig. 25–5). They enter the cerebellum via the restiform body and terminate as mossy fibers in the cortex of the intermediate zone and the vermis of the anterior and posterior lobes (see page 188).

The afferent fibers to the nucleus dorsalis originate from muscle spindles (I_a- and II-fibers) and tendon corpuscles (I_b-fibers) of the lower extremities and the lower part of the trunk.

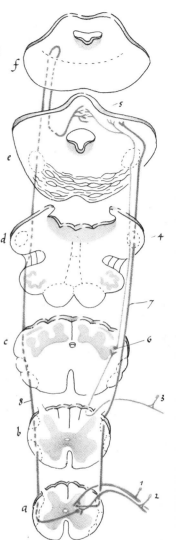

Figure 25–5 Course of the ascending spinocerebellar systems: *right*, the posterior spinocerebellar tract and *left*, the anterior spinocerebellar tract. The latter fibers enter the cerebellum via the superior cerebellar peduncle.

a,b spinal cord
c,d medulla oblongata
e pons
f caudal part of the mesencephalon
1 dorsal root fiber from muscle spindle
2 dorsal root fiber from Golgi's tendon corpuscle
3 dorsal root fiber from muscle spindle
4 inferior cerebellar peduncle
5 vermis cerebelli
6 external cuneate nucleus
7 posterior spinocerebellar tract
8 anterior spinocerebellar tract

Table 25–1   OLIGOSYNAPTIC AND MULTISYNAPTIC SYSTEMS

Lemniscal System	Extralemniscal System
Small receptive fields	Large receptive fields
Modality-specific	Multisensory convergence
Few synapses (2)	Multisynaptic
Limited supraspinal regulation	Pronounced supraspinal regulation
Somatotopic	Not somatotopic
Low sensitivity to anesthetics	High sensitivity to anesthetics (due to the many synapses)
Projects to ventral posterolateral and mediolateral nuclei	Projects to intralaminar thalamic nuclei

CUNEOCEREBELLAR TRACT

The cuneocerebellar tract is a homologue of the posterior spinocerebellar tract and serves to transport proprioceptive impulses from the upper extremities. The fibers ascend in the fasciculus cuneatus and synapse in the external nucleus cuneatus, which consists of cells that closely resemble those of Clarke's nucleus dorsalis. These fibers (posterior external arcuate fibers) reach the cerebellum via the restiform body and terminate as mossy fibers in the ipsilateral cortex of the anterior and posterior lobes, close to the primary fissure.

ANTERIOR SPINOCEREBELLAR TRACT

These fibers arise from the lateral part of the anterior horn (laminae VI and VII). They are thick and not very numerous. After crossing the midline they ascend in the lateral funiculus and brain stem, to reach the cerebellum via the superior cerebellar peduncle. They terminate as mossy fibers, mainly in the anterior lobe.

The fibers of the anterior spinocerebellar tract transport information on the position and movement of the entire lower extremity. The cuneocerebellar and posterior spinocerebellar fibers, however, are thought to transport information on the movement and position of individual muscles.

Other Ascending Systems

The spinotectal tract is localized ventral to the anterior spinothalamic tract, from which it is not readily distinguishable. The fibers arise on the contralateral side, cross the midline, and ascend in the lateral funiculus. At the level of the mesencephalon, they leave the spinothalamic tract and terminate in the lemniscal layer of the superior colliculus. These fibers probably transport pain stimuli.

The spino-olivary tract arises from cells in laminae VII and VIII; the fibers cross the midline, ascend in the lateral funiculus, and synapse in the dorsal accessory olivary muscles. The fibers transport proprioceptive information that originates from muscle spindles and tendon corpuscles.

Chapter 26

The Long Descending Systems

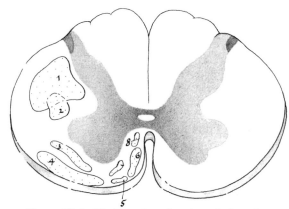

Figure 26–1 Horizontal section through the spinal cord with localization of the descending systems.

1 lateral corticospinal tract
2 rubrospinal tract
3 lateral reticulospinal tract
4 vestibulospinal tract
5 tectospinal tract
6 anterior corticospinal tract
7 medial reticulospinal tract
8 medial longitudinal fasciculus

Despite its relatively small weight, the spinal cord plays an important role as control center of most skeletal muscles and as a site of origin of part of the ANS. The spinal cord itself comprises the anatomic substrate of many mechanisms active in the regulation of muscular activity.

Recent studies, in fact, indicate that the spinal cord contributes far more to the production of complicated movements than has generally been thought. In higher mammals, however, the spinal cord loses some of its autonomy and more and more becomes subject to supraspinal influence. This influence is exerted via fiber systems that arise at higher levels of the CNS and synapse with the spinal neurons.

The Final Common Pathway

The activity of the CNS is ultimately expressed somatically in contractions of muscles (or secretion of glands), and these are a result of the activity of motoneurons in the spinal cord or of comparable cells in the nuclei of the cranial nerves. All impulses to the skeletal muscles, be they phasic or tonic, consciously or unconsciously initiated, originate from these cells.

Because the motoneurons with their axons extending to the periphery constitute the only route through which the nervous system controls the muscles, it is evident that the nervous system focuses on regulation of the firing frequency of the motoneurons.

From various areas of origin, fibers converge (sometimes directly, sometimes via inter-

neurons) on the spinal motoneurons, which are thus subject to diverse influences. The α-motoneuron is the final common pathway (Sherrington) on which all efferent impulses from the CNS converge. It should be borne in mind, however, that some of these impulses are inhibitory and that consequently the activity of the motoneuron is determined by the sum of all arriving impulses.

Corticospinal Tracts

The cortex can influence the spinal cord via two different fiber tracts: the pyramidal tract (corticospinal tract) and the corticosubcorticospinal system (COEPS). The two systems have some cortical areas of origin in common. The great difference, however, lies in the fact that the pyramidal tract establishes a *direct* connection between cortex and spinal cord, whereas the COEPS (formerly known as the extrapyramidal system) is interrupted by numerous synapses. The two systems, however, are inseparable both functionally and anatomically.

THE PYRAMIDAL TRACT

The pyramidal tract derives its name from a particular intumescence (pyramid) which these fibers cause in the ventral part of the medulla oblongata, on either side of the midline (see Fig. 14–1). At this site the pyramidal tract has a very superficial course and is grossly visible.

Phylogenetically it can be regarded as a young system, which attains its maximal development in primates. The hypothesis that this system has developed in connection with the complicated hand and finger movements of primates is probably wrong; in many marine mammals the pyramidal tract is well developed, although these animals lack fingers.

Fiber Pattern. The tract comprises about a million fibers: 3 per cent are thick (10 to 20 μm), 8 per cent are 4 to 10 μm, and 89 per cent are very thin (0.4 to 3 μm). Microscopic examination reveals that some 92 per cent of the fibers are myelinated.

Fiber Origin. The thick fibers are probably axons of the so-called "giant cells" of Betz, located in the inferior part of area 4 (see page 247). Most of the fibers, however, arise from areas 4 and 6 (frontal lobe) and areas 3, 1 and 2 (parietal lobe). Areas 40 and 43 (second somatosensory area) also make an important contribution to this fiber system. The axons of the pyramidal tract originate from cells located in lamina V of the cerebral cortex. There are slow and fast conducting fibers. The neurons that belong to the "fast" fibers are large and located in lamina V_b (see page 241); the neurons with thin axons are smaller and located in lamina V_a. The cells in lamina V_b mostly innervate distal extremity muscles and facial muscles, and show a phasic firing pattern. The cells in lamina V_a innervate postural muscles and show a tonic firing pattern, characterized by a virtually constant, low discharge frequency.

Fiber Course. The fibers descend from the cortex through the posterior limb of the internal capsule (Fig. 26–2) and the cerebral peduncle crus, in which they occupy the central two-thirds. Here, the pyramidal tract is accompanied by the corticopontine fibers (Fig. 26–3). The pyramidal fibers then extend through the pons, where the bundle is divided into numerous groups of fibers that cross the horizontally running pontocerebellar fibers. In the medulla, the pyramidal fibers unite again to form the pyramid. In the transition between medulla and spinal cord, some 80 per cent of the fibers cross the midline (pyramidal decussation). As a result, two tracts descend in the spinal cord: the (crossed) lateral corticospinal tract in the lateral funiculus, and the (uncrossed) anterior corticospinal tract in the anterior funiculus. It should be emphasized that the corticospinal fibers run through the posterior limb of the internal capsule together with many other fibers (COEPS, thalamocortical fibers, etc.). The frequently observed vascular disorders of the internal capsule, therefore, cause symptoms that are *not exclusively* attributable to interruption of the corticospinal fibers!

Termination of the Pyramidal Fibers. In experimental animals, silver staining techniques reveal that the corticospinal fibers do not terminate directly on the motoneurons but on interneurons in laminae IV to VII. A closer look at the components of the corticospinal system shows that the fibers from the parietal cortex ("sensory" corticospinal fibers) terminate in

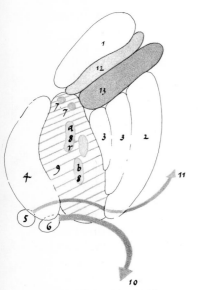

a	arm
r	trunk
b	leg
1	caudate nucleus
2	putamen
3	pallidum
4	thalamus
5	medial geniculate body
6	lateral geniculate body
7	corticobulbar tract
8	corticospinal tract
9	thalamocortical and striatothalamic fibers
10	optic radiation
11	acoustic radiation
12	corticopontine tract
13	thalamocortical fibers

Figure 26–2 Horizontal section through the internal capsule. The corticopontine and corticospinal fibers are colored gray.

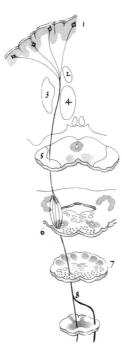

Figure 26–3 Schematic representation of the course of the pyramidal tract.

1 cerebral cortex
2 caudate nucleus
3 putamen
4 thalamus
5 crus cerebri (cerebral peduncle)
6 pons
7 medulla oblongata
8 pyramidal decussation

corticopontocerebellothalamocortical circuit, to mention only two.

The pyramidal tract is not confined to the regulation of the spinal neurons. This is evident especially in its connection with the sensory ascending systems. Recent research has demonstrated that axon collaterals of the pyramidal fibers play an important role in the transformation of the impulse code in the medial lemniscus, via presynaptic inhibition of the fibers of the posterior funiculus in the nucleus gracilis and nucleus cuneatus.

Morphologically, the pyramidal tract can hardly be regarded as a homogeneous fiber system. Too many facts speak against this: the differences in fiber origin, the varying fiber diameters, and the localization of their terminal synapses. It seems possible that, in future, the pyramidal tract will be divided into several anatomically and functionally different components.

lamina IV, while those from the frontal lobe ("motor" corticospinal fibers) terminate in the lateral part of lamina IV and the dorsal part of lamina VII, with a certain overlap in lamina V (Fig. 26–4). In humans, many corticospinal fibers seem to terminate directly on the long dendrites of the α-motoneurons. The pyramidal influence is exerted both on the α- and on the γ-neurons.

Functional Significance

The pyramidal tract is involved in particular in controlling the distal musculature of the extremities during the execution of precision movements. Since over 50 per cent of the fibers terminate at cervical levels, it is understandable that the pyramidal influence on the upper extremity exceeds that on the lower extremity.

As evident from the efferent connections of the neocerebellum and the striatum (see Chapters 28 and 36), the pyramidal tract not only serves to transmit cortical impulses to the spinal cord but also constitutes the principal route via which the activity of the cerebral control circuits is expressed. This means that the activity in the pyramidal tract is a result of the integration of the corticostriopallidothalamocortical circuit and the

Disorders of the Pyramidal Tract

Total interruption of the pyramidal fibers is rarely observed in clinical medicine; experimen-

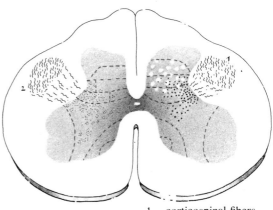

Figure 26–4 Topography of the terminal synapses of the corticospinal and the rubrospinal tract in the gray matter of the spinal cord (according to Brodal).

1 corticospinal fibers
2 rubrospinal fibers
termination of corticospinal fibers from "motor" cortex
termination of corticospinal fibers from "sensory" cortex
termination of rubrospinal fibers

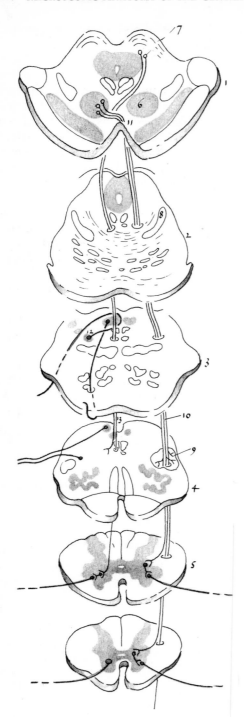

Figure 26–5 Schematic representation of the course of the rubrospinal and tectospinal fibers (according to Carpenter, modified).

1 mesencephalon
2,3 pons
4 medulla oblongata
5 spinal cord
6 red nucleus
7 superior colliculus
8 medial lemniscus
9 lateral reticular nucleus
10 rubrospinal tract
11 ventral tegmental decussation
12 nucleus of facial nerve
13 tectospinal tract

tally, the consequences of bilateral severance have been studied in monkeys. They showed only paresis of the distal musculature of the extremities, associated with a Babinski reflex and loss of skin reflexes. When interruption of the pyramidal tract is associated with dysfunction of the COEPS, other symptoms occur (for example, spasticity and hyperreflexia). These situations are not uncommon in clinical medicine.

THE CORTICOSUBCORTICOSPINAL SYSTEM (COEPS)

The fibers of this system arise from the motor cortex (areas 4 and 6) and from the somatosensory cortex (see page 248). Pyramidal tract and COEPS run a joint course as far as the superior part of the metencephalon, where the COEPS leaves the pyramidal tract and takes its course through the tegmentum.

Three components are distinguished in the COEPS:

Corticorubrospinal Tract. The corticorubrospinal tract is best known in experimental animals. Recent studies have shown that, in humans, the rubrospinal fibers are more numerous than has been generally accepted. The fibers of this system arise from the "motor" cortex. Without decussation, the fibers reach the red nucleus via the internal capsule (distinct somatotopic arrangement). From the red nucleus many fibers arise which cross the midline and descend through the tegmentum to the spinal cord (see page 215 and Figs. 26–1, 26–4, and 26–5), where they extend in the heterolateral lateral funiculus as far as lumbosacral levels. The terminations are found in the lateral part of laminae V, VI, and VII, and here too there are no direct connections with the motor cells of the anterior horn. The red nucleus is an important link in the transmission of cerebellar impulses (from the nucleus interpositus) to the spinal cord. Since the pyramidal tract and the corticorubrospinal tract have the same origin in the cortex, it is understandable that the two tracts are complementary in the intact nervous system. Excitation of the red nucleus facilitates contralateral spinal neurons (α- and γ-neurons) that innervate flexors and inhibit extensor neurons. The red nucleus is probably involved in the regulation of the tone of flexor muscles.

Lateral Corticoreticulospinal Tract. The (indirect) connections between cortex and spinal cord with their wayside station in the reticular formation are ensured by two separate bundles: the lateral and the anterior corticoreticulospinal tracts. Cortical fibers for the reticular formation mainly originate from the "sensorimotor" cortex (see page 248). They extend through the internal capsule along with the corticospinal fibers and reach the brain stem. At several levels in the brain stem fiber bundles leave the corticospinal tract on their way to nuclei of the reticular formation. Some of these fibers synapse on medial reticular nuclei; others synapse on lateral nuclei. The *lateral reticulospinal tract* largely arises in the gigantocellular reticular nucleus, an accumulation of large cells in the medulla. The fibers of this system have varying diameters and extend in part through the ipsilateral and in part through the contralateral lateral funiculus (Fig. 25–4).

Anterior Reticulospinal Tract. The anterior reticulospinal tract arises mainly in the caudal pontine reticular nucleus, whence the fibers descend in the ipsilateral anterior funiculus (Fig. 25–4). The anterior reticulospinal tract terminates mainly in lamina VIII and adjacent parts of lamina VII; the fibers of the lateral reticulospinal tract synapse mainly in lamina VII. Both systems terminate both on α-neurons and on γ-neurons.

The anterior or pontine-originating reticulo-fibers facilitate volitional activity, while the med-ullary or lateral reticulospinal fibers are inhibitory. Pontine reticulospinal fibers facilitate the antigravity muscles of the body, and medullary reticulospinal fibers inhibit these muscles. Transmission in the spinal reflex circuits and in the sensory systems can be influenced by the reticular fibers, which are involved also in controlling muscle tone.

Vestibulospinal Tracts

The vestibular nuclei and the spinal cord are connected by the lateral and the medial vestibulospinal tracts (Fig. 26–6). The lateral vestibular nucleus can be regarded as a relay station for impulses from the cerebellum; here, the fibers of the lateral vestibulospinal tract arise. They take their course through the medulla medially and dorsally in relation to the nucleus ambiguus (Fig. 26–6), and reach their final position in the ipsilateral anterior funiculus. The fiber terminations are found in laminae VIII and VII. The lateral vestibulospinal fibers run through the entire spinal cord.

The anterior vestibulospinal tract arises from the vestibular nucleus of the same designation. The fibers run through the medial longitudinal fasciculus. They are localized in the anterior funiculus close to the anterior median fissure and terminate in lamina VII. They do not extend beyond T1–T2.

The vestibulospinal tracts conduct stimuli from the vestibular apparatus and from certain parts of the cerebellum to the spinal cord. Impulses through the lateral vestibulospinal tract facilitate extensor reflexes in the lower extremity and flexors in the upper extremity and increase the tone of the extensors in the lower extremity and that of flexors in the upper extremity. The increased extensor tone obtained after severance of the mesencephalon (decerebration stiffness) disappears immediately after selective destruction of the lateral vestibular nucleus.

Tectospinal Tract

This bundle arises in the superior colliculus of the mesencephalon. The fibers cross the mid-

Figure 26–6 The vestibulospinal tract and the medial longitudinal fasciculus (according to Carpenter).

1 vestibular nerve
2 medial vestibular nucleus
3 superior vestibular nucleus
4 lateral vestibular nucleus
5 nucleus of the spinal tract of the trigeminal nerve
6 lateral vestibulospinal tract
7 medial vestibulospinal tract

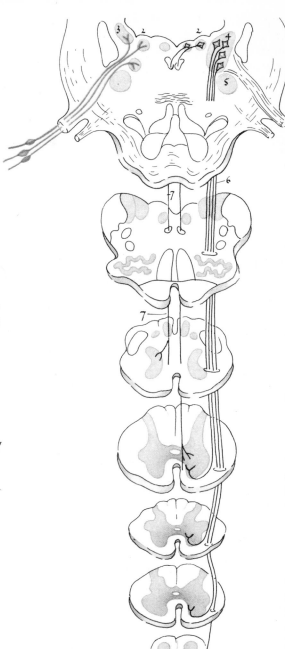

line in the so-called dorsal tegmental decussation and then extend on either side of the midline, ventral to the medial longitudinal fasciculus.

In the spinal cord, the bundle remains in a parasagittal position beside the ventral median fissure (Fig. 26–5). The bundle descends to the approximate level of C6 or C7, the fibers synapsing with interneurons in laminae VII and VIII. It is assumed that the tectospinal tract regulates the influence of optical reflexes on the muscles of the neck.

The Monoaminergic Descending System

Noradrenergic connections between the brain stem and spinal cord have been detected by the fluorescence technique. The cells of origin are localized in the caudal part of the medulla, lateral to the hypoglossal nucleus. These fibers run through the anterior funiculus and innervate the anterior horn. Other (serotonergic) fibers arise from the nucleus raphe pallidus in the ventral part of the medulla oblongata. The fibers descend in the anterior funiculus and synapse in the anterior horn.

Organization of the Supraspinal Systems

The topography of the terminations of the descending fibers in the spinal cord shows that supraspinal influences on motor cells of the anterior horn are exerted via interneurons and via presynaptic inhibition of the dorsal root fibers. In humans, some of the large α-motoneurons are believed to be under direct cortical influence via direct corticospinal fibers.

The interneurons that activate flexors and inhibit extensors are localized *laterally* in laminae V, VI, and VII; neurons that produce the opposite effect are found for the most part *medially* in laminae VII and VIII.

Viewing the position of the large descending systems in relation to their terminations, we observe that the tracts in the lateral funiculus (lateral corticospinal, rubrospinal, and lateral reticulospinal tracts) terminate mostly in laminae V and VI and the dorsal part of lamina VII, largely laterally.

Chapter 27

The Cranial Nerves

General Characteristics

Spinal cord nerves and cranial nerves are homologues; the cranial nerves, too, consist of efferent motor fibers arising from certain nuclei of origin in the brain stem, and afferent sensory fibers from cells of origin in the corresponding peripheral ganglia. Unlike the spinal cord nerves, however, the cranial nerves have no separate dorsal root. The ganglia of the cranial nerves are located close to the cranial aperture through which the nerve leaves the cranial cavity; the central extensions of the sensory ganglion cells accompany the motor fibers and, along with them, enter the brain stem.

Some cranial nerves — the hypoglossal nerve and the group of eye muscle nerves — show marked reduction of their sensory component and therefore appear to be purely somatomotor nerves. In some instances the hypoglossal nerve has a small ganglion (Froriep's ganglion) in which the sensory neurons that ensure the afferent innervation from the tongue muscles are located. In other instances sensory cells are found scattered along the hypoglossal nerve, and these assume the role of Froriep's ganglion.

The eye muscles are likewise provided with an abundance of muscle spindles; the afferent cells that innervate these muscle spindles are located *within the CNS* (nucleus of the mesencephalic tract of the trigeminal nerve). A new situation arises here: an accumulation of primary sensory unipolar cells that has remained within the CNS. The three eye muscle nerves receive fibers from the ophthalmic nerve to ensure the proprioceptive innervation of the eye muscles.

Of the twelve cranial nerves traditionally distinguished, three should be eliminated: the olfactory, the optic, and the spinal accessory nerves. The first is a plexus of thin fibers that ultimately unite in about 20 small bundles (fila olfactoria); the second is nothing but a central fiber system like the medial lemniscus, etc.; the spinal accessory nerve is, in fact, a complex of the three upper spinal cord nerves, which are included within the skull.

The complicated development of the head and the presence of sense organs (taste, hearing, equilibrium) determine the complicated composition of the cranial nerves. The corresponding nuclei in the medulla, pons, and mesencephalon are arranged in columns (Fig. 5–3). As the lateral walls of the rhombencephalon unfold, the sensory nuclei are no longer found dorsally, as in the spinal cord, but laterally; the motor nuclei are no longer found ventrally but medially (Fig. 5–4). Compared with the spinal cord nerves, the cranial nerves have nuclei without equivalents in the spinal cord: They are the special somatic afferent (SSA, sensory) nuclei, the special visceral afferent (SVA, taste) nuclei, and the special visceral efferent (SVE, branchiomotor) nuclei.

The cranial nerves can be divided into three groups: somatomotor nerves (oculomotor, trochlear, abducens, and hypoglossal), branchial nerves (trigeminal, facial, glossopharyngeal, vagus, and accessory) and a special somatic afferent nerve (vestibulocochlear).

This section discusses the 3rd through 12th cranial nerves.

Somatomotor Nerves

The nuclei of these nerves are located quite near the midline. In view of the lack of sensory components, they can be compared with the ventral root of a spinal nerve.

HYPOGLOSSAL (12th CRANIAL) NERVE

The hypoglossal nerve is a purely somatomotor nerve that innervates three myotomes which, although located in the tongue, are occipital in origin. The nucleus lies beneath the hypoglossal trigone and extends from the level of the striae medullares to the boundary between medulla oblongata and spinal cord. The neurons of the nucleus are arranged in a few groups, each of which innervates a separate tongue muscle. The axons extend in ventrolateral direction, cross the reticular formation and the inferior olivary nucleus and appear at the surface of the medulla oblongata via the ventrolateral sulcus, between olive and pyramid (see Fig. 30–2). The nerve roots (about 10 to 14) then unite in a trunk that leaves the cranial cavity via the hypoglossal canal.

Afferent Fibers. In the nucleus of the hypoglossal nerve, fibers from the cortex synapse (corticobulbar fibers). It is via these fibers that voluntary movements of the tongue can be executed. Other fibers come from the reticular formation, the trigeminal nuclei, and the solitary nucleus. It is via these fibers that reflex movements like sucking and swallowing are executed.

Peripheral Innervation. The hypoglossal nerve innervates the intrinsic muscles of the tongue as well as the genioglossus, hyoglossus, and styloglossus muscles.

Dysfunction of the Hypoglossal Nerve. A unilateral lesion of the hypoglossal nerve causes paralysis of the ipsilateral half of the tongue (when protruded, the tongue deviates to the affected side). In addition, unmistakable atrophy of the tongue muscles occurs, sometimes with fibrillations.

ABDUCENS (6th CRANIAL) NERVE

The abducens nerve is one of the three nerves that innervate the extrinsic eye muscles. The nucleus of origin of this nerve is located in the floor of the fourth ventricle (Fig. 27–2), surrounded medially and dorsally by a loop of facial nerve fibers (the internal genu of the facial nerve). The fibers of the abducens nerve leave the brain stem on either side of the cecal foramen and then extend cranially. The nerve enters the orbit via the superior orbital fissure, where it innervates the lateral rectus muscle.

Afferent Fibers. Afferent fibers that originate from the vestibular nuclei and take their course via the medial longitudinal fasciculus synapse in the nucleus of the abducens nerve. Cortical fibers reach the nucleus mainly via the contralateral side (corticobulbar fibers).

Dysfunction of the Nerve. Dysfunction of the nerve causes paralysis of the lateral rectus muscle and prevents lateral movements of the eyeball.

TROCHLEAR (4th CRANIAL) NERVE

The nucleus of the trochlear nerve is located in the caudal part of the mesencephalon at the level of the inferior colliculus. The exiting fibers leave the brain stem dorsal to the aqueduct and on the contralateral side. They extend laterally and cranially, pass through the sinus cavernosus, and reach the orbit via the superior orbital fissure. The trochlear nerve innervates the superior oblique muscle.

Afferent Fibers. Afferent fibers to the nucleus of the trochlear nerve originate from the cortex (corticobulbar fibers) and from the medial longitudinal fasciculus (from the vestibular nuclei).

Dysfunction of the Nerve. Lesions confined to the trochlear nerve are rare. The superior oblique muscle controls lateroinferior eye movements, and dysfunction of the nerve causes diplopia when looking down: The patient has difficulties when going down a flight of stairs.

OCULOMOTOR (3rd CRANIAL) NERVE

The nucleus of the oculomotor nerve is located at the level of the superior colliculus, ventral to the gray matter (see Fig. 30–7). The nucleus has a somatomotor (GSE) part and a parasympathetic (GVE) part. The former part innervates the superior palpebral levator muscle, the superior, inferior, and medial rectus muscles and the inferior oblique muscle on the ipsilateral side.

In the mesencephalon, the axons of the oculomotor nerve pass through the red nucleus and exit on the medial side of the cerebral peduncle. They continue between the superior cerebellar and the posterior cerebral artery, past the posterior communicating artery to the poste-

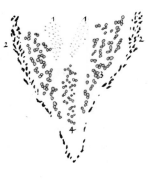

Figure 27–1 Schematic representation of the principal cell groups of the nuclei of origin of the oculomotor nerve (according to Ranson).

1 Edinger-Westphal nucleus
2 medial longitudinal fasciculus
3 lateral nucleus of the oculomotor nerve
4 medial nucleus (of Perlia)

rior clinoid process, where they enter the sinus cavernosus (see Fig. 17–2), in which the nerve divides into a superior and an inferior branch, which reach the orbit via the orbital fissure.

In the somatomotor part of the nucleus, cell groups that innervate the separate eye muscles can be distinguished. Proprioceptive fibers that innervate the extrinsic eye muscles originate from the pseudounipolar cells of the nucleus of the mesencephalic tract of the trigeminal nerve.

The parasympathetic part of the nucleus consist of smaller, multipolar cells from which preganglionic fibers arise that synapse in the ciliary ganglion. The parasympathetic cells are found in the Edinger-Westphal nucleus rostral and dorsal to the somatomotor part; in caudal direction, this parasympathetic nucleus divides into two oblong parts (Fig. 27–1). The parasympathetic fibers innervate the intrinsic eye muscles (pupillary sphincter muscle and ciliary muscle).

Ciliary Ganglion. This ganglion is located lateral to the ophthalmic artery, between the optic nerve and the lateral rectus muscle. The preganglionic fibers arise from the Edinger-Westphal nucleus and accompany the oculomotor branch for the inferior oblique muscle; beyond the synapse, postganglionic fibers innervate the ciliary muscle and the pupillary sphincter muscle via the short ciliary nerves. Impulses via these nerves cause the pupil to contract and the convexity of the lens to increase (accommodation).

Besides the parasympathetic innervation of the intrinsic eye muscles there is a sympathetic innervation that takes place from the ciliospinal center (Budge). At the level of the cervical

intumescence (C7–T1), sympathetic cells produce preganglionic fibers which, via the sympathetic trunk, reach the superior cervical ganglion where they synapse. Postganglionic sympathetic fibers extend via the carotid plexus through the ciliary ganglion (without synapsing in it) to the eyeball via the short ciliary nerves. These nerves have fibers of several kinds (Fig. 27–3): postganglionic parasympathetic fibers (after synapsing in the ciliary ganglion); postganglionic sympathetic fibers (vasomotor fibers) from the superior cervical ganglion, which pass through the ciliary ganglion but do not synapse in it; and sensory fibers from the cornea, iris, and choroid membrane, which pass through the ganglion and then join the nasociliary nerve.

The long ciliary nerves are branches of the nasociliary nerve; they join the short ciliary nerves and, with them, perforate the sclera around the optic nerve.

Secondary Oculomotor Nuclei. This term applies to three nuclei localized in the immediate vicinity of the oculomotor nucleus: Cajal's interstitial nucleus, the nucleus of Darkschevich, and the nucleus of the posterior commissure. Other, more distant nuclei are the pontine oculomotor center and the hypoglossal nucleus prepositus. The interstitial nucleus is localized beside the medial longitudinal fasciculus (see Fig. 30–7) and consists of large multipolar cells. Fibers arising from this nucleus cross the midline in the posterior commissure and synapse with cells of the oculomotor, the trochlear, and the medial vestibular nuclei. Damage to these fibers causes vertical ophthalmoplegia. The nucleus of Darkschevich consists of small cells within the gray matter. Their axons cross the midline in the posterior commissure. The nucleus of the posterior commissure consists of scattered cells between the fibers of the commissure. The final destination of the axons from this nucleus is obscure.

The so-called pontine oculomotor center is of great importance in controlling horizontal eye movements. This center is localized in the pontine reticular formation; it projects to the abducens nucleus and the hypoglossal nucleus prepositus, thus controlling horizontal eye movements. The nucleus prepositus projects to all eye muscle nuclei, both ipsilateral and contralateral. Fibers from Cajal's nucleus and from the

Figure 27–2 The course of the fibers of the facial nerve and the abducens nerve (according to Crosby, Humphrey, and Lauer).

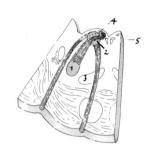

1 nucleus of the facial nerve
2 nucleus of the abducens nerve
3 medial lemniscus
4 internal genu of the facial nerve
5 medial longitudinal fasciculus

vestibular nuclei synapse on this nucleus, which functionally seems to be involved in the production of rapid horizontal and vertical eye movements.

Afferent Fibers.   Homolateral and heterolateral fibers from the cerebral cortex extend via the reticular formation to synapses on the nucleus of the oculomotor nerve. Other fibers come from the vestibular nuclei via the medial longitudinal fasciculus; fibers from the superior colliculus and the reticular formation likewise synapse on this nucleus.

Dysfunction of the Nerve.   Dysfunction of the oculomotor nerve causes ptosis of the upper eyelid. The eye is in abduction (by the lateral rectus muscle) and turned down (by the superior oblique muscle). Dysfunction of the parasympathetic part of the nerve causes mydriasis and loss of the pupillary light reflex. Accommodation is impossible.

Functional Aspects of Eye Movements

Eye movements are very complicated. Sharp vision demands that the light rays emitted by the object fall on the fovea centralis of the retina. This is ensured by exact coordination of the movements of both eyes. When the eyes simultaneously move in the same direction so that the angle between the visual axes remains unchanged, the movement is called conjugate movement. Movement in the horizontal plane follows simultaneous contraction of the lateral rectus muscle of one eye and the medial rectus muscle of the other. Movement in the vertical plane is much more complicated. Binocular vision of an object at a short distance demands that the two visual axes are aimed at the same point, enabling the images on the right and the left retina to be centrally fused into a single image. The eyes converge to make the two visual axes meet in the fixation point. Eye movements are seldom executed without corresponding movements of the head. This means that the activity of the neck muscles and the labyrinthine reactions are essential to eye movements. Coordination of these movements is effected mainly via the medial longitudinal fasciculus.

The *optic reflexes* can be divided into cortical and subcortical reflexes: the reflex arc of the former extends via the cortex, whereas that of the latter does not. We confine ourselves to a discussion of a few reflexes that are of fundamental clinical importance: the light reflex and the accommodation reflex.

Light Reflex.   The pupil reacts to incident light by contraction. When one pupil is illuminated, the contralateral pupil reacts as well (consensual light reflex). In some afflictions of the CNS (syphilis, tabes dorsalis), the so-called Argyll Robertson pupil is found (a non-light-reactive pupil that shows an intensified reaction to convergence). The light reflex takes the following course:

retina → optic nerve → lateral geniculate body → brachium of superior colliculus → pretectal region (synapse?) → posterior commissure → medial longitudinal fasciculus → Edinger-Westphal nucleus → ciliary ganglion → short ciliary nerves → pupillary sphincter muscle.

The light reflex thus described should be regarded as a subcortical reflex; it has been experimentally demonstrated, however, that stimulation of area 19 also causes the pupil to contract. The fibers from area 19 synapse in the pretectum and in the superior colliculus.

Accommodation Reflex.   Objects within six meters of the eye cannot be sharply depicted on the retina unless the curvature of the lens is changed. In near vision, the visual axes must converge to meet in the plane of the object perceived. Accommodation and convergence normally are associated. The reflex arc for accommodation extends via the occipital cortex.

Fibers probably extend from the calcarine area (areas 17, 18, 19) to the pretectal region and then to the nucleus of the oculomotor nerve. The parasympathetic fibers for the ciliary muscle accompany the oculomotor nerve and synapse in the ciliary ganglion.

Branchial Nerves

The branchial nerves are the trigeminal (5th cranial), facial (7th cranial), glossopharyngeal (9th cranial), vagus (10th cranial), and accessory (11th cranial) nerves, which ensure both the sensory and the motor innervation of that which has developed from the original branchial arches. Each branchial nerve shows a characteristic ramification. The nerve first divides into a dorsal and a ventral branch. The former disappears in higher mammals. The latter divides in relation to the branchial cleft into a pretrematic branch, a posttrematic branch, and a dorsal pharyngeal branch (Fig. 27–4).

The *pretrematic branch* extends past the anterior side of the branchial cleft and thus enters the area of the preceding nerve, which it joins. The pretrematic branch comprises only sensory fibers.

The *posttrematic branch* is the largest branch of the branchial nerve and comprises motor and sensory fibers. It innervates the skin, the muscles, and the mucosa of the corresponding branchial arch.

The *small dorsal pharyngeal branch* innervates the dorsal wall of the primitive pharynx. In humans this branch is markedly reduced.

TRIGEMINAL (5th CRANIAL) NERVE

The trigeminal nerve is the nerve of the first branchial arch; functionally it comprises branchiomotor and branchiosensory components. The motor part (SVE) innervates the masseter, tensor tympani, tensor veli palatini, and mylo-hyoid muscles and the anterior belly of the digastric muscle. The perikaryons of these cells (masticatory nucleus) are localized in the dorsolateral part of the pons (see Fig. 30–5). The sensory part of the nerve (portio major) is much larger (about 140,000 fibers) than the motor part (about 9000 fibers) and connects the lateral surface of the pons with the trigeminal (semilunar)

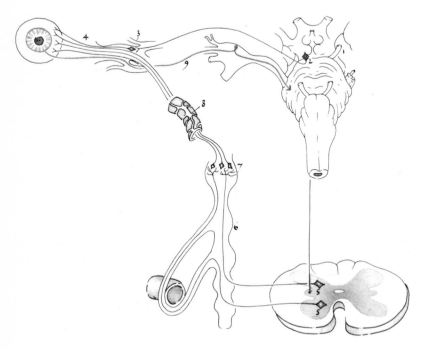

Figure 27–3 Innervation of the intrinsic eye muscles. The parasympathetic fibers from the Edinger-Westphal nucleus synapse in the ciliary ganglion; the sympathetic fibers from the ciliospinal center synapse in the superior cervical ganglion. The perikaryons of the sensory fibers that innervate cornea, iris, and choroid membrane are located in the trigeminal ganglion.

1 oculomotor nerve
2 Edinger-Westphal nucleus
3 ciliary ganglion
4 short ciliary nerves
5 ciliospinal center
6 sympathetic trunk
7 superior cervical ganglion
8 carotid plexus
9 nasociliary nerve

Figure 27–4 Fiber arrangement of the branchial nerves: pretrematic, posttrematic, dorsal, and pharyngeal branches (according to Clara).

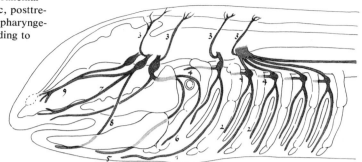

1 posttrematic branch
2 pretrematic branch
3 dorsal branches
4 pharyngeal branches
5 pretrematic branch of facial nerve
6 posttrematic branch of facial nerve
7 maxillary nerve
8 mandibular nerve
9 ophthalmic nerve

ganglion, which lies against the apex of the petrosal bone pyramid. In a dura-lined skull this ganglion is not visible because it is concealed in a dural duplicature.

In the trigeminal root we distinguish a proximal (compact) part and a distal (plexiform) part, which is located near the ganglion. The motor part (portio minor) crosses the underside of the ganglion and joins the mandibular nerve.

The peripheral (GSA) fibers of the nerve arise from the unipolar neurons of the ganglion. There are three principal branches:

(a) *ophthalmic nerve* (pretrematic branch): sensory innervation of the forehead, eyes and nose;

(b) *maxillary nerve* (pretrematic branch): innervates the maxilla (and upper teeth), the mucosa of the upper lip, cheeks and palate, and the maxillary sinus;

(c) *mandibular nerve* (posttrematic branch): innervation of the tongue, mandible (and lower teeth), lower lip, part of the cheek, and part of the external ear; this is a mixed nerve. The motor fibers for the masseter muscles, etc. also extend here.

There is little overlap between the territories of the three principal branches. In addition the trigeminal nerve innervates the receptors in the masseter muscles, the mandibular joint, and the receptors in the ocular muscles.

Trigeminal Ganglion

The sensory neurons of the ganglion are arranged in accordance with the areas they inner-

vate. The cell bodies of the ophthalmic nerve are arranged medially, and those of the mandibular nerve are grouped laterally, the neurons of the maxillary nerve being localized between the two other cell groups. The three principal branches diverge from the periphery of the ganglion and leave the skull immediately: the ophthalmic nerve through the orbital fissure, the maxillary nerve through the foramen rotundum, and the mandibular nerve through the foramen ovale (see Fig. 17–2).

Mesencephalic Nucleus

The proprioceptive impulses from the muscle spindles and teeth are transmitted through fibers from the cells of the so-called mesencephalic nucleus. This nucleus is characteristic inasmuch as the shape of its cells closely resembles that of spinal ganglion cells. The mesencephalic nucleus can be regarded as a sensory ganglion that has remained in the CNS. The axons of some of the cells of the mesencephalic nucleus synapse in the masticatory nucleus. Other axons extend to the superior colliculus and the cerebellum, where they synapse.

Trigeminal Nuclei

Sensory Nuclei. The primary trigeminal nerve fibers synapse in an extensive nuclear complex that covers the area between the pons and the transition from medulla to spinal cord. The sensory fibers of the portio major divide into an ascending and a descending branch. The thick

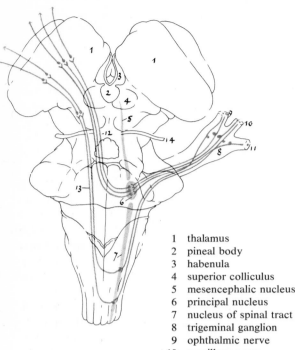

1	thalamus
2	pineal body
3	habenula
4	superior colliculus
5	mesencephalic nucleus
6	principal nucleus
7	nucleus of spinal tract
8	trigeminal ganglion
9	ophthalmic nerve
10	maxillary nerve
11	mandibular nerve
12	dorsal trigeminal lemniscus
13	trigeminal lemniscus
14	trochlear nerve

Figure 27–5 Schematic representation of the trigeminothalamic connections (according to Clara, slightly simplified).

spinal nucleus. This bundle is known as the spinal tract of the trigeminal nerve. The spinal tract shows a distinct somatotopic arrangement: The ophthalmic nerve fibers are most ventrally localized, the mandibular nerve fibers are localized dorsally, and the maxillary nerve fibers in between. The fibers of the spinal tract synapse with cells of the spinal tract nucleus and transmit pain, temperature, and pressure stimuli from the facial region. The pain stimuli probably travel to the caudal nucleus, and temperature stimuli to the interpolar nucleus.

Motor Nucleus (Masticatory Nucleus). This is the most cranially located branchiomotor nucleus. It lies in the pons, medial to the principal nucleus, and contains large multipolar cells (see Fig. 30–5).

Afferent Fibers to the Trigeminal Nuclei

Apart from the direct trigeminal nerve fibers, fibers from the 9th and 10th cranial nerves and posterior funiculus fibers from the first four cervical spinal cord nerves synapse in the trigeminal nuclear complex. The cerebral cortex, especially the primary somatosensory area, projects onto the entire nuclear complex. The masticatory nucleus also receives afferents from the cortex via the corticobulbar fibers. Afferent fibers from other cranial nerves reach this nucleus via the reticular formation.

Efferent Fibers

Efferent fibers from the trigeminal complex synapse in the thalamus, the cerebellum, and the reticular formation. Efferent fibers from the spinal tract nucleus cross the midline and join the medial lemniscus, together with which they reach the thalamus.

The principal nucleus gives rise to crossed as well as uncrossed ascending fibers (dorsal trigeminal lemniscus). The former join the contralateral medial lemniscus; the latter extend alongside the central gray matter in the mesencephalon (Fig. 27–5). All trigeminothalamic fibers except those from the caudal nucleus synapse in the ventral posteromedial (PVM) nucleus of the thalamus. Fibers from the caudal nucleus

fibers are usually shorter than the thin fibers and synapse with the most cranial parts of the nucleus; other (thinner) fibers sometimes descend to the spinal cord and enter Lissauer's marginal zone. The sensory trigeminal complex comprises two nuclei:

PRINCIPAL NUCLEUS. This is an oval accumulation of cells, localized lateral to the incoming fibers. In this accumulation, the ascending branches of the dividing fibers synapse, as do the thick afferent fibers. The nucleus receives mainly touch and pressure stimuli from the face.

SPINAL TRACT NUCLEUS. This nucleus (Fig. 27–5) is located caudal to the principal nucleus and extends to the spinal cord, where it continues in the substantia gelatinosa. The spinal nuclear complex is divided into three components: the oral, the interpolar, and the caudal nuclei. The descending trigeminal nerve fibers constitute a long bundle that runs parallel to the terminate in the intralaminar thalamic nuclei and the medial geniculate body.

Efferent fibers from the mesencephalic nucleus pass through the superior cerebellar peduncle and synapse in the dentate and the emboliform nucleus. They transmit proprioceptive impulses from the masseter muscles and teeth to the cerebellum. Fibers extend from the spinal tract nucleus to the cerebellum via the inferior cerebellar peduncle and terminate in the vermis and the declive.

Efferent fibers to the reticular formation are collaterals of the secondary trigeminothalamic fibers; they synapse in the lateral part of the reticular formation and in the gigantocellular reticular nucleus.

Functional Aspects

Lesions of the spinal tract (or nucleus) are manifested by reduction or loss of the pain and temperature sense in the face; tactile and pressure sensibilities, however, remain intact. Pain and temperature stimuli are processed by the spinal tract nucleus, whereas tactile and pressure stimuli go to the principal nucleus.

Of the many reflexes in which the trigeminal nerve is involved, the corneal reflex merits special attention. Irritation of the cornea causes contraction of the orbicularis oculi muscle and closure of the eyes. This effect is based on impulses that bilaterally reach the nucleus of the facial nerve; it is therefore evident that efferent secondary fibers of the trigeminal nuclei synapse in the facial nerve nucleus. Lesions of the ophthalmic nerve cause ipsilateral loss of tactile and pain sensibility in the cornea; irritation of the contralateral cornea causes both eyes to close, proving that the efferent part of the reflex arc is intact. In the case of a lesion of the facial nerve, however, corneal sensibility remains intact although the corneal reflex is disturbed.

Facial (7th Cranial) Nerve. The facial nerve is a mixed nerve that innervates the second branchial arch. Grossly, one can distinguish a main component, which consists of SVE fibers (facial nerve in the strict sense), and a smaller component, which consists of parasympathetic and sensory fibers (intermediate nerve).

Main Nucleus of the Facial Nerve. The main (motor) nucleus of the facial nerve is an accumulation of cells (about 4 mm long) that is the cranial continuation of the nucleus ambiguus (see Fig. 5–3). The ambiguus, the facial, and the masticatory nuclei are the links of a chain of nuclei for the innervation of muscles of branchial origin.

The nucleus of the facial nerve is located in the pons, lateral to the reticular formation and immediately dorsal to the superior olive (Fig. 27–2). The nucleus comprises a few cell groups that innervate the various facial muscles. These are the muscles of facial expression: orbicularis oculi, zygomatic, buccinator, orbicularis oris, and labial muscles. The nucleus also innervates the platysma, the stylohyoid, and the stapedius muscles, and the posterior venter of the digastric muscle.

The course of the facial nerve fibers is highly characteristic. The fibers first extend to the floor of the ventricle, curve around the abducens nucleus (internal genu), and emerge from the brain stem quite near the inferior margin of the pons (Fig. 27–2). The facial nerve and the intermediate nerve then enter the internal auditory meatus and extend through the facial canal of the petrosal bone. Finally, the nerve leaves the skull through the stylomastoid foramen. Part of its course through the facial canal is quite near the tympanic cavity, and consequently the nerve can be involved in pathologic processes in the middle ear.

Afferent Fibers. The motor nucleus of the facial nerve receives afferents from the spinal tract nucleus, the superior colliculus, the reticular formation, and the cerebral cortex. There are direct corticobulbar fibers that synapse in the so-called intermediate part (upper part of the nucleus), and indirect cortical fibers that conduct impulses to the facial nerve nucleus via the reticular formation. The intermediate part innervates the orbicularis oculi, the frontal, and the corrugator muscles.

Lesions of the Facial Nerve. Lesions confined to facial nerve fibers (peripheral paralysis, Bell's palsy) cause ipsilateral paralysis and atrophy of the muscles of facial expression. The patient is unable to close the eyes, whistle (pursed lips), or frown. The corneal reflex is lost, but corneal sensibility remains intact. Central lesions of the corticobulbar fibers that synapse in the facial nerve nucleus cause contralateral paralysis of the labial and buccal muscles; closing the eyes or frowning, however, are hardly affected because the cell groups that innervate these muscles (intermediate part) are innervated bilaterally.

INTERMEDIATE NERVE

The intermediate nerve is the parasympathetic sensory root of the facial nerve. Grossly it is located between the facial and the vestibular nerve (Fig. 27–6). The sensory ganglion of this nerve (geniculate ganglion) is located in the first curvature (external genu) of the facial canal. The intermediate nerve is composed of efferent (GVE) and afferent (GSA and SVA) components.

Efferent Fibers. The efferent fibers originate from the superior salivatory nucleus, a diffuse cellular area dorsolaterally localized in the reticular formation. The fibers innervate the submandibular, sublingual and lacrimal glands. Some of these (parasympathetic) fibers extend in the chorda tympani, while others extend in the greater petrosal nerve:

intermediate nerve → chorda tympani → lingual nerve → submandibular ganglion (synapse) → submandibular and sublingual gland;

intermediate nerve → greater petrosal nerve → pterygopalatine ganglion (synapse) → lacrimal nerve → lacrimal gland.

The postganglionic fibers of the submandibular and the pterygopalatine ganglion are vasomotor and secretory fibers that ensure increased secretion of these glands.

Afferent Fibers. These fibers have their perikaryons in the geniculate ganglion. Two groups are distinguished:

(a) general afferent (FSA) fibers, which in-

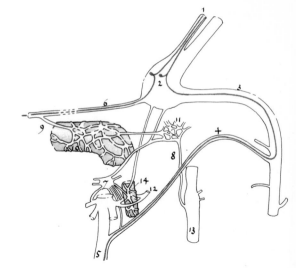

Figure 27–6 Ramification of the intermediate nerve in the petrosal bone (according to Gray).

1 intermediate nerve
2 geniculate ganglion
3 facial nerve
4 chorda tympani
5 lingual nerve
6 greater petrosal nerve
7 otic ganglion
8 caroticotympanic nerve
9 deep petrosal nerve
10 internal carotid artery
11 tympanic plexus
12 auriculotemporal nerve
13 glossopharyngeal nerve
14 middle meningeal artery

nervate part of the external auditory meatus and a small area behind the external ear;

(b) special visceral afferent (SVA) fibers, which originate from the taste buds on the anterior two-thirds of the tongue and first join the lingual nerve and then the chorda tympani (pretrematic branch) and the facial nerve. The central process of the geniculate ganglion extends with the intermediate nerve to the solitary tract of the medulla oblongata. The first synapse of these (gustatory) fibers is in the nucleus of the solitary tract.

Dysfunction of the Nerve. Lesions of the intermediate nerve cause ipsilateral loss of gustatory function in the anterior two-thirds of the tongue and reduced salivation.

Figure 27–7 Arrangement of the nuclei of the glossopharyngeal nerve.

1 glossopharyngeal nerve
2 superior ganglion
3 inferior ganglion
4 nucleus ambiguus
5 nucleus solitarius
6 hypoglossal nucleus
7 nucleus of the spinal tract of V
8 inferior salivatory nucleus
9 inferior cerebellar peduncle
10 otic ganglion
11 parotid gland
12 carotid nerve

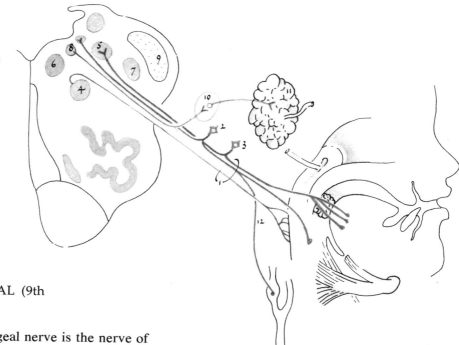

GLOSSOPHARYNGEAL (9th CRANIAL) NERVE

The glossopharyngeal nerve is the nerve of the third branchial arch; anatomically and functionally it is very closely related to the vagus nerve. Both nerves leave the brain stem behind the inferior olive and emerge from the skull through (separate parts of) the jugular foramen. The glossopharyngeal nerve innervates part of the pharynx, the tympanic cavity, and the auditory tube and has gustatory fibers from the posterior one-third of the tongue. The perikaryons of the sensory neurons are located in two ganglia (superior and inferior ganglia) at the level of the jugular foramen or slightly below it. The inferior ganglion of the glossopharyngeal nerve is only partly comparable to a spinal ganglion because it contains motor (parasympathetic) neurons as well.

Afferent Fibers. Functionally, the following fibers are distinguished: (a) general somatic afferent (GSA) fibers (superior ganglion): nucleus of the spinal tract of the trigeminal nerve; (b) general visceral afferent (GVA) fibers (inferior ganglion); and (c) special visceral afferent (SVA) fibers (gustatory fibers, inferior ganglion): nucleus of the solitary tract.

The GSA fibers innervate a small retroauricular skin area; their perikaryons are located in the superior ganglion and they synapse in the nucleus of the spinal tract of the trigeminal nerve, which has taken over the entire sensibility of the facial region.

The GVA fibers innervate parts of the oropharynx, the palatoglossal arch, the dorsal part of the tongue, the auditory tube, and the tympanic cavity. These fibers are important also for the palatal (swallowing) reflex.

The SVA fibers originate from the posterior one-third of the tongue and conduct gustatory stimuli. They synapse in the upper part of the nucleus of the solitary tract.

Special mention should be made of the carotid nerve, which comprises fibers from the carotid sinus (Fig. 27–7). These fibers synapse in the nucleus solitarius, from which secondary fibers extend to the "vasomotor center" (see page 200) and to the dorsal nucleus of the vagus nerve. This nucleus produces vagus fibers that inhibit the heart; from the vasomotor center, fibers descend to the lateral horn of the spinal cord. Impulses from the nucleus tractus solitarius activate the dorsal nucleus and inhibit the vasomotor center. Increased blood pressure increases the firing rate of the pressure receptors in the carotid sinus; impulses from the nucleus tractus solitarius cause deceleration of heart action and vasodilatation, with a result of a decrease in blood pressure. In the case of decreased blood pressure the pressure receptors are less stimulated, the firing rate in the carotid nucleus and the solitary tract nucleus diminishes, and the blood pressure rises. This is the so-called carotid sinus reflex, which constantly controls the blood pressure.

Tractus Solitarius. Among the fibers found in this tract are the following: fibers from the 9th cranial nerve (taste, posterior one-third of the tongue), from the 7th cranial nerve (taste, anterior two-thirds of the tongue), and from the 10th cranial nerve (viscerosensory impulses from the mucosa of the respiratory and the digestive system).

Efferent Fibers. GVE: inferior salivatory nucleus → tympanic nerve → tympanic plexus → lesser petrosal nerve → otic ganglion → auriculotemporal nerve → facial nerve → parotid gland;

SVE: nucleus ambiguus → superior pharyngeal constrictor and stylopharyngeal muscle.

Dysfunction of the Nerve. Unilateral dysfunction causes reduced salivation associated with disturbed sensibility in the posterior part of the tongue and the superior part of the pharynx. Bilateral dysfunction causes disorders of deglutition, especially for liquid food.

VAGUS (10th CRANIAL) NERVE

The vagus nerve is a complicated complex of morphologically different components. In principle, two parts are grossly distinguishable: a branchial part, which is involved in the innervation of branchial arch derivatives, and a parasympathetic visceral part, which innervates the viscera (respiratory and digestive system, heart, and blood vessels) as far as the descending colon. The branchial part of the vagus nerve terminates in the inferior laryngeal nerve; caudal to this, the vagus nerve comprises exclusively parasympathetic and sensory fibers for the viscera.

Branchial Part

The branchial part innervates the fourth and subsequent branchial arches and can therefore be regarded as an aggregate of branchial nerves. The posttrematic branch of the fourth branchial arch is the superior laryngeal nerve; the posttrematic branch of the sixth branchial arch (the fifth soon disappears) is the recurrent laryngeal nerve. The pretrematic branches of the vagus nerve, together with those of the glossopharyngeal nerve, form a network of nerve fibers called the pharyngeal plexus. In addition to the original sensory fibers of the pharyngeal plexus there are motor fibers and autonomic fibers that innervate the muscles of the pharyngeal wall (pharyngeal constrictor muscles).

Afferent Fibers. General somatic (GSA): superior ganglion → nucleus of the spinal tract of the trigeminal nerve; general visceral (GVA): superior and inferior ganglion → nucleus solitarius tractus.

There are two vagal ganglions: (a) the superior (jugular) ganglion for somatosensory impulses from the retroauricular skin and the posterior wall of the external auditory meatus and (b) the inferior (nodose) ganglion for viscerosensory impulses and, to a lesser extent, gustatory impulses. Multipolar (parasympathetic motor) cells are found scattered among the pseudounipolar neurons.

The sensory fibers of the branchial derivatives come from the epiglottis, the laryngeal part of the pharynx as far as the level of the infraglottic cavity.

Efferent Fibers. General viscera (GVE): dorsal nucleus of the vagus nerve (parasympathetic vagus nucleus); special visceral (SVE): nucleus ambiguus (branchiogenic musculature of the 4th and 6th branchial arches).

The nucleus ambiguus is situated between the spinal nucleus of the trigeminal nerve and the inferior olive (Fig. 27–8). It innervates the laryngeal and pharyngeal muscles (striated muscles that originate from branchial arch mesenchyma). This nucleus receives impulses from the cortex (corticobulbar fibers), the trigeminal and the

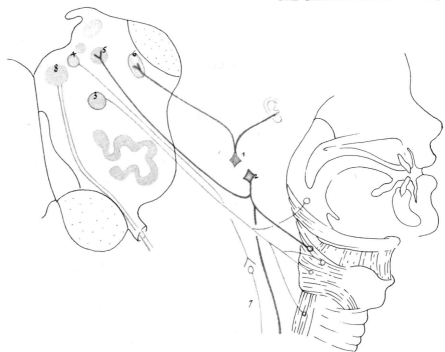

Figure 27–8 Arrangement of the nuclei of the vagus nerve.

1 superior ganglion
2 inferior ganglion
3 nucleus ambiguus
4 dorsal nucleus of the vagus nerve
5 nucleus solitarius
6 nucleus of the spinal tract of V
7 intestinal branch
8 hypoglossal nucleus

glossopharyngeal nerves, and other nuclei of the vagus nerve. The nucleus ambiguus is important for reflexes like swallowing, coughing, and vomiting.

Parasympathetic Visceral Part (Intestinal Branch, Pneumogastric Branch)

The intestinal branch innervates the smooth muscles of the gastrointestinal tract, the respiratory system, and the myocardium. This nerve can be regarded as a cranial part of the autonomic nervous system (parasympathetic). The corresponding ganglion is the nodose ganglion.

Afferent Fibers. General visceral (GVA): inferior ganglion → nucleus of the solitary tract (sensory fibers from the viscera).

Efferent Fibers. General visceral (GVE): dorsal nucleus of vagus nerve (intestinal nucleus) → parasympathetic vagal nuclei.

Dysfunction of the Nerve. A lesion at a low level (lesion of the recurrent nerve due to a disturbance in the mediastinum) gives rise to hoarseness due to paresis of the laryngeal muscles. Bilateral dysfunction of the recurrent nerve

causes dyspnea and asphyxia; the vocal cords are sucked together.

ACCESSORY (11th CRANIAL) NERVE

The accessory nerve is a motor nerve that arises from the anterior horn cells at C6 and upward, to a level halfway through the pyramidal decussation. The root fibers combine to form the spinal accessory nerve, which enters the skull via the foramen magnum and leaves it again via the jugular foramen; it innervates the sternocleidomastoid muscle and the trapezius muscle, together with small branches from the cervical plexus (C2–C3).

Special Somatic Afferent Nerves

VESTIBULOCOCHLEAR (8th CRANIAL) NERVE

The vestibulocochlear nerve has two components: the vestibular nerve (equilibrium) and

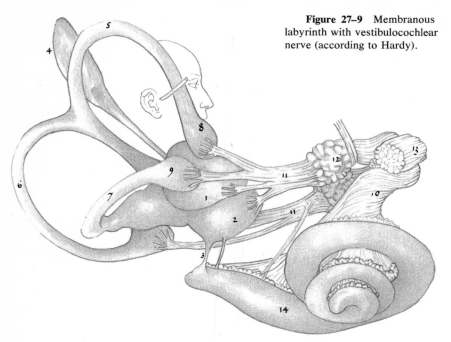

Figure 27–9 Membranous labyrinth with vestibulocochlear nerve (according to Hardy).

1 utricle
2 saccule
3 ductus reuniens
4 endolymphatic sac
5 superior semicircular canal
6 posterior semicircular canal
7 lateral semicircular canal
8 superior ampullary crista
9 lateral ampullary crista
10 cochlear nerve
11 vestibular nerve
12 vestibular ganglion
13 facial nerve
14 cochlea

the cochlear nerve (hearing). Both nerves comprise mainly afferent fibers from the labyrinth. The vestibular nerve is phylogenetically older and is subservient to proprioceptive sensibility, while the cochlear nerve is involved in exteroceptive sensibility.

The Labyrinth

The peripheral receptors of the vestibulocochlear nerve are localized in a complex of communicating, fluid-filled epithelial tubes situated in the bony labyrinth of the petrosal bone. The receptors of the vestibular nerve are localized in specialized parts of the semicircular canals, utricle, and saccule. The receptors of the cochlear nerve are localized in the organ of Corti, in the cochlea.

The three semicircular canals are arranged at right angles to each other (Fig. 27–9). The lateral (horizontal) canal lies in the horizontal plane when the head is inclined 30° in an anterior direction; the plane of the right anterior vertical canal roughly parallels that of the left posterior vertical canal; inversely, the plane of the left anterior canal parallels that of the right posterior canal (Fig. 27–9).

Sensory Epithelium in the Vestibular Labyrinth. The specific sensory elements of the semicircular canals (cristae) are localized in parts of the canals that are distended as ampullae. The three ampullae are of virtually the same size and shape (Fig. 27–9). The crista ampullaris is a kind of crest that protrudes into the lumen: situated above the crest is a gelatinous mass, the cupula, which extends to the opposite side of the ampulla (Fig. 27–10). In this way the lumen of the canal is closed as if by a valve. The cristae are innervated by the superior, the posterior, and the lateral ampullary branches, respectively.

Sensory epithelium is also found in the utricle and the saccule; it is confined to relatively small parts of the wall: the utricular macula and the saccular macula. These specialized structures are likewise covered by a gelatinous mass, in which small crystals of $CaCO_3$ (statoconia) are

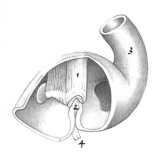

Figure 27–10 Opened ampulla of a semicircular canal. The gelatinous cupula closes the lumen of the canal (according to Werner).

1 cupula
2 ampullary crista
3 semicircular canal
4 ampullary nerve

found. Their specific gravity significantly exceeds that of the surrounding endolymph.

STRUCTURE OF THE SENSORY EPITHELIUM. Two types of receptor cells are distinguished in the sensory epithelium: type I (bottle-shaped) and type II (cylindrical). The innervation of these two types differs: type I is enclosed by a large, cup-shaped nerve ending (calyx), while type II is innervated only on the underside of the cell by bud-like endings. The surface of the receptor cells has 60 to 100 so-called stereocilia, which are embedded in the cupula. At one side of the brush plate stands a kinocilium, that is a true cilium. The five specialized sensory epithelia (three cristae and two maculae) are innervated by six branches of the vestibular nerve. These fibers are the peripheral extensions of the bipolar cells of the vestibular ganglion (Scarpa's ganglion); their central extensions make up the vestibular nerve (SSA).

At rest, the sensory hairs or cilia are perpendicular to the brush plate, and the receptor cell fires at a certain resting frequency. When the head is turned, the endolymph with its mass inertia exerts pressure on the cupula. This causes the cupula to bend in a direction opposite to that of the movement of the head. The bending of the cupula causes the cilia to bend likewise as a result of the tangential force that acts on them. It has been found that movement of the cupula toward the cilium causes an increase in firing frequency, whereas movement of the cupula in the opposite direction reduces the firing rate.

The cilia in a crista all have the same direction of polarization. Of each pair of parallel

semicircular canals, one is excited and the other is inhibited during rotation. Rotation perpendicular to the plane of the semicircular canal has no effect.

Function of the Vestibular Labyrinth. The cristae ampullares function as angular acceleration meters; particularly changes in the direction of the head movements act as a stimulus. Due to the spatial arrangement of the three semicircular canals, angular accelerations can be registered in three orthogonal directions. The crista of each semicircular canal reacts especially to rotation of the head in its own plane. After about 20 seconds, endolymph and wall of semicircular canal rotate at the same speed, and the cupula returns to its rest position. Uniform movements (movements of constant speed and direction) are not perceived.

The cristae ampullares have a dynamic function: Each rotation can be resolved into three mutually perpendicular components, and consequently each of the semicircular canals can make its own contribution to the perception. However, the left and right canals support each other.

The maculae in the utricle and saccule register the static effect of gravity as well as linear accelerations, utilizing the specific gravity of the statoconia. In linear accelerations the statoconia lag behind in relation to the macula, and the resultant bending of the cilia is the adequate stimulus. The utricle is sensitive to accelerations in anterior and posterior directions, while the saccule registers vertical accelerations.

Vestibular Nuclei

After entering the brain stem, the vestibular fibers divide into an ascending branch (from the semicircular canals) and a descending branch (from utricle and saccule). Some of the vestibular fibers project directly the cerebellum (nodulus, uvula) via the juxtarestiform body. Most vestibular axons, however, synapse in the vestibular nuclei. The four vestibular nuclei are localized immediately beneath the floor of the fourth ventricle, in the vestibular area. Lateral to this area is found the inferior cerebellar peduncle. The four vestibular nuclei are the following:

(a) *Inferior Vestibular Nucleus.* This is localized between the fibers of the inferior cerebellar peduncle and the floor of the ventricle; the nucleus is fairly long and tapered caudally (Fig. 27–11). Its ventrolateral part carries large cells on which no vestibular fibers synapse.

(b) *Medial Vestibular Nucleus.* The cells of this nucleus are localized beneath the floor of the fourth ventricle, medial to the cells of the inferior vestibular nucleus. In a rostral direction, the nucleus gradually merges into the lateral vestibular nucleus.

(c) *Superior Vestibular Nucleus.* This nucleus is localized in the angle between the floor and the lateral wall of the fourth ventricle, adjacent to the superior cerebellar peduncle, and ventrally alongside the spinal tract nucleus.

(d) *Lateral Vestibular Nucleus.* This nucleus (Deiters' nucleus) is localized beneath the ventricular floor at the level of the entry of the vestibular fibers (Fig. 27–11). This nucleus is characterized by large multipolar cells, with macrogranular Nissl bodies. The nucleus receives few vestibular afferents (only in its central part).

Afferent Vestibular Fibers. The distribution of the nerve endings in the vestibular nuclei is irregular. Each of the four nuclei shows areas in which vestibular axons are absent. The synapses are mostly on small and medium-size cells. Fibers from the semicircular canals terminate in the superior vestibular nucleus and the rostral part of the medial vestibular nucleus. Other fibers, from utricle and saccule, extend through the juxtarestiform body and end in the inferior vestibular nucleus and the caudal part of the medial vestibular nucleus (Lorente de Nó, 1933). Direct vestibulocerebellar fibers run through the juxtarestiform body and end as mossy fibers in the ipsilateral cortex of the nodulus, uvula, and flocculus.

Nonvestibular Afferent Fibers. Nonvestibular afferent fibers, which likewise synapse in the vestibular nuclei, are fibers from Cajal's interstitial nucleus (via the medial longitudinal fasciculus), from the cerebellum and from the reticular formation. The lateral vestibular nucleus (Deiters' nucleus) receives many Purkinje cell axons from the intermediate zone of the anterior lobe. That is why this nucleus can be regarded as a cerebellar nucleus that has migrated in a ventral direction. Other cerebellar afferents from the flocculonodular lobe and the fastigial nuclei descend in the juxtarestiform body and end in the "true" vestibular nuclei (medial, superior, and inferior). From the pontine and bulbar reticular formations, too, come fibers that synapse in the vestibular nuclei.

Efferent Fibers. Efferent fibers from the vestibular nuclei can be divided into the following groups:

(a) *Descending vestibulospinal fibers,* which belong to two different systems: the lateral and the medial vestibulospinal tract. The former is an ipsilateral, somatotopically organized fiber system that extends in the lateral part of the anterior funiculus of the spinal cord (see page 161). The fibers run through the entire spinal cord, and impulses via these fibers facilitate antigravity muscle reflexes. The medial and the inferior vestibular nucleus produce vestibulospinal fibers (medial vestibulospinal tract), which extend to the spinal cord via the medial longitudinal fasciculus. These fibers do not descend beyond the level of T6–T8; it is via these fibers that the vestibular nuclei control the muscles of the neck.

(b) *Vestibulocerebellar fibers,* which arise mainly from the inferior and the medial vestibular nucleus and enter the cerebellum via the juxtarestiform body. They synapse in the cortex of the nodulus, uvula, flocculus, and fastigial nucleus.

(c) *Vestibulomesencephalic fibers,* which connect the vestibular nuclei with the nuclei of the ocular muscles. These fibers mostly arise from the superior and the medial vestibular nuclei. Fibers from the former project mainly to the trochlear and the oculomotor nuclei (ipsilaterally). Fibers from the latter project contralaterally to the trochlear and the oculomotor nuclei. The abducens nucleus seems to receive fibers from the ventral part of the lateral vestibular nucleus.

(d) *Vestibulothalamic fibers*. The anatomic substrate of these fibers is still obscure. Physiologic experiments point to the posterior ventral inferior (PVI) nucleus of the thalamus (part of the posterior ventral nucleus) as a relay station of a possible vestibulocortical tract.

(e) *Efferent fibers in the vestibular nerve*. A few of the fibers of the vestibular nerve are *efferent*; they arise mostly from an ipsilateral cell group localized lateral to the abducens nucleus. These fibers inhibit the hair cells and thus reduce the sensitivity of the peripheral receptors.

Medial Longitudinal Fasciculus

The medial longitudinal fasciculus is a complex bundle of ascending and descending fibers of widely diverse origin. In the medulla oblongata, this fasciculus is located ventral to the hypoglossal nucleus, beside the raphe; in the pons and the mesencephalon it is always situated quite near the midline, at a short distance from the lumen (Fig. 27–11).

Ascending fibers in this fasciculus are, for the most part, vestibular fibers, especially from the superior and the medial vestibular nuclei. These fibers innervate the nuclei of the ocular muscles, while other fibers ascend to Cajal's interstitial nucleus.

Descending fibers can be either vestibular or nonvestibular. The former arise from the medial vestibular nucleus and extend to the medulla oblongata (medial vestibulospinal tract). Nonvestibular fibers come from Cajal's interstitial nucleus and extend to the spinal cord. From the tectum and the reticular formation, too, fibers descend to the spinal cord via the fasciculus. Fibers of a third group (internuclear component) correlate the nuclei of origin of the 3rd, 4th, and 6th cranial nerves and also extend to the 7th and 10th cranial nerves. (The medial longitudinal fasciculus is of importance also for coordination of chewing and swallowing.)

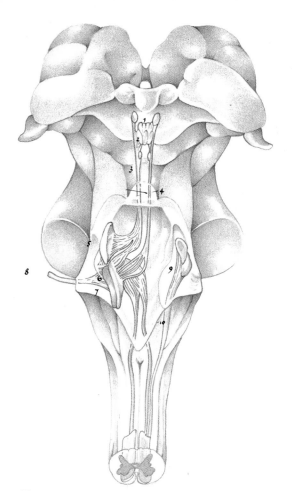

Figure 27–11 Vestibular nuclei and medial longitudinal fasciculus (according to Nieuwenhuys, Voogd, and Van Huijzen).

1 Cajal's interstitial nucleus
2 nucleus of oculomotor nerve
3 nucleus of trochlear nerve
4 medial longitudinal fasciculus
5 superior vestibular nucleus
6 medial vestibular nucleus
7 inferior vestibular nucleus
8 vestibular nerve
9 lateral vestibular nucleus
10 lateral vestibulospinal tract

Functional Aspects of the Vestibular Nerve

The vestibular apparatus is involved in spatial orientation, reflex movements of the eyes, and equilibrium in general. It makes an important contribution to the orientation of the head in relation to the horizontal and the vertical planes. The latter is important because the median plane of the body has to be kept vertical to ensure equilibrium; the former is important in view of the relation between this plane and the visual direction.

The labyrinthine reactions are closely correlated with the muscles of the neck (via the medial vestibulospinal tract). In this way the head is kept in its normal position. A distinction has to be made between labyrinthine and cervical righting reflexes: The former are induced by impulses from both laryrinths (utricle and saccule), concerning the position of the head in relation to gravity; the latter result from stimulation of proprioceptors in the neck muscles and in the joints and ligaments of the cervical vertebrae (Magnus and De Kleyn's neck reflexes). A cat falling from a height first turns its head to the normal position (labyrinthine righting reflex) and then corrects the position of its trunk (cervical righting reflex) in order to land on its feet.

Reflex Movements of the Eyes

When the gaze is fixed on a particular object, the eyes continue to aim at this object, regardless of any movements of the head. This can be verified in an individual who shakes his head to indicate "no": the eye movements are opposed to the movements of the head. When the head rotates to the left in the horizontal plane, a flow of endolymph is generated in the horizontal semicircular canals. The firing rate in the right ampullary crista increases, while that in the left crista diminishes. The impulses from the cristae are conducted to the vestibular nuclei (superior and medial), where certain cells are excited; via the medial longitudinal fasciculus, impulses travel to the nuclei of the ocular muscles, causing the lateral rectus muscle (6th cranial nerve) to contract while the medial rectus muscle (3rd cranial nerve) relaxes on the right side. On the left side, the opposite muscles are activated and inhibited, respectively.

The influence of the vestibular nuclei on equilibrium and regulation of posture is exerted in close cooperation with the cerebellum. The efferent tracts are the medial and the lateral vestibulospinal tracts; the latter exerts a facilitating influence on the tone of the extensors. This is demonstrable in experiments in which the brain stem is severed between the superior and inferior colliculi: The experimental animals show stiffness of the extensors (anti-gravity muscles) in the extremities (decerebrate rigidity). Selective destruction of the lateral vestibular muscle almost immediately remedies this stiffness.

COCHLEAR NERVE

Structure of the Sound Receptors

The sound receptors that form part of the auditory apparatus are localized in a special part of the labyrinth, the cochlear duct. As viewed from the bony labyrinth, part of the cochlear duct rests on the bony spiral lamina; from its free edge, the basilar membrane extends (Fig. 27–12). This membrane attaches to the opposite wall of the cochlea by means of the spiral ligament. The space of the bony cochlea is divided into an upper level (scala vestibuli) and a lower level (scala tympani). The membranous cochlear duct occupies part of the space of the scala vestibuli (Fig. 27–12).

The scala vestibuli begins in the vestibule, whence it can be followed over two and one-half turns as far as the apex of the cochlea. Beyond the helicotrema, one enters the scala tympani, through which one descends to the round window (cochlear fenestra); this gives access to the tympanic cavity, but the aperture is always sealed by the secondary tympanic membrane.

Basilar Membrane

This membrane bridges the space between the margin of the spiral lamina on the inside and

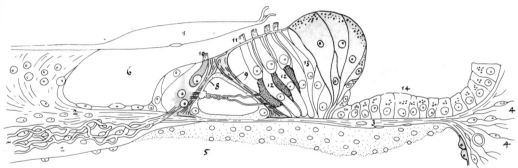

Figure 27–12 Structure of the organ of Corti (according to Retzius).

1	tectorial membrane	8	inner pillar cell
2	bony spiral lamina	9	outer pillar cell
3	basilar membrane	10	inner hair cells
4	spiral ligament	11	outer hair cells
5	scala tympani	12	Deiters' cells
6	internal spiral sulcus	13	Hensen's cells
7	fibers of the cochlear nerve	14	Claudius' cells

the basilar crest on the outside. The organ of Corti rests on the basilar membrane (Fig. 27–12). The membrane is divided into a medial (tectal) and a lateral (pectinate) part. The former extends from the margin of the spiral lamina to below the free margin of the tectorial membrane and carries the organ of Corti. The latter lies adjacent to the spiral ligament.

The basilar membrane consists of radial keratinized fibers, beneath which a second, thin membrane of connective tissue is situated. Its tympanic surface is lined with a layer of loosely packed connective tissue cells. The basilar membrane has a width of 0.5 mm at the apical end while at the basal end its width is only 0.04 mm. Its length is 34 mm.

Organ of Corti

The specific sensory epithelium known as the organ of Corti rests on the basilar membrane. As viewed from the internal spiral sulcus (Fig. 27–12), the following components can be distinguished: pillar cells; inner hair cells; outer hair cells; Deiters', Hensen's and Claudius' cells; the reticular lamina, and the tectorial membrane.

Pillar cells are arranged in two rows, an inner and an outer row. Together they form a kind of arch which, viewed in three dimensions, traverses the entire cochlea like a tunnel (Fig. 27–12). The inner pillar cells have a thin, flat midportion and two ends. The lower end (base) is markedly widened and rests on the tectal part of

the basilar membrane; the upper end shows a small indentation in which the outer pillar cell fits. The outer pillar cell has a virtually cylindrical midportion (Fig. 27–12) with widened ends. Each inner pillar cell unites with the corresponding outer pillar cell in such a way that the roof plate of the inner pillar cell lies above the phalanx of the outer and virtually covers it.

Cochlear receptors consist of hair cells, from whose free surface several stereocilia (modified microvilli) arise. The ends of the stereocilia are embedded in the tectorial membrane (Fig. 27–12). In view of their situation relative to the tunnel of Corti, the hair cells are divided into inner and outer hair cells.

The *inner* hair cells (about 3500) are arranged in a single row associated with the inner pillar cells. The free ends of these hair cells are enclosed by the reticular membrane, which continues in the roof plates of the pillar cells. These hair cells are shaped like a pear. The apex of the cell shows 50 to 60 microvilli; there is no kinocilium, but a basal corpuscle is located close to one of the margins of the cell. The bases of the stereocilia are narrowed. With the electron microscope, numerous microfilaments can be seen which are connected with the terminal web of the hair cell. Viewed from above, the stereo-

Figure 27-13 Innervation of the hair cells of the organ of Corti (according to Benninghoff and Goerttler). The afferent fibers are yellow, while the efferent fibers are black.

1 tectorial membrane
2 outer hair cells
3 inner hair cells
4 inner pillar cell
5 outer pillar cell
6 tunnel of Corti
7 afferent fibers of cochlear nerve
8 efferent fibers of cochlear nerve

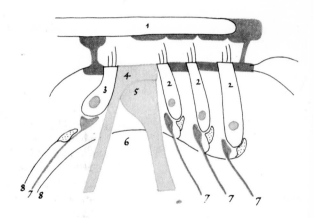

cilia invariably are arranged in the shape of a horseshoe.

The *outer* hair cells number about 12,000 and are arranged in three or four rows lateral to the outer pillar cells. The rows are separated by the extensions of Deiters' cells. The outer hair cells are much longer than the inner; their free ends are flat, and each end has about 100 stereocilia. Viewed from above, the stereocilia are arranged in the shape of a W. The ends of these stereocilia are embedded in the tectorial membrane.

Deiters' cells are fusiform cells with a thickened midportion and two thin extensions. The basal extension (Fig. 27-12) rests on the basilar membrane, while the apical extension reaches as far as the free surface of the hair cells, where it ends in an elongated, finger-like process. These processes (phalanges) are especially conspicuous when the organ of Corti is viewed from above after removal of the tectorial membrane.

The tectorial membrane can be compared to a roof that extends over the organ of Corti. Its inner margin attaches to the limbus of the spiral lamina; laterally, the tectorial membrane is much thicker. It ends above the outer hair cells in a sharp free margin (Fig. 27-13). The structure of the tectorial membrane is a network of very delicate fibers embedded in a jelly-like, highly refringent matrix.

Structure of the Nerve Endings. The lower part of the cytoplasm of the inner hair cells is in touch with endings of the cochlear nerve. There are afferent and efferent nerve endings. The former contain many electron-dense inclusions, lamellae, etc.; the latter contain mitochondria, microtubules and synaptic vesicles. The efferent endings synapse on the afferent end-feet (not on the hair cells).

The pattern of innervation of the inner hair cells differs from that of the outer hair cells. Of the approximately 30,000 fibers of the cochlear nerve, about 18,000 are in contact with the 3500 inner hair cells (divergence). For the outer hair cells the situation is reversed (no more than about 4000 fibers are in touch with at least 12,000 cells). The cytoplasm of these cells is covered largely by the surrounding cells of Deiters, except where synaptic junctions with cochlear nerve fibers are situated. The efferent fibers synapse directly with the cytoplasm of the outer hair cells (which in this respect differs from the inner hair cells).

Functional Aspects of the Cochlea

The vibrations of the tympanic membrane are transmitted to the oval window by the auditory ossicles. The movements of the foot plate of the stapes causes the perilymph to vibrate, thus transforming air vibrations to fluid vibrations. Since the perilymph is not compressible, an inward deviation of the stapes (to the vestibule) has to be compensated by an outward deviation of the secondary tympanic membrane (in the round window) toward the tympanic cavity. The vibrations in the perilymph have a small amplitude and a high pressure variation.

The vibrations in the perilymph in the scala vestibuli and the scala tympani cause the cochlear duct to vibrate as well; the basilar membrane begins to move in a plane perpendicular to its surface. Relative movements of the tectorial and the basilar membranes cause the auditory hairs to bend in response to the shearing force. This bending is the stimulus that gives rise to the action potentials in the auditory nerve. The production of the action potentials coincides with the site of the maximal excursion of the basilar membrane: High-pitched tones excite receptors in the basal turns of the cochlear duct, whereas low-pitched tones excite receptors near the apex.

Fibers of the Cochlear Nerve

The fibers of the cochlear nerve are central extensions of the bipolar cells located in the spiral ganglion. Immediately after entering the brain stem, these fibers divide into an ascending and a descending branch; the former synapses in the ventral cochlear nucleus and the latter in the dorsal cochlear nucleus.

Central Acoustic Pathway

The neuronal circuits involved in the function of hearing constitute a complicated linkage of rhombencephalic, mesencephalic, diencephalic, and cortical centers. The afferent sensory pathway is assisted by an efferent olivocochlear tract (Rasmussen, 1946, 1953), which inhibits the hair cells of the organ of Corti.

Rhombencephalic Centers. The dorsal cochlear nucleus is an elevation in the most lateral part of the floor of the fourth ventricle; in many mammals this nucleus is a layered structure. The ventral cochlear nucleus comprises medium-size cells with a fair amount of cytoplasm; there are some local structural changes, but the neurons are never arranged in layers. Fibers from the basal part of the cochlea (high-pitched tones) synapse in the dorsal part of both nuclei, whereas fibers from the apex (low-pitched tones) synapse in ventral parts of the nuclei. Fibers that arise from the cochlea nuclei project ipsilaterally and heterolaterally to the next nuclei in the rhombencephalon.

(a) Fibers from the dorsal cochlear nucleus extend past the superior aspect of the inferior cerebellar peduncle, traverse the reticular formation, cross the midline, and join the lateral lemniscus. These fibers are arranged in two bundles: the dorsal and the intermediate acoustic striae (Fig. 27–14). Many fibers of these striae synapse in the superior olive and the trapezoid nucleus.

(b) Fibers from the ventral cochlear nucleus extend (as ventral acoustic striae) through the ventral part of the tegmentum (trapezoid body), cross the midline, and in part synapse in the reticular formation, the trapezoid nucleus, and the superior olive. Other fibers show a sharp upward bend at the level of the superior olive and ascend in the so-called lateral lemniscus.

The superior olive is a group of nuclei localized between the medial lemniscus and the spinal tract of the trigeminal nerve. A principal and an accessory olivary nucleus are distinguished. The superior olive receives afferent fibers (bilaterally) from the cochlear nuclei; its efferent fibers extend to the lateral lemniscus.

The trapezoid nucleus comprises cells lying scattered among the fibers of the trapezoid body. In it fibers from the bundle of the same name and from the acoustic striae synapse.

LATERAL LEMNISCUS. This term is applied to the complex of crossed and uncrossed fibers from the cochlear nuclei and from the superior olive, which extend in the lateral part of the tegmentum (Fig. 27–14) to the inferior colliculus. Scattered among these fibers are neurons on which some of the fibers synapse (nucleus of the lateral lemniscus). The lateral lemniscus is the most important acoustic pathway in the brain stem.

Mesencephalic Nuclei. The principal nucleus of the acoustic pathway in the mesencephalon is the inferior colliculus. The morphology of this nucleus shows a central part with cells of several types and a cortical part in which the cells are arranged in four layers.

Afferent fibers to the inferior colliculus originate from: (a) the lateral lemniscus; these fibers synapse in the central part and the lower two

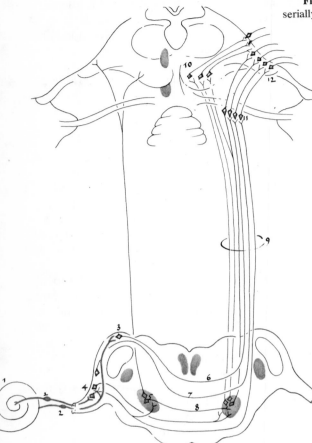

Figure 27–14 The central acoustic pathway. Note the numerous serially connected nuclei that characterize this pathway.

1 cochlea
2 spiral ganglion
3 dorsal cochlear nerve
4 ventral cochlear nerve
5 superior olivary nucleus
6 dorsal acoustic stria
7 intermediate acoustic stria
8 trapezoid body
9 lateral lemniscus
10 inferior colliculus
11 nucleus of lateral lemniscus
12 medial geniculate body

frequencies being projected laterally and the high frequencies medially.

Cortical Projection. Cells of the medial geniculate body project to the upper temporal gyrus (areas 41 and 42) via the geniculotemporal tract. In animals, a tonotopic localization has been demonstrated in the acoustic cortex. The basal turns of the cochlea (high frequencies) project onto the anterior part of area 41, while the apical turns (low frequencies) project onto the posterior part. Each cochlea is represented bilaterally in the acoustic cortex, although there are differences between left and right.

The above shows that numerous hearing centers are linked in the acoustic system. Some of these "stations" (superior olive, inferior colliculus, medial geniculate body) are for the most part connected "in series." Other centers, however (trapezoid nucleus, reticular formation, nucleus of the lateral lemniscus), are connected "in parallel." Evidently these centers play a much more important role than the simple "relay stations"; aspects of hearing such as discrimination of pitch, sound intensity, and discrimination between significant and indifferent ("noise") sounds by means of so-called lateral inhibition are governed by these intercalated acoustic centers.

layers of the cortical part; (b) the contralateral colliculus; and (c) the cerebral cortex; these fibers synapse in the upper layers of the cortical part.

Efferent fibers from the inferior colliculus extend via the brachium of the inferior colliculus (Fig. 27–14) to the medial geniculate body of the thalamus. Other fibers extend to the contralateral inferior colliculus or descend to the rhombencephalic acoustic nuclei.

Diencephalic Centers. The fibers from the inferior colliculus synapse in the medial geniculate body, in which a parvocellular and a magnocellular part must be distinguished. The fibers from the colliculus synapse in the parvocellular part; we observe a tonotopic projection, the low

Efferent Fibers in the Acoustic Pathway

The nervous system can exert a regulatory influence on incoming acoustic information. Descending "efferent" fibers arise from all acoustic nuclei and synapse on the next underlying nucleus. The olivocochlear tract is the best known of these efferent connections. This tract arises from the superior olive and comprises a homolateral and a contralateral component. The homolateral component arises from the principal olivary nucleus, while the (larger) contralateral component arises from the accessory olivary nucleus. The fibers of the olivocochlear tract are not numerous (about 500). They accompany the vestibular nerve and leave it in the labyrinth, via the vestibulocochlear anastomosis. These fibers terminate on hair cells.

Chapter 28

The Olivocerebellar System

The development of the inferior olive parallels that of the cerebellum. Functionally and anatomically, too, these structures are closely related. On the basis of these relationships, the inferior olive and the cerebellum are not discussed separately but as components of a functional unit.

The Olive

The inferior olive can be divided into a medial and a dorsal accessory olive and a principal olive. The latter (see Fig. 30–2) is a strongly folded, phylogenetically young nucleus which, in transverse sections through the medulla, has the shape of a horseshoe. The accessory olives and the principal olive differ both in structure and in connections.

Structure.   The medium-size to small neurons of the olive are arranged in layers within a zone of gray matter. The dendrite tree, abundantly ramified and facing the hilus of the olive, is a dense, diffuse plexus. Numerous synaptic clusters are found scattered among the neurons.

The accessory olives are characterized by neurons with long dendrites, without many ramifications. The rostral part of both accessory olives, however, comprises cells that resemble those of the principal olive.

Afferent Fibers.   Descending fibers to the inferior olive originate from the red nucleus, the cerebral cortex, the periaqueductal gray matter, and the cerebellar nuclei. Ascending fibers come mostly from the spinal cord. From the parvicellular part of the red nucleus and from the

central gray matter, fibers arise that extend to the ipsilateral olive via the central tegmental fasciculus. Before they terminate in the dorsal lamella of the principal olive, these fibers form a kind of capsule around it (olivary amiculum). The corticoolivary fibers originate from all four lobes of the brain but mainly from their motor areas. These fibers join the corticospinal tract and synapse on the ventral zone of the principal olive and the dorsal accessory olive.

The medial accessory olive receives fibers from the central (periaqueductal) gray matter and, via the central tegmental fasciculus, from the nucleus of Darkschevich. The dorsal accessory olive receives fibers from the spinal cord (spinoolivary tract), from the trigeminal nerve, and from the cerebral cortex (area 6). It serves as a kind of "mixing station" for cortical and spinal stimuli on the way to the cerebellum.

From the dentate nucleus of the cerebellum, too, fibers arise that synapse in the dorsal and ventral zones of the principal olive. Studies reported by Gerebtzoff (1939), Hand and Liu (1966), and Groenewegen, Boesten and Voogd (1975) have shown that there are connections between the nuclei of the posterior funiculus and the contralateral accessory olives.

Efferent Fibers.   The efferent fibers from the olive extend to the cerebellum (climbing fibers). They traverse the medial lemniscus, cross the midline, traverse the contralateral olive and the trigeminal complex, and reach the inferior cerebellar peduncle, with which they enter the cerebellum (Fig. 28–1). Efferents from the accessory olive terminate exclusively in the vermis and the intermediate zone; efferents from the principal olive terminate exclusively in the hemisphere.

Microscopic Structure of the Cerebellum

The cerebellum can be regarded as a superimposed center that exerts a regulatory influence on other parts of the CNS: vestibular nuclei, reticular formation, and thalamocortical system. It exerts this influence largely indirectly. One of the most typical characteristics of this organ is that there is no direct contact between efferent cerebellar fibers and motoneurons, either in the spinal cord or in the brain stem.

Functionally, the cerebellum can be re-

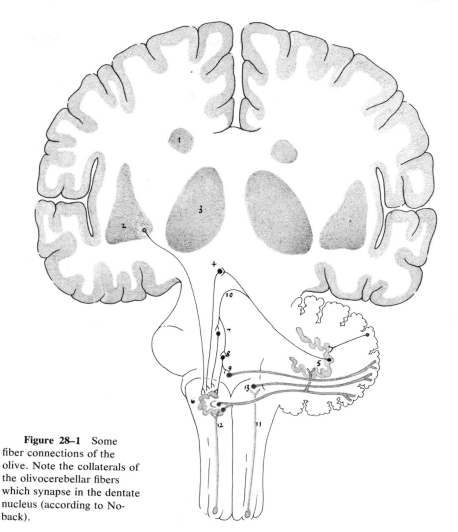

1 caudate nucleus
2 lentiform nucleus
3 thalamus
4 red nucleus
5 dentate nucleus
6 inferior olivary nucleus
7 pontine tegmental reticular nucleus
8 gigantocellular reticular
   nucleus
9 paramedian reticular
   nucleus
10 descending fibers of the
    superior cerebellar pe-
    duncle
11 spinoreticular tract
12 spinoolivary tract
13 lateral reticular nucleus

Figure 28–1 Some
fiber connections of the
olive. Note the collaterals of
the olivocerebellar fibers
which synapse in the dentate
nucleus (according to No-
back).

garded as an information processing system, the
input of which comprises two different fiber
types: mossy fibers and climbing fibers. The
fluorescence technique, moreover, has demonstrated relatively small numbers of noradrenergic
fibers that enter the cerebellum. These fibers
originate from the locus ceruleus and extend via
the superior cerebellar peduncle.

The output channels of the cerebellum are
the Purkinje cell axons and the axons of the
cerebellar nuclei that synapse with them.

MOSSY FIBERS

Mossy fibers are thick, myelinated fibers
that repeatedly divide in the white matter of the
cerebellum. Even within the granular layer of the
cortex they produce collaterals. They terminate
in the granular layer with a terminal enlargement
known as a rosette; the rosettes are localized in
the so-called cerebellar glomeruli (see page
190).

Mossy fibers transmit information to the
cortex from the following sources:

(a) *Vestibular system:* Vestibular fibers from
the vestibular nuclei or directly from the vestibular nerve (via the juxtarestiform body) terminate in the cortex of the flocculonodular lobe
and the fastigial nucleus;

(b) *Spinal cord:* Via the posterior spinocerebellar, the anterior spinocerebellar, and the
cuneocerebellar tract, the spinocerebellar fibers
extend to the vermis and intermediate zone of

Figure 28–2 Cortical projection of the afferent fiber systems of the cerebellum (according to Snider).

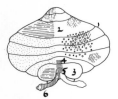

pontocerebellar fibers
spinocerebellar fibers
vestibulocerebellar fibers
. cortex sensitive to visual stimuli
° cortex sensitive to auditory stimuli
cortex sensitive to tactile stimuli
1 primary fissure
2 anterior lobe
3 cerebellar tonsil
4 pyramis
5 uvula
6 flocculonodular lobe

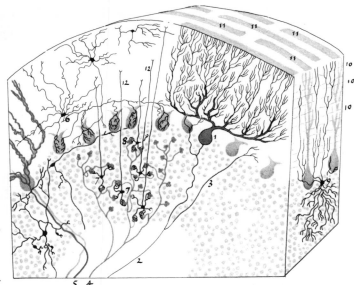

Figure 28–3 The structure of the cerebellar cortex in sagittal and frontal views.

1 Purkinje cell (P-cell)
2 axon of P-cell

3 recurrent axon collateral of P-cell
4 mossy fiber
5 climbing fiber
6 basket cell
7 granule cells
8 glomerulus
9 Golgi cell
10 parallel fibers
11 cortical zones corresponding with the dendrite ramification of a P-cell
12 axons of the granule cells

the anterior lobe and to the pyramid and uvula of the posterior lobe; fibers from the cuneocerebellar tract terminate in the intermediate zone on either side of the primary fissure (Fig. 28–2);

(c) *Cerebral cortex:* A thick bundle of fibers from the frontal and temporal cortex (corticopontine tract) synapse in the ipsilateral pontine nuclei; the axons of these nuclei cross the midline (middle cerebellar peduncle) and synapse in the cortex of the contralateral hemisphere and the midportion of the vermis, immediately behind the primary fissure;

(d) *Reticular formation:* These fibers terminate in an area similar to that of the external cuneate nucleus (Fig. 28–2); the reticular fibers arise from the lateral reticular nucleus, the paramedian reticular nucleus, and the pontine red nucleus and extend via the inferior cerebellar peduncle;

(e) *Tectum:* Fibers from the tectum extend via the superior cerebellar peduncle and conduct optic and acoustic impulses to the cerebellum;

(f) *Trigeminal nuclei:* Fibers from the tri-

geminal nuclei likewise reach the cerebellum via the superior and the inferior cerebellar peduncles.

This enumeration shows that the mossy fibers transmit most of the information destined for the cerebellum.

CLIMBING FIBERS

The climbing fibers originate mainly from the inferior olive; all other afferent fibers of the cerebellum are mossy fibers. The origin of the climbing fibers is yet to be established with certainty. The view that they arise exclusively from the inferior olive seems to have become obsolete; they probably arise in part from the inferior olive and in part from the reticular formation and the pontine nucleus.

The climbing fibers pass through the inferior cerebellar peduncle into the white matter of the cerebellum, where they arrange themselves in longitudinal (sagittal) bundles. Each climbing fiber produces a number of collaterals that remain in the same sagittal plane but extend to several cerebellar folia (gyri). The fibers extend through the granular layer, pass the Purkinje cell (P-cell) perikaryons, and ascend along the dendrite tree of the P-cell to the tertiary branches, immediately beneath the pial lining (the "smooth" part of the ramification), where they end in series of "synapses en passage" (Fig. 28–3). Each terminal climbing fiber synapses with a single P-cell; terminal branches of a terminal climbing fiber can also synapse with adjacent Golgi cells and granule cells, but the main synapse is with one particular P-cell. Climbing fibers have a diameter of 1 to 5 μm and form a relatively slowly conducting system.

LONGITUDINAL ORGANIZATION OF THE WHITE MATTER

The sagittal division of the cerebellum into vermis, intermediate zone, and hemisphere (proposed by Jansen and Brodal, 1940, 1942) was further analyzed and detailed by Voogd (1964, 1969) on the basis of studies of corticonuclear fiber projections. Moreover, Groenewegen and Voogd (1976) demonstrated that the white matter of the cerebellar folia is divided into compartments by three or four thin fiber bundles called raphes. These raphes are nothing but groups of climbing fibers arranged in a sagittal or parasagittal plane. The climbing fibers ultimately leave the raphes in order to "seek" the individual P-cells with which they synapse.

A good understanding of the three-dimensional organization of the cerebellum requires insight into the contrast between the sagittal arrangement of the climbing fibers and corticonuclear fibers, and the horizontal arrangement of the mossy fibers and parallel fibers (see below).

CORTICAL STRUCTURE

The cerebellar cortex is characterized by a regular structure with few local variations. The most characteristic cortical neurons are of the following types:

Purkinje Cells (P-cells). These are arranged in single-cell rows on the boundary between the molecular and the granular layers. They have an extensive dendrite tree (Fig. 28–3) that arises from the peripheral part of the perikaryon, usually from one or two primary dendrites.

The thin terminal branches of the dendrites extend to a level immediately beneath the superficial lining of the pia. The dendrite tree extends in only one plane, perpendicular to the longitudinal axis of the folia. The width of a P-cell is about 30 μm, and its vertical diameter is 70 μm. The distance between two P-cells in the frontal plane varies from 50 to 100 μm.

The primary and secondary dendrites are smooth; the thinner tertiary and higher-order dendrites have numerous gemmules. According to Braitenberg and Atwood (1958), each P-cell has an average of 180,000 gemmules. The receptive surface area of the dendrites is thus markedly enlarged. Human P-cells are estimated to number about 15 million.

The axon arises from the underside of the P-cell. Its initial segment is hardly distinguishable from the adjacent perikaryon. The myelin sheath begins at some distance from the cell body; the axon extends to the white matter of the cerebellum and synapses in one of the central cerebellar nuclei. The P-cell axons produce collaterals that synapse with the dendrites of the Golgi cells and basket cells.

Golgi Cells. Golgi cells are localized in the periphery of the granular layer (Fig. 28–3). They have long, radial dendrites in all directions. Most of these dendrites enter the molecular layer. The few remaining dendrites extend in the granular layer. The axon of the Golgi cell arises from the bottom part of the perikaryon and immediately divides into a dense bundle of delicate branches that extend through the entire thickness of the granular layer. These axon branches terminate in the so-called cerebellar glomeruli together with the moss fibers and the dendrites of the granule cells. Impulses are conducted to the Golgi cells chiefly through the parallel fibers in the molecular layer and through collaterals of the P-cell axons.

Granule Cells. Granule cells are the smallest cells of the entire CNS. Enormous numbers of closely packed granule cells are localized in the deep layer of the cerebellar cortex (granular layer, granule cell layer). These cells have a diameter of 5 to 7 μm; the nucleus is round, easily stainable, and surrounded by a thinner layer of cytoplasm. Each cell has 4 to 7 dendrites radiating in several directions. The claw-shaped end-feet of these dendrites terminate in the cerebellar glomeruli, where they synapse with the rosettes of the mossy fibers. Each mossy fiber extends branches to about 20 to 30 glomeruli. Each glomerulus comprises dendrites from about 15 different granule cells. The divergence within the folium, therefore, amounts to at least 300 granule cells per mossy fiber.

The axons of the granule cells ascend perpendicularly to the molecular layer and there dichotomize; the resulting branches (parallel fibers) extend parallel to the transverse grooves of the cerebellum over some distance (2 to 3 mm). The axons of the deep granule cells divide in the deeper areas of the molecular layer and synapse with the gemmules of the most proximal dendrites of the P-cells (Fig. 28–4); the axons of the superficial granule cells are thinner and synapse with the peripheral branches of the dendrite trees of the P-cells (Fig. 28–4).

In the molecular layer, the parallel fibers are arranged like thick bundles of telephone wires, suspended from the perpendicular dendrite trees of the P-cells (Fig. 28–4). Each parallel fiber passes about 220 P-cells; each P-cell in turn is "perforated" by 300,000 to 400,000 parallel fibers.

Basket Cells and Stellate Cells. Basket cells and stellate cells are located in the molecular layer. The dendrites, like those of the P-cells, are localized in a sagittal plane. The axon arises at the base of the perikaryon and extends in a sagittal plane, parallel to the dendrite ramification of the P-cells. At some distance from the perikaryon, the axon produces descending branches that enclose the initial segment of the

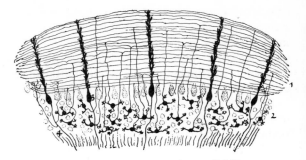

Figure 28–4 Granule cells and parallel fibers (according to Cajal).

1 parallel fibers
2 granule cells
3 P-cells
4 P-cell axons

P-cell axon like a kind of basket before terminating the numerous synapses. In a sagittal direction, a basket cell establishes contact with about 12 P-cells; perpendicular to it, there are contacts with two to three P-cells.

Layers of the Cortex

The cerebellar cortex has three layers: the granular (granule cell) layer, the P-cell layer, and the molecular layer (Fig. 28–5).

Granular Layer. The granular layer is about 100 μm thick in the depth of the sulci, and about 400 μm at the apex of the folia. This layer comprises granule cells and Golgi cells, mossy fibers and climbing fibers, granule cell axons, Golgi cell axons, and P-cell axons. According to Braitenberg and Atwood (1958), the number of granule cells per cubic millimeter is 3.7×10^6. The so-called *glomeruli* are an interesting component of the granular layer. Routine histologic techniques reveal them as "empty" spots between the closely packed nuclei of the granule cells. By the Golgi technique it can be established that the center of the glomerulus is occupied by the terminal enlargement (rosette) of a mossy fiber. It is surrounded by the terminations of a number (about 15) of dendrites of granule cells and the terminals of Golgi cell axons. A glial capsule encloses the glomerulus and isolates it from the surrounding granule cells. In the glomerulus is found the synaptic junction between the afferent mossy fibers and the cerebellar cortex. Apart from the axodendritic (excitatory) synapses between mossy fiber rosettes and granule cell dendrites, there are axodendritic (inhibitory) synapses between Golgi cell axons and granule cell dendrites. The functional significance of the synapses between rosette and Golgi cell dendrite is still obscure.

P-cell Layer. The P-cell layer is composed of the pear-shaped perikaryons of the P-cells. Between the cells, we observe a dense plexus of collaterals of P-cell axons (Fig. 28–3).

Molecular Layer. The molecular layer has a thickness of about 500 μm and consists mainly of fibers (dendrite trees of P-cells, parallel fibers, dendrite trees of basket cells, and Golgi cells) and neurons, which are mainly found in the deeper part of the layer (basket cells and stellate cells). The molecular layer is a synaptic region with numerous synapses. Its components are microscopically visible only by the Golgi method; the routine histologic techniques reveal only a diffuse, virtually "empty" region.

Synaptic Circuits

The P-cell axons are the sole output channels of the cerebellar cortex. Impulses from many sources (parallel fibers, climbing fibers, basket cell axons, stellate cell axons) converge on these cells. Most of the cellular surface is occupied by many thousands of synapses. The interaction of these incoming (excitatory and inhibitory) impulses ultimately determines the firing pattern of the P-cell.

Physiologic experiments have shown that mossy fibers, climbing fibers, and parallel fibers are excitatory, whereas the cells with short axons (Golgi cells, basket cells, and stellate cells) are inhibitory. The P-cell likewise proves to exert an inhibitory influence on the central cerebellar nuclei. On the other hand, these nuclei are constantly activated by collaterals of the olivocerebellar fibers and fibers from the lateral reticular nucleus. The activity in the cerebellar cortex is evidently aimed at modulation of the firing pattern of the cerebellar nuclei via delicately differentiated inhibition by the P-cell. Two factors play a role in this respect: (a) the spatial distribution of this inhibition over the cerebellar nuclei and (b) the timing of the inhibition within a given movement.

Figure 28–6 gives an impression of a simplified microcircuit of the cortex. The afferent information enters the cerebellum mainly via mossy fibers; the granule cells are excited in the glomeruli, and this activates parallel fibers. A particular train of impulses through the fast

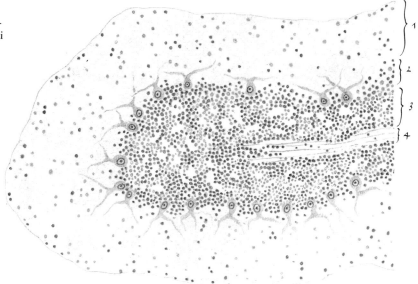

Figure 28–5 Cross-section through a folium of the cerebellum. The light, colorless spots in the granular layer are the cerebellar glomeruli (according to Clara).

1 molecular layer
2 layer of P-cells
3 granular layer
4 medullary radius

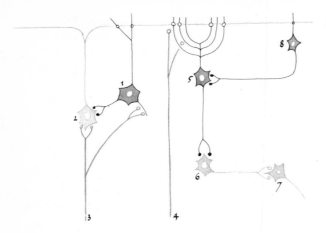

Figure 28–6 Synaptic circuits of the cerebellar cortex.

1 Golgi cell
2 granule cell
3 mossy fiber
4 climbing fiber
5 P-cell
6 central cerebellar nucleus
7 thalamus
8 basket cell

fibers causes — if the excited granule cells are closely packed — activation of parallel fibers within a zone of about 2 mm width (Fig. 28–7). The depth and length of this zone depend on the localization of the excited granule cells. In many cases, however, a varying number of zones of parallel fibers are activated.

The impulses in these zones excite the P-cells within the zone. The P-cells outside the zone are vigorously inhibited by the basket cells and stellate cells within this zone because the terminals of the basket axons are localized lateral to the parallel fibers that extend through the dendrites of the basket involved (Fig. 28–7). The activity of the mossy fibers thus leads to the formation of transverse zones of activated cerebellar cortex, isolated on either side by two "fringes" of lateral inhibition. The P-cells of the activated cortical zone are "primed" as a result of the spatial facilitation by the parallel fibers; when large numbers of parallel fibers within a zone are excited, the P-cells fire as a result of summation.

The localization of the activated cortical zones depends entirely on the afferent mossy fiber projection to the cerebellar cortex. This projection covers extensive cortical areas, in which unmistakable convergence occurs; impulses from various different regions activate common cortical areas (see page 195).

Another circuit that functions in close collaboration with the above is the microcircuit of the Golgi cell. This circuit utilizes the negative feedback principle in the following way: via parallel fibers the Golgi cell is facilitated and made to fire. The (inhibitory) impulses travel through the axon to the same glomeruli from which the granule cells were activated. In this way the transmission of information from the mossy fibers to the cerebellar cortex is inhibited. This, in turn, exerts a distinct influence on the size and topographic localization of the zones of excited parallel fibers.

The third important microcircuit is that formed by the synapses between climbing fibers and P-cells. Each impulse traveling through a climbing fiber causes vigorous excitation of the P-cell, which cannot be blocked by inhibition of the basket cells or stellate cells. As a result of this excitation, the P-cell produces one to four action potentials, depending on the degree of facilitation of the cell.

The arrangement of the climbing fibers and their branches in a sagittal plane means that activation of the olivocerebellar fibers causes selected P-cells to fire within a narrow sagittal "disk" that extends through many folia and even through lobules. As a consequence, many P-cells on which afferents from different regions converge are integrated and start to exert a joint influence on the cerebellar nuclei.

CEREBELLAR NUCLEI

The dentate nucleus is a horseshoe-shaped lamella of gray matter that is reminiscent of the inferior olive. The cells are multipolar, and among these large cells some smaller neurons (Golgi type II) are localized. The hilus faces

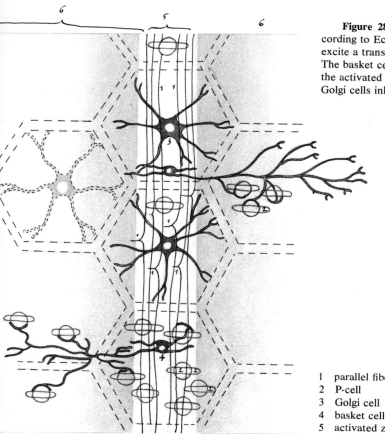

Figure 28–7 Activated cerebellar cortex (partly according to Eccles, Ito, and Szentágothai). The parallel fibers excite a transverse strip of P-cells that is about 3 mm long. The basket cells ensure "lateral inhibition" and thus separate the activated zone from adjacent parts. Activation of the Golgi cells inhibits the granule cells in the glomeruli.

1 parallel fibers
2 P-cell
3 Golgi cell
4 basket cell
5 activated zone
6 inhibited zone

rostrally and medially; through it, the fibers leave the nucleus (superior cerebellar peduncle).

The emboliform nucleus is located quite near the hilus of the dentate nucleus (see Fig. 30–3). The globose nucleus likewise comprises large multipolar as well as small cells. The fastigial nucleus is the most medially located of all nuclei; its cells are of various types and are closely packed.

Afferent Fibers

A distinction is made between cerebellar and noncerebellar afferent fibers.

Cerebellar Afferent Fibers. Cerebellar afferent fibers consist of P-cell axons from the cerebellar cortex. In the cortex of the cerebellum, several longitudinal zones are distinguished from which fibers extend to one of the nuclei. Fibers from the vermis project to the fastigial nucleus and, in this nucleus, retain their craniocaudal order of arrival. The fibers of the intermediate zone project to the globose and the emboliform nuclei. The fibers of the hemispheres project to the dentate nucleus and parts of the globose nucleus. The corticonuclear fiber projection follows the sagittal pattern of distribution that characterizes the radiation of the climbing fibers.

Noncerebellar Afferent Fibers. The central nuclei also receive afferent fibers from some nuclei of the brain stem (inferior olive, lateral reticular nucleus). Some of these fibers are axon collaterals, while others are direct axons. This noncerebellar fiber projection is excitatory.

Figure 28–8 Efferent connections of the cerebellum (according to Brodal).

1 thalamus (LV)
2 red nucleus
3 dentate nucleus
4 emboliform nucleus
5 globose nucleus
6 fastigial nucleus
7 superior vestibular nucleus
8 medial vestibular nucleus
9 lateral vestibular (LV) nucleus
10 inferior vestibular nucleus
11 floccule
12 nodule
13 Russell's uncinate fasciculus

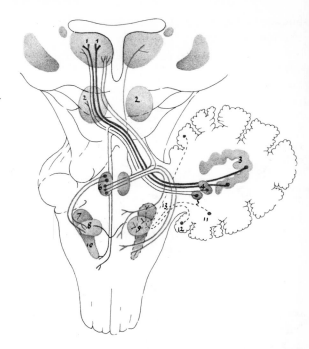

Efferent Fibers

The efferent fibers of the cerebellum originate from the central cerebellar nuclei, which include the lateral vestibular nucleus. The efferent fibers extend in two main bundles: the superior cerebellar peduncle and the juxtarestiform body.

Fastigial Nucleus. Fibers from the basal part of this nucleus cross the midline, curve around the brachium conjunctivum (Fig. 28–8), and divide into an ascending and a descending bundle. The ascending fibers project to the thalamus, while the descending fibers (Russell's uncinate fasciculus) synapse in the heterolateral vestibular nuclei and in the reticular formation. Fibers from the rostral pole of the fastigial nucleus descend in the ipsilateral part of the juxtarestiform body to the ipsilateral vestibular nuclei where they synapse. However, there is hardly any overlap between the terminations of the crossed and uncrossed fastigiovestibular fibers.

Nuclei Emboliformis and Globosus. Fibers from this nucleus cross the midline in the caudal part of the mesencephalon and mostly end in the magnocellular part of the red nucleus. Descend-

ing fibers from the red nucleus synapse in the spinal cord (rubrospinal tract), and via these fibers the cerebellum can influence the spinal cord (almost) directly.

Dentate Nucleus. The fibers from the dentate nucleus cross the midline at the level of the inferior colliculus; they circumvent the red nucleus. Some of these fibers synapse in the parvicellular part of this nucleus, but others leave the main bundle, descend in the tegmentum, and synapse in the paramedian reticular nucleus. Most of the fibers, however, ascend and synapse in the thalamus (lateral-ventral and anterior ventral nucleus, LV and AV), from which other fibers project to areas 4 and 6 (Fig. 28–8).

Part of the lateral strip of the vermis of the cerebellum projects directly to the rostrodorsal part of Deiters' nucleus. From this nucleus arises the vestibulospinal tract, which can be regarded as the most direct connection between the cerebellum and the motoneurons of somatic muscles. The lateral vestibular nucleus can be regarded as a slightly displaced cerebellar nucleus.

The axons from the P-cells of the flocculonodular lobe mostly end in the vestibular nuclei but not in the lateral vestibular nucleus.

The above enumeration shows that the influence of the cerebellum on motor activity is exerted only indirectly, via the following systems: (a) The cerebellar hemisphere acts via the contralateral cortex on the ipsilateral spinal cord via the corticospinal tract; (b) The intermediate zone acts via the red nucleus on the ipsilateral spinal cord via the rubrospinal fibers; (c) The vermis influences the vestibular nuclei and the reticular formation via Russell's uncinate fasciculus and the juxtarestiform body.

FUNCTIONAL ASPECTS

Although knowledge of the structure and synapses of the cerebellar cortex is far advanced, the exact function of the cerebellum still poses questions that have not been answered satisfactorily. However, understanding has been enhanced by intensive research in recent years, making use of the most modern techniques. The cerebellum has long been associated with the processing of proprioceptive stimuli (muscle spindles, tendon corpuscles) that generally remain outside the conscious mind. This view has changed: Reports by Dow and Moruzzi (1958), Snider (1944), and Eccles and co-workers (1967) have shown that not only proprioceptive but virtually all sensory information (exteroceptive and interoceptive) is transmitted to the cerebellum. It is an established fact, however, that lesions of the cerebellum have never caused sensibility disorders. So far as we know, the function of the cerebellum is to regulate motor activity; it ensures proper coordination of the various groups of muscles involved in movement; it regulates muscle tone and makes corrections in the course of a movement, thus minimizing directional deviations or oscillations.

One of the remarkable morphologic aspects of the cerebellum is the structural uniformity of its cortex. So far as function and structure are correlated, this means that there are no local differences in cerebellar function. Such an organization might mean that as the complexity of the movement to be controlled increases, increasingly large areas of the cerebellar cortex are "recruited."

For a better understanding of the function of the cerebellum the following considerations, derived from morphology, are of importance:

(a) The afferent mossy fiber systems project to fairly large, rather diffuse cortical areas that extend mostly in a frontal (transverse) plane.

(b) There is convergence between the cortical projections of the various moss fiber systems. This applies, for instance, to Larsell's fourth, fifth, and sixth lobes (declive, folium, tuber), to which the cuneocerebellar tract and the corticopontocerebellar fibers project.

(c) The information that enters the cerebellum via the spinocerebellar and vestibulocerebellar mossy fibers probably cannot be compared with that coming via the pontocerebellar system. The former is modality-specific and has a low level of integration, whereas the latter is not modality-specific and is far more integrated.

(d) The cerebellar cortex is assumed to receive a continuous flow of information from the locomotor apparatus so that the situation of muscles, joints and tendons is registered from second to second. The cerebellum, however, has no memory; the data from the periphery are extinguished within a few milliseconds to be replaced by fresh data.

(e) Mossy fibers facilitate strips of P-cells via parallel fibers. This facilitation leads to firing (after spatial summation) or to a brief transient state of subliminal excitation.

(f) Via reticulocerebellar fibers, the cerebellum receives integrated information on changes or events within the CNS.

(g) The role of the integrated corticopontocerebellar information is little known. The information generally projects to the hemisphere and, more specifically, to the ansiform lobe (superior and inferior semilunar lobules).

(h) P-cells are made to fire via climbing fibers. After a climbing fiber impulse, a P-cell produces one to four action potentials, depending on its excitatory state. This state is determined by the activity in the mossy fiber system.

(i) Olivocerebellar fibers (climbing fibers) activate sagittal cortical zones that "incise" the transversely directed mossy fiber areas. In this way they select sagittally arranged strips of P-cells and, via these, sagittal slices of the central cerebellar nuclei. The olivocerebellar input is highly integrated by the convergence on the olive of impulses from the spinal cord, nuclei of the posterior funiculus, cerebral cortex, red nucleus, etc.

The functional role of the climbing fibers is still a moot point. The problem is that almost as many impulses come from the P-cells as climbing cells supply, albeit with a very special spatial arrangement. The spatial arrangement of the P-cell inhibition on the central nuclei is probably a factor that plays an important role in the function of the cerebellum.

Chapter 29

The Reticular Formation

The reticular formation is localized in the tegmentum of the medulla oblongata, pons, and midbrain. This area is characterized by a diffuse, seemingly unorganized structure with interlacing cells and fibers. Scattered through the reticular formation lie some cell accumulations with ill defined boundaries (reticular nuclei). Most reticular neurons are fairly large (20 to 70 μm), and it is notable that the larger neurons are found more medially while the smaller ones are located more laterally.

These neurons are of class I and, therefore, have gemmules and a long axon with a T-shaped division into a long ascending and a long descending branch (Fig. 29–1). In view of this, reticular neurons should be able to exert both an ascending and a descending influence. The reticular axons produce many collaterals; the dendrites extend in a plane perpendicular to the longitudinal axis of the brain stem. Synapses number many thousands per cell.

Reticular Nuclei

The nuclei of the reticular formation are arranged in three longitudinal columns in a mediolateral direction: raphe nuclei (unpaired), medial nuclei (paired), and lateral nuclei (paired). The raphe nuclei are localized in the mediosagittal plane; the medial nuclei are found centrally in each half of the tegmentum; the lateral nuclei are in a lateral position (Fig. 29–2).

MEDIAL RETICULAR NUCLEI

These nuclei are found in the central part of each half of the tegmentum and comprise medium to large cells with long axons (effector part of the reticular formation). Another conspicuous feature is that not only the reticular dendrites but also the preterminal axons with which they synapse are arranged perpendicular to the longitudinal axis of the brain stem. In view of these facts, the reticular formation can be regarded as a chain of successive dendritic segments.

The principal medial nuclei are the ventral reticular nucleus, the paramedian reticular nucleus and the gigantocellular reticular nucleus (medulla oblongata), the caudal and the oral pontine reticular nucleus and the reticulotegmental nucleus (Fig. 29–3) in the pons. The mesencephalon has chiefly lateral reticular nuclei.

Figure 29–1 General schematic representation of a cell of the reticular formation. Note the distribution of the axonal branches.

1 pons
2 medulla oblongata
3 midbrain
4 axon

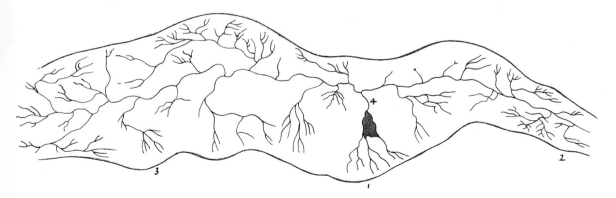

Figure 29–2 Nuclei of the reticular formation (according to Delmas).

1 midbrain
2 pons
3 medulla oblongata
4 transition to spinal cord
5 red nucleus
6 substantia nigra
7 raphe nuclei
8 medial reticular nuclei
9 lateral reticular nuclei

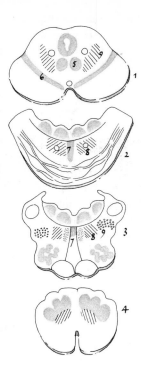

LATERAL RETICULAR NUCLEI

The lateral nuclei generally consist of smaller cells and are of a more associative character. The principal lateral nuclei are the parvicellular reticular nucleus and the lateral reticular nucleus (medulla oblongata), the parabrachial nuclei in the pons, and the pedunculopontine and cuneiform nuclei in the mesencephalon.

Some authors maintain that the reticular formation is not confined to the brain stem but extends further rostrally; some include the intralaminar thalamic nuclei, the zona incerta (subthalamus), and the septal nuclei as well as the substantia innominata (telencephalon) in the reticular formation.

RAPHE NUCLEI

The word "raphe" indicates a fiber structure (seam, interlacing) that is localized in the median plane. The median cell accumulations (raphe nuclei) are usually separated from the other nuclei of the tegmentum by dense fiber bundles. The principal raphe nuclei are the nucleus raphe obscurus and the nucleus raphe pallidus in the medulla oblongata (see Fig. 30–2), the nucleus raphe magnus, the pontine raphe nucleus, and the ventral tegmental nucleus (Fig. 29–3) in the pons, and the dorsal raphe nucleus and superior central nucleus (Fig. 29–3) in the mesencephalon.

The raphe nuclei are characterized by a high concentration of serotonin (5-hydroxytryptamine). It is currently assumed that all serotonin-synthesizing neurons are grouped in the raphe nuclei of the brain stem. However, not all cells of these nuclei synthesize serotonin.

Ascending fibers from the raphe nuclei project to various components of the limbic system (see page 200), and descending fibers extend to the cerebellum, the spinal cord, or to other brain stem nuclei.

AFFERENT FIBERS

To the Reticular Formation. Afferent fibers to the reticular formation (RF) originate from

Figure 29–3 Schematic representation of the topography of the reticular nuclei. The SVE nuclei are colored darker (according to Nieuwenhuys, Voogd, and Van Huijzen).

1 dorsal raphe nucleus
2 superior central nucleus
3 nucleus raphe pontis
4 nucleus raphe magnus
5 nucleus raphe obscurus
6 cuneiform nucleus
7 oral pontine reticular nucleus
8 pontine reticulotegmental nucleus
9 caudal pontine reticular nucleus
10 gigantocellular nucleus
11 inferior colliculus

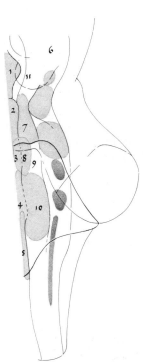

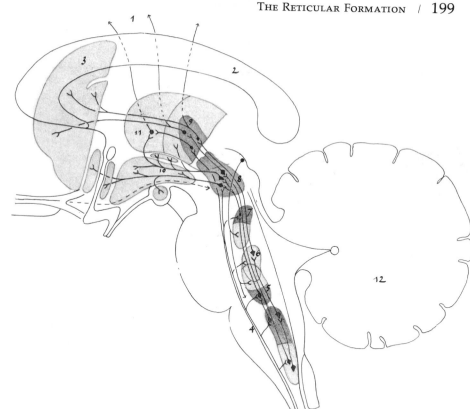

Figure 29-4 Ascending reticular fiber systems (according to Nieuwenhuys, Voogd, and Van Huijzen, modified).

1   neocortex
2   corpus callosum
3   striatum
4   spinoreticular tract
5   gigantocellular nucleus
6   caudal pontine reticular nucleus
7   oral pontine reticular nucleus
8   mesencephalic part of the reticular formation
9   nonspecific thalamic nuclei
10 telencephalic medial fasciculus
11 ventral lateral and ventral anterior nuclei
12 cerebellum

several different sources; a characteristic feature of the RF is the *convergence* of impulses from the spinal cord, cranial nerves, cerebellum, red nucleus, tectum, hypothalamus, limbic system, and neocortex. The dendritic ramification of the reticular neurons extends virtually perpendicular to the longitudinal fiber systems and is thus able to obtain information on the activity in these systems. The input is integrated in the reticular formation to influence complex motor patterns and facilitation or inhibition of distant centers. The following afferent systems are distinguished: (a) afferents from the spinal cord via the spinoreticular tract; (b) axon collaterals of secondary sensory systems (spinothalamic fasciculus, ventral spinocerebellar fasciculus, etc.); (c) afferents from the sensory nuclei of the cranial nerves; (d) afferents from the cerebral cortex via the corticoreticular tract and collaterals of the corticospinal tract; (e) afferents from the hypothalamus via the medial telencephalic fasciculus, the mamillotegmental fasciculus, and the dorsal longitudinal fasciculus of Schütz, and (f) afferents from the cerebellum via Russell's uncinate fasciculus.

The spinoreticular tract synapses in the medial (effector) part of the RF with the large neurons of the gigantocellular nucleus and the oral and caudal pontine reticular nucleus. An interesting feature is that these nuclei also extend fibers to the thalamus (intralaminar nuclei). Nearly all ascending secondarily sensory systems (except the medial lemniscus) extend collaterals to the RF. This also applies to the nuclei of the cranial nerves, particularly the trigeminal nuclei, and the vestibular system, as well as to the acoustic and optic systems, which likewise exert a marked influence on the RF. The cortical fibers terminate on the cells of the lateral reticular formation (Kuypers, 1973).

To the Raphe Nuclei. These fibers originate from the prefrontal cortex (areas 8, 9, and 10) from the spinal cord, cerebellum, lateral hypothalamic region and, particularly, from the lateral habenular nucleus. The projection habenular nucleus → mesencephalic raphe nuclei (dorsal raphe nucleus, medial raphe nucleus) is believed to be of special significance as "dorsal limbic-mesencephalic pathway," which connects the amygdala, hippocampus, and septum with the mesencephalic raphe nuclei. The circuit is as follows: hippocampus, amygdala, septum → stria medullaris → lateral habenular nucleus → fasciculus retroflexus → raphe nuclei.

EFFERENT FIBERS

From the Reticular Nuclei. Since the reticular axons have an ascending and a descending branch, ascending and descending pathways are distinguished. The principal descending pathway is the reticulospinal tract (see page 161). The ascending fibers likewise arise from the medial part of the RF, partly in pons and medulla (for example, in the oral and the caudal pontine reticular nucleus) and partly in the mesencephalon. The two ascending fiber systems project to different areas of the prosencephalon (Fig. 29–4).

The pontine and medullary ascending fibers are localized in the central tegmental fasciculus. Physiologic data would seem to suggest that these fibers are interrupted several times by numerous synapses. The fibers terminate in the nonspecific thalamic nuclei. They are the anatomic substrate of the ARAS (ascending reticular activating system), which projects to the cerebral cortex via the thalamus.

The ascending mesencephalic fibers extend in the dorsal longitudinal fasciculus of Schütz to the hypothalamus, and via the telencephalic medial fasciculus to the lateral hypothalamic area, the dorsomedial (DM) nucleus of the thalamus, and the septal area. The ascending mesencephalic fibers preferably terminate in the limbic system.

Other efferent fibers extend to the cerebellum via the inferior cerebellar peduncle. These fibers arise from the paramedian reticular and the lateral reticular nuclei. The latter projects to the neocerebellum and the central cerebellar nuclei, while the former is involved in a reticulocerebelloreticular circuit.

From the Raphe Nuclei. These fibers are not arranged in well defined bundles but are scattered among other fibers in composite fiber systems. The projection from the raphe nuclei is very extensive. Three groups of fibers are distinguished: ascending projections to telencephalon and diencephalon, cerebellar projection, and descending projections to other brain stem nuclei and the spinal cord.

The *ascending* projections arise mainly from the dorsal raphe nucleus and the medial raphe nucleus. The fibers ascend in the tegmentum and synapse in the substantia nigra, the interpeduncular nucleus, and the habenula via the fasciculus reflexus. Other fibers terminate in nonspecific nuclei of the thalamus, via the internal medullary lamina, and in the caudate nucleus and the putamen. Many fibers extend in the telencephalic medial fasciculus (medial forebrain bundle) and innervate the amygdala and the infundibulum of the neurohypophysis. The rostral part of the serotonergic projection synapses in the hippocampus, cingulum, parts of the cerebral cortex, and the olfactory bulb. It can be deduced from the above that the efferent ascending projections are not very specific, although they show a predilection for the limbic system.

The *cerebellar* projection arises from the pontine raphe nucleus; the fibers extend via the brachium pontis and synapse in the cerebellar cortex and the central cerebellar nuclei.

The *descending* projections arise from the superior central nucleus and the nucleus raphe magnus; they synapse in the locus ceruleus and in the reticular formation. From the nucleus raphe obscurus and the nucleus raphe pallidus fibers extend to the spinal cord.

Functional Significance of the Reticular Formation

Morphologic data seem to indicate that the reticular cells react to stimuli from diverse sources (such as light, pain, and vestibular and auditory stimuli). There must, therefore, be marked convergence on the reticular cells, but these cells can also exert an influence in rostral and caudal directions by means of their dividing axons. Their numerous synaptic contacts enable the cells to influence areas that are spaced far apart (divergence).

The reticular formation (RF) is able to regulate the impulse activity of the afferent fibers via marked inhibition or facilitation of the corresponding neurons. In this way the impulse transmission in many sensory fibers can be suppressed or enhanced by the RF. The RF also controls important autonomic functions such as respiration, cardiac function, and blood pressure. Certain areas in the medulla oblongata are responsible for the regulation of inspiration and expiration and for increase or decrease of the blood pressure. The boundaries of these areas are ill defined; it seems that the ''inspiratory center'' can be divided into a ventral and a dorsal group of neurons. The latter group is localized in the nucleus of the solitary tract; the former group is localized near the nucleus ambiguus and comprises inspiratory as well as expiratory neurons. The latter do not become active until the former cease firing.

The serotonergic cells of the raphe nuclei are involved also in the regulation of the sleep-wake rhythm. Several phases of sleep are distinguished, of which the most important are the non-REM phase and the REM (rapid eye movements) phase. A high serotonin level prolongs the non-REM phase and abbreviates the REM phase. Lesions in the pontine raphe nuclei lead to a state of constant waking.

The RF is involved also in controlling the tone and reflex activity of the striated muscles. This control is exerted by the pontine and medullary centers. Excitation of the medullary part (gigantocellular reticular nucleus) has an inhibitory effect on the monosynaptic stretch reflex and facilitates the polysynaptic reflexes. Excitation of the pontine part facilitates reflex activity in general. These effects are achieved by influencing the α- and γ-neurons.

Interaction of Reticular Formation and Cerebral Cortex

Electric stimulation of the reticular formation causes a characteristic change in the electroencephalogram. The α-rhythm (8 to 12 waves per second), which is typical of rest with closed eyes, is replaced with another rhythm (higher frequency and lower voltage, β-rhythm) that is characteristic of the so-called arousal or attention response. These responses can also be evoked indirectly by means of an increased sensory input, more specifically by trigeminal, pain, optic, and acoustic stimuli. All modalities of sensory stimuli of a given intensity can alter the activity of the cortex.

The reticular formation exerts influence on the cortex via the ascending reticular activating system (ARAS). The morphologic substrate is provided by the medullary and pontine reticular nuclei with their ascending reticulothalamic fibers, which extend in the central tegmental fasciculus. The reticular impulses reach the cerebral cortex via the nonspecific thalamic nuclei. The importance of the reticular formation for the regulation of the level of consciousness is evident from the observation that denervation of part of the RF can cause a state of profound unconsciousness (coma). On the other hand, electric stimulation of other reticular areas can cause arousal from sleep.

Chapter 30

Internal Configuration of the Brain Stem

The topography of nuclei and tracts in the brain stem is best studied on the basis of a number of transverse sections. Attention will be focused on the structure and fiber projections of some brain stem nuclei not yet discussed. The few levels portrayed cannot possibly show all of the important structures present in the region. Consequently, the discussion of each level will intentionally include some important structures that lie either somewhat caudal or rostral to the section shown.

The Medulla Oblongata

(1) LEVEL OF THE PYRAMIDAL DECUSSATION

The area of transition between medulla oblongata and spinal cord still shows unmistakable structural similarities to the spinal cord (Fig. 30–1), but there are no dorsal roots; ventral roots are represented by the axons of the so-called supraspinal nucleus (first cervical nerve).

The anterior horn of the spinal cord is markedly reduced and confines itself to the cells of origin of the 11th cranial nerve and the supraspinal nucleus. A striking feature is the decussation of the pyramidal fibers: Some 90 per cent of these fibers cross the midline and come to occupy a lateral position in the future lateral funiculus.

Around the dorsal end of the decussating pyramidal fibers is found a horseshoe-shaped area (central reticular nucleus) with scanty cells (reticular formation). The changes in the posterior horn are drastic: The nucleus of the trigeminal spinal tract is highly developed and separated from the surface by the trigeminal spinal tract. At lower levels the nucleus becomes the substantia gelatinosa of the posterior horn (lamina II), while the tract becomes Lissauer's marginal zone. The continuity of the posterior horn is interrupted by the decussating pyramidal fibers (Fig. 30–1).

The superficial fiber systems of the anterolateral funiculus (posterior spinocerebellar, anterior spinocerebellar, and spinotectal tracts) have hardly changed their position. The lateral spinothalamic tract is adjacent to the lateral reticular nucleus.

The posterior funiculus is very extensive; the available space is partly occupied by the neurons of the nucleus gracilis, in which the fibers of the fasciculus gracilis end. The nucleus cuneatus develops at a slightly higher level than the nucleus gracilis.

(2) LEVEL MID-OLIVE

The central canal is in part displaced dorsally and constitutes the floor of the fourth ventricle. The nuclei of the olivary complex are clearly visible. The aperture, the hilus, of the principal olive faces medially. Here, many fibers emerge which extend to the midline and cross it ventral to the decussation of the lemniscus (olivocerebellar fibers). These fibers join the spinocerebellar systems that come from the spinal cord and, with them, form the restiform body. The medial accessory olive lies medial to the olive, while the dorsal accessory olive lies dorsal to it (Fig. 30–2). Ventral to the olive, on either side of the ventral median fissure, lies the pyramidal tract. Right up against the ventral surface lie the arcuate nuclei, which constitute the caudal part of a group of nuclei whose axons extend to the cerebellum.

In the raphe region we distinguish the ventrally located nucleus raphe pallidus and the dorsally located nucleus raphe obscurus (Fig. 30–2). The area between is occupied by the medial lemniscus. On either side of the nucleus raphe obscurus extends the medial longitudinal

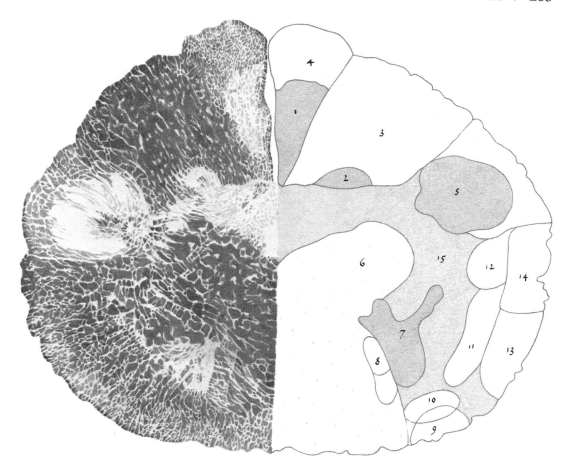

fasciculus, which is not always clearly distinguishable from the medial lemniscus. At this level the medial longitudinal fasciculus comprises the medial vestibulospinal tract, the interstitiospinal fibers (from Cajal's interstitial nucleus), and reticulospinal fibers.

A row of cranial nerve nuclei is found in the floor of the fourth ventricle. The most medial of them is the nucleus of the hypoglossal nerve (12th cranial), while more laterally the dorsal nucleus of the vagus nerve (intestinal nucleus) is found. The nucleus solitarius is located lateral to the sulcus limitans. Further laterally and caudally is found the cuneate nucleus and the accessory cuneate nucleus.

The restiform body is immediately adjacent to the spinal tract of the trigeminal nerve and the corresponding nucleus of the spinal tract. Centrally in the tegmentum lies the nucleus ambiguus, which consists of multipolar cells. A

Figure 30–1 Transverse section through the area of transition from spinal cord to medulla oblongata at the level of the decussation of the pyramidal fibers. The fibers are shown on the left; the outlines of the nuclei (gray) and the fiber tracts (white) are shown on the right.

1 nucleus gracilis
2 nucleus cuneatus
3 fasciculus cuneatus
4 fasciculus gracilis
5 nucleus of the spinal tract (of the trigeminal nerve)
6 pyramidal fibers (decussating)
7 accessory nucleus
8 medial longitudinal fasciculus
9 anterior spinothalamic tract
10 lateral vestibulospinal tract
11 lateral spinothalamic tract
12 rubrospinal tract
13 anterior spinocerebellar tract
14 posterior spinocerebellar tract
15 reticular formation

large part of the tegmentum is occupied by the gigantocellular reticular nucleus, lateral to which lies the lateral reticular nucleus.

Topography of the Fiber Systems. Little has changed in the position of the long fiber systems. The lateral spinothalamic tract is still at a considerable distance from the medial lemniscus; the spinocerebellar tracts have begun to diverge. These tracts still occupy a fairly superficial position on the lateral side of the medulla oblongata.

(3) LEVEL OF THE COCHLEAR NERVE

The central canal has widened to become the fourth ventricle. The olivary complex and the pyramidal tract are unchanged; the nucleus

raphe pallidus and the nucleus raphe obscurus are still visible in the median plane. Lateral to them, the medial lemniscus and the medial longitudinal fasciculus are seen (Fig. 30–3).

Of the cranial nerves, the nucleus of the spinal tract of the trigeminal nerve, the nucleus ambiguus, and the nucleus solitarius are visible. The hypoglossal nucleus and the dorsal nucleus of the vagus nerve have disappeared. In the area between the inferior cerebellar peduncle and the fourth ventricle, the nuclei of the posterior funiculus and the external cuneate nucleus have likewise disappeared. Instead, one finds components of the vestibular nuclear complex (lateral, inferior, and medial vestibular nucleus). Very superficially, against the outside of the peduncle, the ventral and the dorsal cochlear nuclei are localized (Fig. 30–3).

Figure 30–2 Transverse section through the caudal part of the medulla oblongata. Note the nuclei of origin of the hypoglossal and vagus nerves.

1 nucleus of the hypoglossal nerve
2 medial longitudinal fasciculus
3 tectospinal tract
4 nucleus raphe obscurus
5 fourth ventricle
6 gigantocellular nucleus
7 dorsal nucleus of vagus nerve
8 medial vestibular nucleus
9 inferior vestibular nucleus
10 accessory cuneate nucleus
11 inferior cerebellar peduncle
12 spinal tract of the trigeminal nerve
13 nucleus of the spinal tract
14 nucleus ambiguus
15 lateral reticular nucleus
16 dorsal accessory olivary nucleus
17 nucleus of the inferior olive
18 corticospinal tract
19 arcuate nucleus
20 medial accessory olivary nucleus
21 medial lemniscus
22 nucleus raphe pallidus
23 lateral spinothalamic tract
24 posterior spinocerebellar tract
25 rubrospinal tract
26 solitary tract and nucleus
27 vagus nerve

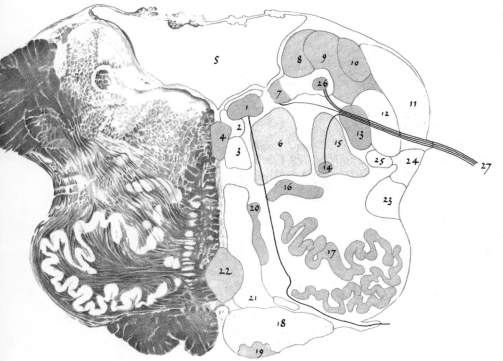

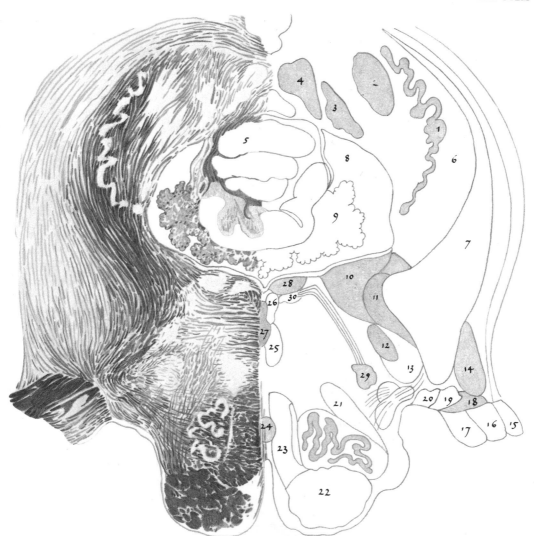

Figure 30–3 Transverse section through the transition from medulla oblongata to pons. Note the central cerebellar nuclei around the wall of the fourth ventricle.

1 dentate nucleus
2 emboliform nucleus
3 globose nucleus
4 fastigial nucleus
5 cerebellar lingula
6 inferior cerebellar peduncle
7 middle cerebellar peduncle
8 fourth ventricle
9 choroid plexus
10 medial vestibular nucleus
11 inferior vestibular nucleus

12 nucleus of spinal tract of V
13 spinal tract of V
14 inferior cochlear nucleus
15 vestibular nerve
16 cochlear nerve
17 facial nerve
18 pontobulbar nucleus
19 lateral spinothalamic tract
20 anterior spinothalamic tract
21 central tegmental tract
22 corticospinal tract

23 medial lemniscus
24 nucleus raphe pallidus
25 tectospinal tract
26 medial longitudinal fasciculus
27 nucleus raphe obscurus
28 abducens nucleus
29 facial nerve nucleus
30 ascending fibers of facial nerve

The large reticular cells of the gigantocellular nucleus are located centrally in the tegmentum. Lateral to them there is an extensive area with few cells and numerous, rather widely dispersed, fibers; this is the area of the parvicellular nucleus, which is difficult to demarcate.

Topography of the Fiber Systems. On either side of the midline, the same fiber systems are found as in the previous section, namely, the medial lemniscus and the medial longitudinal fasciculus. The central tegmental fasciculus is localized centrally in the tegmentum, well within the area of the parvicellular reticular nucleus. This fairly diffuse bundle consists of short fibers that synapse with other reticular cells. In the lateral part of the medulla, an evagination is seen which is caused by the inferior cerebellar peduncle. The spinal tract of the trigeminal nerve lies snugly against the peduncle (Fig. 30–3).

It can be stated, in general, that the long fiber systems have two sites of predilection in the medulla oblongata. One site is the area on either side of the midline where, apart from the pyramidal tract, the medial lemniscus, medial longitudinal fasciculus, and dorsal longitudinal fasciculus are stacked. This space is divided between the aforementioned tracts and the raphe nuclei (nucleus raphe pallidus and nucleus raphe obscurus). The second site of predilection is the angle between the inferior cerebellar peduncle and the inferior olive. Here is found, closely packed, the spinothalamic, anterior spinocerebellar, lateral vestibulospinal, and rubroolivary tracts and, in a slightly more medial position, the rubrospinal tract (Fig. 30–3).

The Pons

(4) LEVEL OF THE FACIAL NERVE

At this level there is a marked difference between tegmentum and base. The base comprises transverse fiber bundles (pontocerebellar fibers), among which the pontine nuclei are localized. The pontocerebellar fibers cross the midline and enter the cerebellum via the middle cerebellar peduncle. In the base, the pyramidal tract is divided into many bundles that cross transversely arranged pontocerebellar fibers.

The tegmentum comprises the nuclei of origin of a few cranial nerves and other nuclei that are specific to the pons. Nuclei of the cranial nerves include the abducens nucleus, the nucleus of the facial nerve, and the nucleus of the trigeminal spinal tract. The abducens nucleus is located immediately beneath the floor of the fourth ventricle (Fig. 30–4), while the nucleus of the facial nerve lies deeper, as a SVE nucleus should. The nucleus of the spinal tract has not changed its position.

Of the specific nuclei of the pons, the pontine nuclei should be mentioned first. In addition we find the superior olivary nucleus and the nucleus of the trapezoid body (both of which are links in the acoustic pathway). The superior olive lies ventromedial to the facial nerve nucleus and consists of fusiform cells. The nucleus of the trapezoid body is small and not readily demarcated because it lies among the fibers of the trapezoid body (Fig. 30–4). Immediately beneath the floor of the ventricle, dorsal to the abducens nucleus, is found the nucleus prepositus of the hypoglossal nerve. Lateral to it lie the vestibular nuclei: the medial, inferior, and lateral vestibular nuclei.

Topography of the Fiber Systems. On either side of the midline we see the dorsal longitudinal fasciculus of Schütz, the medial longitudinal fascilus, and the tectospinal tract (Fig. 30–4). The medial lemniscus rotates 90° and becomes a transverse fiber band between the tegmentum and the base of the pons. Ventral to it extend the fibers of the trapezoid body. The spinothalamic and the spinotectal tracts leave their superficial position and come to lie lateral to the medial lemniscus. At this level the spinothalamic and the spinotectal tracts, together with the rubrospinal tract, are localized between the medial lemniscus and the superior olive. The central tegmental fasciculus joins the rubrospinal tract and fills the space between the medial lemniscus and the facial nucleus. The trigeminal tract has not changed its position.

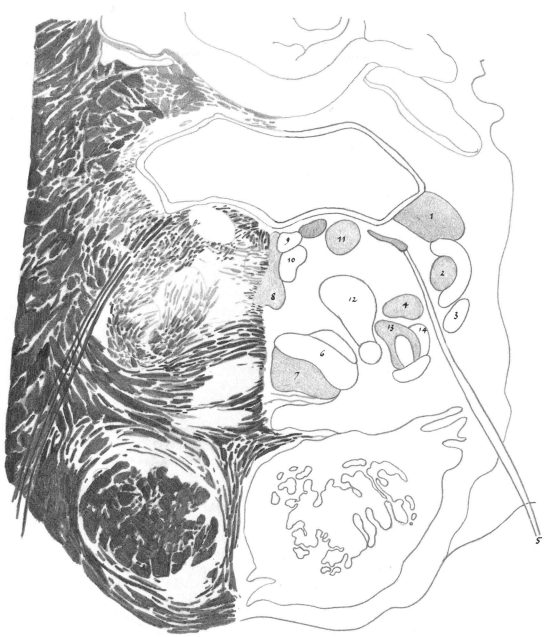

Figure 30–4 Transverse section through the pons, with the nuclei of origin of the facial and abducens nerves. The trapezoid body marks the boundary between the tegmentum and the base.

1 superior vestibular nucleus
2 nucleus of spinal tract of V
3 anterior spinocerebellar tract
4 facial nerve nucleus
5 facial nerve
6 medial lemniscus
7 nucleus raphe magnus
8 pontine raphe nucleus
9 medial longitudinal fasciculus
10 tectospinal tract
11 nucleus of the abducens nerve
12 central tegmental tract
13 superior olivary nucleus
14 lateral lemniscus

(5) LEVEL OF THE MASTICATORY NUCLEUS

The base of the pons is well developed; the pontocerebellar fibers run laterally to the cerebellum via the middle cerebellar peduncle. The nuclei of origin of the trigeminal nerve are found in the tegmentum. The nucleus of the spinal tract is a long column that extends from this level to the cervical spinal cord. The masticatory nucleus is found medial to the thickened upper end of the nucleus of the spinal tract (principal nucleus). The nucleus of the mesencephalic tract of the trigeminal nerve can be seen as a column of cells beneath the lateral corner of the fourth ventricle, beneath the superior cerebellar peduncle (Fig. 30–5).

Quite near the nucleus of the mesencephalic tract, against the floor of the corner of the fourth ventricle, is seen a nucleus (locus ceruleus) that comprises dark blue-brown cells of medium size (see below). Medial to the line from masticatory nucleus to locus ceruleus is a large area with scanty cells. This is the reticular formation made up of the oral pontine reticular nucleus and the reticulotegmental nucleus. In the raphe region, the superior central nucleus is located.

Topography of the Fiber Systems. This level is characterized by the massive fiber bundles that arise from the pontine nuclei and extend to the cerebellum via the middle cerebellar peduncle. In the tegmentum, several fiber tracts are arranged on the dorsolateral side of the medial lemniscus (Fig. 30–5). On either side of the midline, immediately beneath the ventricle, the medial longitudinal fasciculus and the tectospinal tract are found. The central tegmental fasciculus lies at the center of the tegmentum, within the area of the oral pontine reticular nucleus. Dorsal to this fasciculus, the dorsal trigeminothalamic fibers extend. The fourth ventricle is bounded laterally by the superior cerebellar peduncle, in which the ventral spinocerebellar tract is found.

(6) LEVEL OF THE RHOMBENCEPHALIC ISTHMUS

This section is through the trochlear nerve nucleus and the inferior colliculus, the area of transition between the pons and the mensencephalon. The fourth ventricle has disappeared, to be replaced by the cerebral aqueduct. The base of the pons and the pontocerebellar fibers are markedly reduced. The tegmentum is slightly larger, and the alar plate (tectum) has increased in size. In the tectum is found the inferior colliculus, separated from the outer surface by the brachium of the inferior colliculus. In the base of the colliculus are the incoming fibers from the lateral lemniscus, which synapse with the neurons of the colliculus.

Here the reticular formation is represented by vestiges of the oral pontine reticular nucleus and, more specifically, by the pedunculopontine reticular nucleus, which receives afferent fibers from the pallidum and from the precentral gyrus of the cortex. The dorsal raphe nucleus is found between the trochlear nucleus and the aqueduct. The interpeduncular nucleus is located ventral to the decussation of the superior cerebellar peduncles.

The nuclei of the cranial nerves are represented at this level by the trochlear nerve nucleus, which consists of large multipolar cells and is located fairly far from the aqueduct, medial to the medial longitudinal fasciculus. The nucleus of the spinal tract has disappeared, but the nucleus of the mesencephalic tract of the trigeminal nerve is still visible (Fig. 30–6).

Topography of the Fiber Systems. Marked changes in the position of the large fiber systems are evident. The base of the section shows similarities to the cerebral peduncles (mesencephalon) and the base of the pons (rhombencephalon). Laterally, the large descending systems are recognizable: the occipitotemporopontine fibers on the dorsal side, the corticospinal fibers in the middle, and the

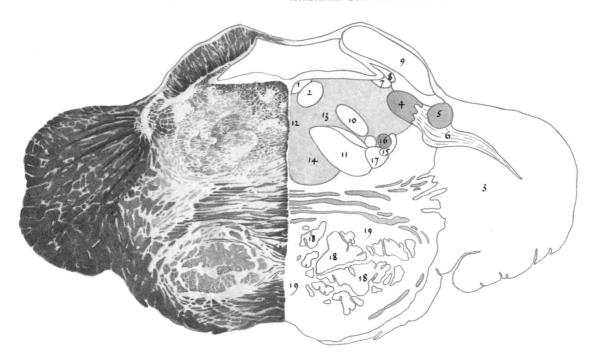

frontopontine fibers on the medial side. The pontine nuclei and the transversely extending pontocerebellar fibers are seen in the medioventral region of the section.

The boundary between tegmentum and base is again formed by the medial lemniscus, together with the basal part of the substantia nigra (Fig. 30–6). The medial lemniscus has increased in size because the spinothalamic and spinotectal fibers have joined it; moreover, it has moved to the periphery and now shows some curvature. The central part of the tegmentum is occupied by the decussation of the superior cerebellar peduncles. Immediately dorsal to the decussation, the fibers of the tectospinal tract are found; ventral to it and on either side of the interpeduncular nucleus lies the rubrospinal tract. The medial longitudinal fasciculus extends between the tectospinal tract and the trochlear nucleus. The dorsal longitudinal fasciculus is located centrally in the central gray matter, immediately beneath the aqueduct.

Figure 30–5 Transverse section through the pons, with masticatory nucleus and locus ceruleus. The pyramidal fibers are divided into numerous bundles.

1 medial longitudinal fasciculus
2 tectospinal tract
3 middle cerebellar peduncle
4 masticatory nucleus
5 principal nucleus
6 trigeminal fibers
7 locus ceruleus
8 nucleus of the mesencephalic tract (of trigeminal nerve)
9 superior cerebellar peduncle
10 central tegmental tract
11 medial lemniscus
12 superior central nucleus
13 oral pontine reticular nucleus
14 reticulotegmental nucleus
15 lateral lemniscus
16 nucleus of lateral lemniscus
17 lateral spinothalamic tract
18 pyramidal fibers
19 pontine nuclei

The not readily definable central tegmental fasciculus (central tegmental tract) lies embedded in the reticular formation; the dorsal trigeminothalamic fibers run beside it, while the ventral trigeminothalamic fibers have joined the medial lemniscus.

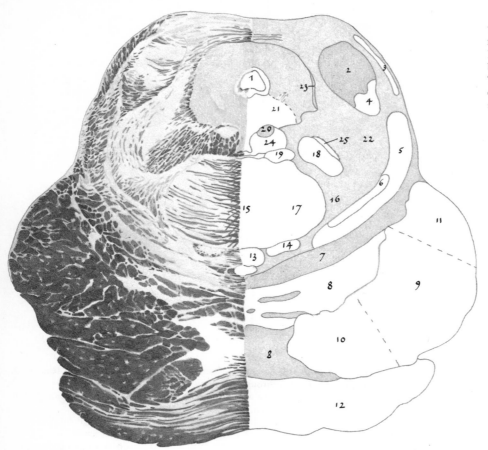

Figure 30–6 Transverse section through the rhombencephalic isthmus. Note the decussating cerebellorubrothalamic fibers. The upper fibers of the middle cerebellar peduncle are still visible.

1	cerebral aqueduct	9	crus cerebri (corticospinal tract)	
2	inferior colliculus	10	crus cerebri (frontopontine tract)	
3	brachium of the inferior colliculus	11	crus cerebri (occipitopontine tract)	
4	lateral lemniscus	12	middle cerebellar peduncle	
5	medial lemniscus	13	interpeduncular nucleus	
6	ventral trigeminothalamic fibers	14	rubrospinal tract	
7	substantia nigra			
8	pontine nuclei			

15	ventral tegmental nucleus
16	pedunculopontile reticular nucleus
17	decussation of superior peduncles
18	central tegmental tract
19	tectospinal tract
20	trochlear nerve nucleus
21	dorsal raphe nucleus

22	oral pontine reticular nucleus
23	nucleus of mesencephalic tract (of trigeminal nerve)
24	medial longitudinal fasciculus
25	dorsal trigeminothalamic fibers

THE LOCUS CERULEUS: STRUCTURE AND FIBER CONNECTIONS

The locus ceruleus is grossly visible as a blue streak in the lateral part of the upper half of the fourth ventricle. The locus ceruleus had long been regarded as a part of the trigeminal nuclei until norepinephrine-containing neurons were discovered in it. The locus ceruleus has since been regarded as an independent structure (Fig. 30–5).

In the rat, the locus ceruleus is surrounded by a plexus of not readily stainable, very thin fibers of obscure origin. On the basis of cytoarchitectonic data, a ventral and a dorsal part can be distinguished. The dorsal part comprises medium-size fusiform cells, localized between the nucleus of the mesencephalic tract of the trigeminal nerve and the superior vestibular nucleus. The ventral part comprises fewer cells, but these are larger and often multipolar. The dendrites of the multipolar cells are long and exceed the boundaries of the locus ceruleus. They have contacts with cells of the nucleus of the mesencephalic tract and of the central gray matter. Locus ceruleus cells are characterized by thin processes that resemble axons and arise directly from the perikaryon (somatic gemmules). The cells contain norepinephrine and the enzyme dopamine hydroxylase, which converts dopamine to norepinephrine. These adrenergic neurons project to extensive areas of the CNS.

Many noradrenergic nerve endings are involved in the innervation of cerebral blood vessels. Modern investigators are inclined to assume that noradrenergic fibers play a role in the regulation of the cerebral blood flow. Moreover, the locus ceruleus seems to be active in physiologic processes like regulation of respiration, micturition, and the sleep-wake rhythm.

Afferent Fibers. These originate from the pontine raphe nucleus, the nucleus raphe magnus, and the ipsilateral part of the substantia nigra. Other fibers originate from the nucleus of the solitary tract and from an area surrounding the facial nerve nucleus.

Efferent Fibers. These are largely localized in the dorsal noradrenergic system; other efferent fibers extend to the cerebellum, medulla oblongata, and spinal cord. The dorsal noradrenergic system is quite extensive. One distinguishes a main group of fibers that ascend in the lateral part of the tegmentum and reach the septal area via the lateral hypothalamic area; these fibers continue in fibers that innervate the cingulum. From the main group, many fibers curve away to extensive areas of the mesencephalon and telencephalon: to the tectum, thalamus, amygdala, hippocampus, and neocortex. It is astonishing that a relatively small number of cells can project to so extensive an area.

The fibers to the cerebellum run through the superior cerebellar peduncle and innervate the central nuclei and the cortex. Fibers to the spinal cord run through its entire length and innervate the anterior horn and the base of the posterior horn.

The Mesencephalon

(7) LEVEL OF THE OCULOMOTOR NERVE

The components of the mesencephalon are clearly distinguishable: the tectum dorsally, the tegmentum centrally, and the crus cerebri ventrally. Around the aqueduct lies a fairly wide layer of gray matter (central gray matter) that lacks myelinated fibers. Lateral to the tegmentum are nuclei that belong to the diencephalon: the lateral geniculate body and the pulvinar.

The superior colliculus shows alternate layers of gray and white matter. From its lateral area a strong bundle of fibers extends between the pulvinar and medial geniculate body (Fig. 30–7); this is the brachium of the superior colliculus, on its way to the lateral geniculate body. The inferior colliculus has already disappeared.

Of the cranial nerves, the nucleus of the oculomotor nerve and the nucleus of the mesencephalic tract of the trigeminal nerve are found. The oculomotor nucleus lies on either side of the midline against the central gray matter. The nucleus is divided into a gigantocellular and a parvicellular part. The former innervates extrinsic eye muscles and consists of large multipolar cells with unmistakable Nissl bodies. The latter (Edinger-Westphal's nucleus and anterior median nucleus) is located medial to the gigantocellular part.

The nucleus of the mesencephalic tract is still in evidence as a thin layer of cells localized at the edge of the central gray matter, on the boundary between tectum and tegmentum (Fig. 30–7).

In the rostral part of the tegmentum, where the aqueduct opens up into the third ventricle, two small nuclei are located between the central gray matter and the reticular formation; these are Cajal's interstitial nucleus and the nucleus of Darkschevich. The former is an accumulation of multipolar cells slightly lateral to the medial longitudinal fasciculus; the latter lies within the central gray matter quite near Cajal's nucleus.

The reticular formation is localized between the red nucleus and medial lemniscus on the one hand and the central gray matter on the other. In it is the cuneiform nucleus, while the raphe nuclei are represented by the linear nucleus. The cells of the central gray matter are rather small and difficult to stain. They continue in a rostral direction in the periventricular gray matter of the third ventricle.

The interpeduncular nucleus is localized against the floor of the interpeduncular fossa, in the midline. Its cells are fusiform and rather

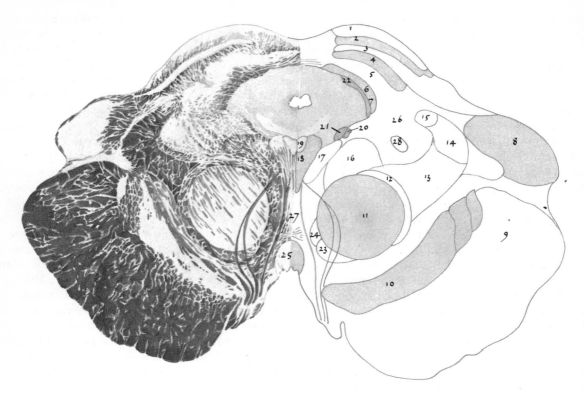

Figure 30–7 Transverse section through the mesencephalon. The stratified structure of the superior colliculus is clearly shown.

1	zonal layer
2,3	optic layer
4,5	lemniscal layer
6,7	deep layer
8	medial geniculate body
9	crus cerebri
10	substantia nigra
11	red nucleus
12	cerebellorubrothalamic fibers
13	medial lemniscus
14	spinothalamic tract
15	spinotectal tract
16	central tegmental tract
17	medial longitudinal fasciculus
18	nucleus of oculomotor nerve
19	Edinger-Westphal nucleus
20	Cajal's interstitial nucleus
21	nucleus of Darkshevich
22	nucleus of mesencephalic tract
23	rubrospinal tract
24	fasciculus retroflexus
25	interpeduncular nucleus
26	cuneiform nucleus
27	linear nucleus
28	trigeminothalamic tract

small, and are closely packed. The habenulointerpeduncular fasciculus (Meynert's fasciculus retroflexus) synapses with these cells.

The largest grossly visible nucleus in transverse sections through the mesencephalon is the substantia nigra. This semilunar area is localized on the boundary between tegmentum and crus cerebri (Fig. 30–7). The lateral margin adjacent to the crus cerebri is crenated, whereas the medial margin is smooth. The ventromedial part of the nucleus is traversed by fibers from the oculomotor nucleus. The substantia nigra extends along the entire mesencephalon; the rostral part almost touches the globus pallidus. The caudal part continues in the pontine nuclei.

The red nucleus localized centrally in the tegmentum is pink on cross-section and can thus be distinguished from adjacent tissue. Fibers of the oculomotor nerve traverse the central part of this nucleus.

Topography of the Fiber Systems. The fiber systems in the mesencephalon comprise fibers that run through the crus cerebri and those that run through the tegmentum. At the base of the mesencephalon, we find almost exclusively fibers. This phylogenetically young area attains maximal development in humans. The fibers arise from the cerebral cortex and extend to the pons, medulla oblongata, and spinal cord. The lateral fibers of the peduncle (Fig. 30–6) come from the occipital and the temporal lobe (Arnold's temporopontine fasciculus) and synapse in the nuclei of the pons; the central area is occupied by the corticobulbar and corticospinal tracts, with synapses in the nuclei of the cranial nerves and in the spinal cord, respectively. The medial area comprises fibers from the frontal lobe (Türck's frontopontile fasciculus), which synapse in the pontine nuclei.

Many ascending, descending, and associative fiber systems run in the tegmentum. The dorsal longitudinal fasciculus of Schütz is located in the central gray matter, quite near the midline. The bundle runs through the entire brain stem as far as the cervical spinal cord, without changing its position. The medial longitudinal fasciculus lies alongside the midline, ventral to the previous fasciculus; it extends from Cajal's interstitial nucleus to about T2 in the spinal cord.

The medial lemniscus still comprises — in addition to the original fibers of the posterior funiculus — the fibers of the spinothalamic and the spinotectal tracts as well as the ventral trigeminothalamic fibers. The entire structure is located lateral to the red nucleus, between this nucleus and the medial geniculate body. Lateral to the medial lemniscus is the brachium of the inferior colliculus, through which the acoustic fibers from (among others) the inferior colliculus reach the medial geniculate body.

Between medial lemniscus and red nucleus, a sickle-shaped layer of fibers is observed; this is the cerebellorubral tract, which is a component of the cerebellorubrothalamic projection from the central cerebellar nuclei, of whose fibers about 50 per cent synapse in the rostral one-third of the red nucleus.

Ventromedial to the red nucleus, the rubrospinal tract and the fasciculus retroflexus extend to the interpeduncular nucleus. Immediately behind the latter nucleus are fibers that cross the midline (Forel's ventral tegmental decussation). Here the rubrospinal fibers cross to the contralateral side. Dorsal to the ventral tegmental decussation, the tectospinal fibers also cross to the contralateral side (dorsal tegmental decussation).

The central tegmental tract still lies in the reticular formation, between the red nucleus and the medial longitudinal fasciculus. Lateral to this tract are the dorsal trigeminothalamic fibers. Descending fibers to the substantia nigra (pallidonigral and corticonigral fibers) are localized more laterally, at the edge of the substantia nigra.

Chapter 31

Structure and Connections of Some Mesencephalic Nuclei

Superior Colliculus

The superior colliculus is grossly visible as a round elevation on the rostral part of the alar plate. The colliculus consists of alternate layers of cells and fibers (Fig. 31–1). Layers 2, 4, and 6 comprise mainly cells, whereas layers 1, 3, 5, and 7 are fiber layers. A distinction is made between the optic layer (2 and 3), the lemniscal layer (4 and 5), and the deep layer (6 and 7). In humans, the optic layer is far less developed than in nonprimates. The superior colliculus with its stratified structure has the character of a cortex.

Afferent Fibers. Most afferent fibers originate from the cerebral cortex (areas 8, 18, and 19). These are homolateral fibers that synapse in the optic and the lemniscal layers (rostral part of the colliculus). Other afferent fibers come from the retina via the optic nerve, optic tract, and brachium of the superior colliculus. They end mostly in the optic layer. In the deep and the lemniscal layers, too, many fibers from the cuneiform nucleus (reticular formation) synapse. Fibers from the spinal cord and lateral lemniscus synapse in the lemniscal layer; on this layer, therefore, impulses from the cerebral cortex, retina, spinal cord, reticular formation, and inferior colliculus converge.

Efferent Fibers. Efferent fibers connect the superior colliculus with the spinal cord, reticular formation, pontine nuclei, and thalamus. The tectospinal fibers cross the midline in the dorsal tegmental decussation and extend to the spinal cord (see page 161). Tectoreticular fibers extend to the cuneiform nucleus and the pedunculopontine tegmental nucleus on the ipsilateral and the contralateral sides. Other fibers terminate in Cajal's interstitial nucleus. Tectopontine fibers synapse in the homolateral rostral pontine nuclei; some investigators maintain that optic impulses reach the cerebellum by this route, but others hold that direct tectocerebellar fibers are located in the superior cerebellar peduncle. Tectothalamic fibers arise from the optic layer and project to the homolateral pulvinar and lateral geniculate bodies.

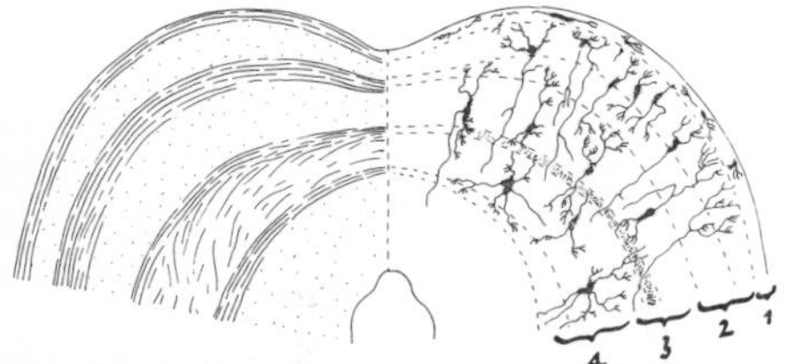

Substantia Nigra

The substantia nigra has two main structural components: the cellular compact part and the fibrous reticular part. The former comprises medium-size cells that contain melanin. The pigment melanin appears in about the fifth year of life and increases in the course of years. The reticular part, however, consists of a dense plexus of fibers with irregularly scattered cells that contain lipofuscin and iron but no melanin. Near the cerebral peduncle, the cells of the reticular part are smaller and resemble pallidal cells.

TYPOLOGY OF THE NEURONS

Using the Golgi technique, three neuron types can be distinguished: large neurons (45 to 65 μm), which characterize the reticular part; medium-size neurons (20 to 45 μm); and small

Figure 31–1 Structure of the superior colliculus (according to Sterzi). Fibers on the left, and neurons on the right (Golgi technique).

1 zonal layer
2 optic layer
3 lemniscal layer
4 deep layer

cells (12 to 26 μm), which are characterized by very thin, radiating dendrites and a short axon. The neurons of the compact part are of medium size; they have one or two long dendrites that can even penetrate the reticular part. The axons of these cells are thin and often arise from a dendrite. The axons of the neurons in the compact part are the characteristic dopaminergic fibers of the substantia nigra. The reticular part seems to be the principal area where afferent fibers to the substantia nigra synapse.

FIBER CONNECTIONS

It is technically difficult to study these, and they are not fully known. It can be stated in summary that this nucleus is closely related to the striatum (see Fig. 36–2).

Afferent Fibers. The known afferent fibers originate from the caudate nucleus, the putamen and, according to recent research (Hattori et al., 1975), from the pallidum.

The strionigral projection shows a topical organization: The head of the caudate nucleus projects to ventrolateral parts of the substantia nigra, and the putamen to its caudal parts. The striatal fibers run through the globus pallidus and produce collaterals to this nucleus; they then leave the pallidum and descend to the substantia nigra, where they synapse in the reticular part. These fibers probably contain GABA as a neurotransmitter. Fibers from the pallidum synapse in the compact part with axodendritic synapses.

Efferent Fibers. Degeneration experiments indicate that the substantia nigra comprises two different neuron populations: one population (reticular part) projects to the thalamus, and the other (compact part) to the striatum. The nigrostriatal projection comprises exceedingly thin, not readily stainable fibers that arise from the compact part. These fibers ascend to above the subthalamic nucleus, traverse the internal capsule, run through the pallidum, and synapse in the caudate nucleus and the putamen. The nigrothalamic projection arises from the rostrolateral part of the reticular part. The fibers ascend through the prerubral field (Forel's field H),

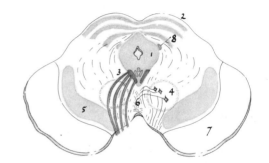

Figure 31–2 Transverse section through the mesencephalon at the level of the nucleus of origin of the oculomotor nerve.

1 central gray matter
2 superior colliculus
3 nucleus of origin of the oculomotor nerve
4 red nucleus
5 substantia nigra
6 ventral tegmental decussation
7 crus cerebri
8 nucleus of the mesencephalic tract of the trigeminal nerve

whence they extend rostrally and dorsally to the ventral anterior (VA) and the ventral lateral (VL) nuclei of the thalamus.

FUNCTIONAL ASPECTS

Nigrostriatal fibers transport dopamine to the cells of the striatum. In patients with Parkinson's disease, the dopamine concentration in the substantia nigra and the striatum is known to be diminished. In modern treatment of Parkinson's disease, L-dopa is combined with decarboxylase inhibitors; in these cases the L-dopa is not converted to dopamine outside the CNS, but almost the entire L-dopa dose is utilized within the CNS.

Red Nucleus

The red nucleus — thus called in view of its light pinkish color in fresh preparations — is located in the ventrolateral part of the tegmentum, dorsal to the substantia nigra. In transverse sections it has a fairly regular round shape. At the level of the superior colliculus this nucleus is perforated by the fibers of the oculomotor nerve; fibers from the superior cerebellar peduncle and fasciculus retroflexus likewise extend among the cells of the red nucleus (see Fig. 30–7). In the three-dimensional view, the nucleus resembles a "column" that extends from the transition between mesencephalon and diencephalon to the level of the superior colliculus.

Structurally distinguishable are an upper part (parvicellular part), which comprises medium-size and small neurons, and a lower part (magnocellular part), which comprises large and very large cells. In humans, the magnocellular part comprises a small group of about 200 cells in the most caudal area of the red nucleus. The neurons of the nucleus contain much iron, and the entire red nucleus is enclosed by a richly fibrous capsule.

CELL TYPES

The large neurons have a central nucleus and numerous Nissl bodies; the medium-size (20 to 30 μm) cells of the parvicellular part are triangular or fusiform in shape. The nucleus in these cells is eccentric, and the Nissl bodies are granular and located at the periphery of the perikaryon. These medium-size cells are often accompanied by glia satellites (oligodendroglia cells). Golgi staining shows that the perikaryon of the red nucleus cells possesses gemmules (somatic gemmules). The dendrites radiate in all directions but do not exceed the boundaries of the nucleus.

The medium-size cells have less ramified, thinner dendrites with scanty gemmules. The small cells have thin but long dendrites and an axon that ends very close to the perikaryon. The nuclei of these cells are relatively large and occupy most of the perikaryon.

FIBER CONNECTIONS

Afferent Fibers. Afferent fibers originate from the cerebellum and the cerebral cortex.

Those from the cerebellum arise from the nucleus interpositus and the dentate nucleus. They cross the midline and synapse in the contralateral red nucleus. The fibers from the nucleus interpositus synapse mainly in the caudal part of the red nucleus. The fibers from the cortex arise mainly from the frontal lobe and run through the internal capsule to the homolateral red nucleus. These fibers are arranged as follows: Fibers from the cortical area that innervates the upper extremity synapse in the dorsal part of the red nucleus, whereas those from the "lower extremity area" of the cortex synapse in the ventral part of the red nucleus.

Efferent Fibers. Efferent fibers extend to the spinal cord, the cerebellum, and the inferior olive. Ascending rubrothalamic projections have not been demonstrated with certainty. The rubrospinal tract arises from the caudal three-fourths of the red nucleus, crosses the midline in the ventral tegmental decussation (Forel), and descends alongside the branchimotor nuclei (Fig. 31–2). Some of these fibers leave the bundle, reach the cerebellum via the superior cerebellar peduncle, and synapse in the nucleus interpositus. Other descending fibers from the red nucleus synapse in the facial nerve nucleus and the lateral reticular nucleus of the medulla oblongata. The rubrospinal fibers extend through the lateral fasciculus of the spinal cord (see Figures 26–1 and 26–4) and terminate on interneurons of the lateral part of laminae V, VI, and VII. The parvicellular part of the red nucleus gives rise to rubroolivary fibers, which are an important component of the central tegmental tract. This bundle is localized centrally in the reticular substance (see Figure 30–4). The rubroolivary fibers terminate on the dorsal lamella of the principal olive.

FUNCTIONAL ASPECTS

The situation of the red nucleus within the cerebellorubro-olivocerebellar circuit makes it difficult to differentiate the function of the red nucleus from that of the other components of the circuit, and especially from that of the cerebellum. In any case, the red nucleus serves as a wayside station via which the cerebellum can exert its influence on the spinal cord. Direct stimulation of the red nucleus causes flexion of the muscles of the contralateral extremity. At the same time, extensor motoneurons are inhibited.

The aforementioned circuit is probably involved in the regulation of the alternate facilitation and inhibition of the flexors during the motor-active and non–motor-active phases, respectively, of the extremity while walking. The rubrospinal tract might function as an efferent pathway of the system.

Chapter 32

Structure and Connections of the Pretectal Area

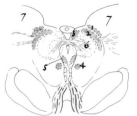

Figure 32-1 Transverse section through the area of transition between mesencephalon and diencephalon; topography of the principal nuclei of the pretectal area (according to Carpenter).

1 lentiform nucleus
2 sublentiform nucleus
3 pretectal nucleus
4 Cajal's interstitial nucleus
5 nucleus of Darkshevich
6 nucleus of the posterior commissure
7 pulvinar

The pretectal area comprises a complex of often ill defined nuclei and fibers, located between the superior colliculus and the habenular nuclei. Some of the pretectal nuclei originate from the epithalamus, while others come from the mesencephalon. Functionally, the pretectum has been related to the optic reflexes.

The area is not fully known. A few of the nuclei in it have different representatives in different mammals; like Kuhlenbeck and Miller (1949), we distinguish between diencephalic and mesencephalic pretectal nuclei.

Diencephalic Nuclei

The principal diencephalic pretectal nuclei are the pretectal nucleus and the interstitial nucleus of the posterior commissure. The pretectal nucleus (Fig. 32-1) extends from the dorsal end of the habenula to the superior colliculus. It comprises small multipolar cells found scattered among myelinated fiber bundles.

The interstitial nucleus of the posterior commissure (Fig. 32-1) comprises cells on either side of and among the fibers of the posterior commissure. A magnocellular and a parvicellular part of this nucleus can be distinguished.

Mesencephalic Nuclei

The principal mesencephalic nuclei of the pretectum are the lentiform nucleus (nucleus of the optic tract), the olivary nucleus of the superior colliculus (pretectal olivary nucleus), and the sublentiform nucleus.

The lentiform (optic tract) nucleus can be observed as a narrow streak of large dark colored cells, extending from the medial margin of the suprageniculate nucleus to the angle between pretectum and pulvinar (Fig. 32-1). Parts of this nucleus are perforated by fibers from the brachium of the superior colliculus.

The pretectal olivary nucleus is a small, well defined nucleus localized rostrolateral to the superior colliculus. The nucleus comprises small and medium-size cells and differs from its surroundings in that it presents a characteristic gelatinous appearance.

In humans, it is difficult to distinguish the sublentiform nucleus from the lentiform nucleus. The former is localized lateral to the nucleus of the posterior commissure and comprises small cells and transversely arranged, thin myelinated fiber bundles.

Fiber Connections

The afferent and efferent fibers of the pretectal area are little known; they are the subject of considerable current research. It can be stated in general that the efferent fibers from the pretectal area take a mainly ascending course and connect the pretectum with the thalamus, among other structures.

Afferent Fibers. Afferent fibers originate

218

from the retina, the ventral thalamus (zona incerta and reticular nucleus), and the reticular formation, dorsolateral to the red nucleus. The lentiform (optic tract) nucleus and the pretectal olivary nucleus also receive fibers from the cerebral cortex (areas 17, 18, and 19). The posterior commissure nucleus receives afferents from the superior colliculus. The afferents from the retina terminate exclusively in the lentiform and the pretectal olivary nuclei.

Efferent Fibers. Research into the efferent projection of the principal nuclei of the pretectum is not yet entirely completed, and the tentative conclusions are not unequivocal. The studies of Carpenter and Pierson (1973) in monkeys and that of Berman (1977) in cats have yielded the following preliminary results. The lentiform and the sublentiform nucleus project to the contralateral nucleus of the posterior commissure and to the homolateral pulvinar and pregeniculate nuclei. The nucleus of the posterior commissure projects to the homonymous contralateral nucleus via fibers of the posterior commissure. According to Berman (1977), this nucleus projects to the contralateral interstitial nucleus of Cajal and the ipsilateral nucleus of Darkschewich, via fibers that extend on the rostral side of the aqueduct. The fibers from the pretectal olivary nucleus cross the midline in the posterior commissure and synapse in the homonymous contralateral nucleus. According to Carpenter and Pierson (1973), fibers from this nucleus synapse in the nuclear complex of the oculomotor nerve.

The pretectal nucleus projects to an extensive area. Ascending fibers extend to the thalamic reticular nucleus and thalamic central nucleus (on the ipsilateral side); other fibers extend to the zona incerta and Forel's fields. Descending fibers synapse in the mesencephalic reticular formation, dorsolateral to the red nucleus.

Functional Aspects

The pretectal area has long been related to optic reflexes and, in particular, to the light reflex, but more recent studies seem to indicate that this area may be of importance also for normal behavior dependent on optic information. The above-described projections within the pretectal area indicate the likelihood that retinal impulses reach the nuclear complex of the oculomotor nerve via a synapse in the lentiform nucleus (and/or a synapse in the pretectal olivary nucleus) and a second synapse in the nucleus of the posterior commissure. The course of the light reflex is probably as follows: retina → optic tract → lentiform nucleus (or pretectal olivary nucleus) → nucleus of the posterior commissure → posterior commissure (or ventral aqueductal fibers) → Edinger-Westphal nucleus → ciliary ganglion → short ciliary nerves → pupillary sphincter muscle.

Chapter 33

Thalamus and Epithalamus

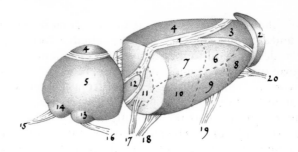

Figure 33-1 The internal medullary lamina divides the thalamus into a lateral, a medial, and a rostral part (according to Brodal).

1 internal medullary lamina
2 reticular nucleus
3 anterior nucleus
4 dorsal medial (DM) nucleus
5 pulvinar
6 lateral dorsal (LD) nucleus
7 lateral posterior (LP) nucleus
8 ventral anterior (VA) nucleus
9 ventral lateral (VL) nucleus

10 ventral posterolateral (VPL) nucleus
11 ventral posteromedial (VPM) nucleus
12 central nucleus or centromedian (CM)
13 lateral geniculate body (LGB)
14 medial geniculate body (MGB)
15 brachium of the inferior colliculus
16 optic tract
17 trigeminothalamic fibers
18 medial lemniscus and spinothalamic fibers
19 cerebellothalamic fibers
20 pallidothalamic fibers

The diencephalon is divided in the ventrodorsal direction into hypothalamus, subthalamus, (dorsal) thalamus, and epithalamus. The hypothalamus is discussed in chapter 39, and the subthalamus (briefly) in chapter 36. This chapter discusses the dorsal thalamus (henceforth called thalamus) and the epithalamus.

The Thalamus

The thalamus can be regarded as an extremely important junction of sensory and integrative systems. All sensory tracts with the exception of the olfactory fibers project to corresponding thalamic areas. The flow of information that travels through the sensory fibers is processed in the thalamus and sent on to the cortex via thalamocortical fibers. The cortex in its turn can influence the processing of these impulses via numerous corticothalamic fibers; thalamus and cerebral cortex thus act as a functional unit (Fig. 33–2). The various sensory modalities (pain sense, temperature sense, tactile sense) each have their own area of projection in which an exact somatotopic localization exists. The "motor" information is transmitted through fibers from the cerebellum and the basal ganglia. More complex information from the integrative systems (limbic system, reticular formation) likewise reaches the thalamus; the latter thus functions as a link between the limbic system and the reticular formation on the one hand, and the neocortex on the other.

ORGANIZATION

The thalamus is a large gray mass that comprises many nuclei that differ in fiber projections and structure. It is a striking fact that the projections to the cortex are more numerous than those between the various thalamic nuclei. The thalamus is incompletely divided by a few fiber lamellae. The internal medullary lamina marks the boundary between the lateral and the medial nuclear complexes. In an anterior direction this lamina divides into two lamellae that bound the anterior nuclear complex (Fig. 33–1).

The external medullary lamina bounds the thalamus on the lateral, ventral, and rostral sides. The "thin" layer of neurons localized in it is known as the thalamic reticular nucleus. The

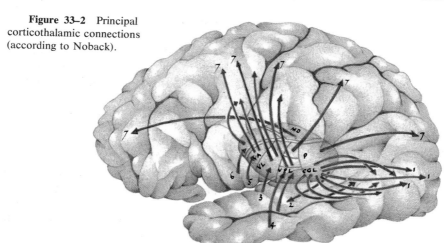

Figure 33–2 Principal corticothalamic connections (according to Noback).

1 geniculocalcarine tract
2 geniculotemporal tract
3 cerebellothalamic fibers
4 medial lemniscus
5 thalamic fasciculus
6 mamillothalamic fasciculus
7 thalamocortical fibers
VA ventral anterior nucleus
VL ventral lateral nucleus
VPL ventral posterolateral nucleus
LGB lateral geniculate body
P pulvinar
DM dorsal medial nucleus

nerve cells in the medial medullary lamina are called intralaminar nuclei.

The lateral nuclear complex is subdivided into a dorsal and a ventral area; the latter comprises important nuclei like the ventral postero-lateral (VPL) nucleus, the ventral lateral (VL) nucleus, and the ventral anterior ventral (VA) nucleus.

According to the nature of the incoming impulses and their further projection to the cortex, the following nuclei can be distinguished in the thalamus: nonspecific and specific nuclei, nuclei involved in motor activity, nuclei involved in the limbic system, and associative nuclei.

NONSPECIFIC THALAMIC NUCLEI

This group comprises usually ill defined agglomerations of mostly small round or fusiform cells. The following are the principal nuclei of this group:

(a) Intralaminar nuclei, which comprise groups of neurons localized between fibers of the fairly broad internal medullary lamina (Fig. 33–3); some of these nuclei are relatively large (central nucleus or centrum medianum, parafascicular nucleus);

(b) Periventricular nuclei, which are groups of pigment-rich small neurons lying against the wall of the third ventricle; the best known are the paratenial nucleus and the periventricular nucleus;

(c) Reticular nucleus, which is a thin layer of cells between the external medullary lamina and the internal capsule; the medium-size cells are multipolar, have long dendrites, and resemble the neurons of the reticular formation.

The nonspecific nuclei are phylogenetically old. They are inconspicuous in humans, with the exception of the central nucleus and the reticular nucleus.

Afferent Fibers. Afferent fibers are little known. The principal afferents originate from the reticular formation of the medulla oblongata and pons, the spinal cord, cerebral cortex, and other thalamic nuclei. Afferents to the central nucleus originate from area 4 of the cerebral cortex, the pallidum, and the reticular formation.

Efferent Fibers. Efferent fibers extend to specific thalamic nuclei like the ventral anterior (VA) and the ventral lateral (VL) nucleus, the striatum, and the hypothalamus. The central nucleus and the parafascicular nucleus project to the putamen; other intralaminar nuclei project to the caudate nucleus. The reticular nucleus projects to the reticular formation of the mesencephalon and is also connected with many other thalamic nuclei via axon collaterals.

Nonspecific Nuclei and the Cortex. There has long been a discrepancy between anatomic and neurophysiologic data on the connections between the nonspecific thalamic nuclei and the cortex. Neurophysiology proceeds from the assumption that excitation of the nonspecific nuclei causes changes in the electrical activity of the

Figure 33–3 Frontal section through the thalamus. *A,* Rostral part; *B,* central part (according to Clara).

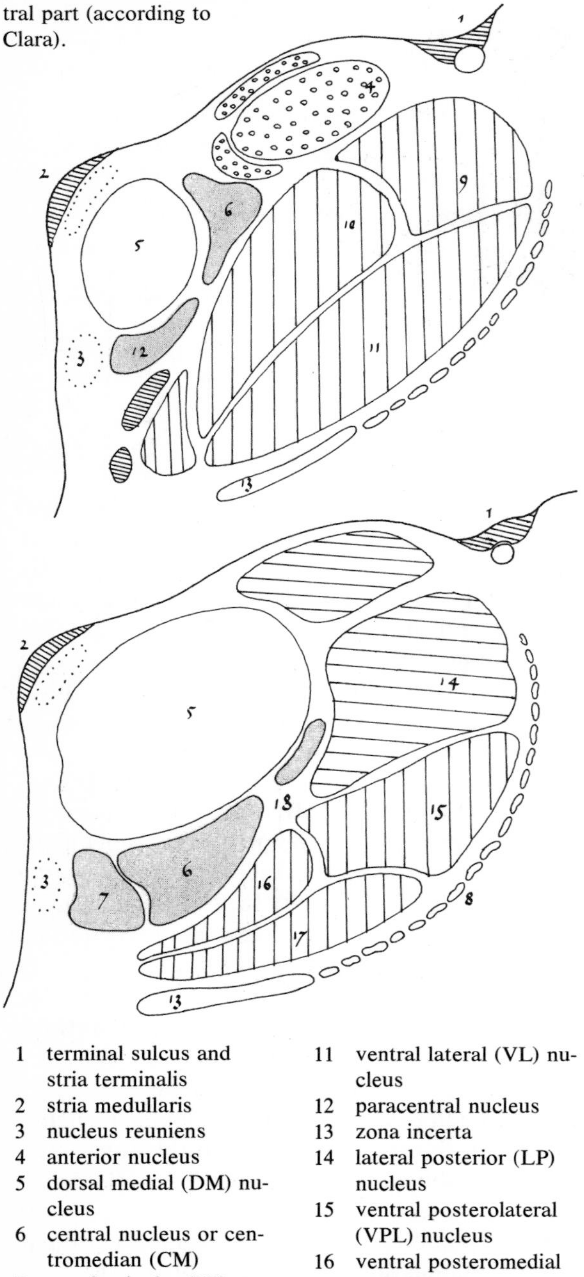

1	terminal sulcus and stria terminalis
2	stria medullaris
3	nucleus reuniens
4	anterior nucleus
5	dorsal medial (DM) nucleus
6	central nucleus or centromedian (CM)
7	parafascicular (PF) nucleus
8	reticular nucleus
9	ventral anterior (VA) nucleus
10	lateral dorsal (LD) nucleus

11	ventral lateral (VL) nucleus
12	paracentral nucleus
13	zona incerta
14	lateral posterior (LP) nucleus
15	ventral posterolateral (VPL) nucleus
16	ventral posteromedial (VPM) nucleus
17	posterior nucleus (ventral posterior inferior, VPI)
18	internal medullary lamina

cortex. Stimulus frequencies of 5 to 10 per second produce the so-called recruiting response, which can be derived from large parts of the cortex. This response consists of waves that slowly increase and then diminish in amplitude (waxing and waning).

Neuroanatomic studies using degeneration methods or the Golgi technique, however, have failed to demonstrate direct connections between nonspecific nuclei and the cortex. According to recent research with the horseradish-peroxidase technique, the nonspecific thalamic fibers project mainly to the striatum. The cortical projection is diffuse and takes place via axon collaterals of the thalamostriatal fibers. Another connection between nonspecific nuclei and cortex might be established via the ventral anterior (VA) nucleus.

SPECIFIC SENSORY THALAMIC NUCLEI

Unlike the nuclei of the previous group, these nuclei project to well defined areas of the cerebral cortex through numerous fibers of somatotopic localization. The following are the principal nuclei:

(a) *Ventral posteromedial (VPM) nucleus,* which receives fibers from the trigeminal system (somatic sensibility of the face) and from the nucleus of the tractus solitarius. It projects to the inferior part of areas 3, 1, and 2 of the cortex (Fig. 33–2).

(b) *Ventral posterolateral (VPL) nucleus,* in which the fibers of the medial lemniscus and the spinothalamic tract synapse. The lemniscal fibers terminate in sharply defined conical telodendria that synapse on the thalamus cells; the spinothalamic fibers terminate in diffuse terminal ramifications. The information is processed, switched over, and conducted to areas 3, 1, and 2 (Fig. 33–2). Spinothalamic fibers also terminate in the posterior thalamic nucleus, the intralaminar nuclei, and the medial geniculate body.

Body Projection to VPL and VPM Nucleus. The VPL and VPM nuclei are wayside stations on the way of somatic sensibility to the cortex. The somatotopic organization of the lemniscal system is maintained in the thalamus. The fibers coming from a caudal area synapse laterally in the nucleus, while those coming from a cranial area synapse medially. Besides this lateromedial spinal projection there is also a dorsoventral division; dorsally in the VPL nucleus corresponds with proximally in the extremities. The cells in the dorsal part of the VPL nucleus are sensitive in particular to kinesthetic stimuli, whereas those in the ventral part of the VPL nucleus respond more readily to somesthetic stimuli (pressure and touch). In a map of the body projection on the VPL nucleus, the face and hands occupy a relatively much larger area than the trunk.

(c) *Medial geniculate body*, which is divided into a magnocellular and a parvicellular part. The former receives spinothalamic fibers that transport pain impulses. The latter receives acoustic fibers from the inferior colliculus and the lateral lemniscus. This part projects to areas 41 and 42 (Fig. 33–2).

(d) *Lateral geniculate body,* which is the transfer station of the optic tract fibers. The nucleus is grossly visible as a rounded thickening on the posterolateral side of the thalamus, close to its boundary with the mesencephalon. The lateral geniculate body has two distinct parts: a dorsal, stratified part in which most of the optic tract fibers synapse, and a ventral part (pregeniculate nucleus) that might be included in the pretectal region (Fig. 33–4). The cells of the dorsal part are arranged in six layers, separated by thin lamellae of myelinated optic tract fibers. In a lateral direction these layers merge. Layers 1 and 2 comprise large nerve cells, while other layers consist of distinctly smaller cells.

The uncrossed temporal fibers of the optic tract terminate in layers 2, 3, and 5, while the crossed nasal fibers synapse in layers 1, 4, and 6 (Fig. 33–5). The optic tract fibers and the dendrites of the cells of the geniculate body form intricate synaptic complexes (glomeruli), which involve terminations of corticofugal fibers as well. In addition to optic tract fibers, other afferent fibers that originate from the visual cortex also terminate in the lateral geniculate body. Efferent fibers from the lateral geniculate body synapse in areas 17, 18, and 19 of the cerebral cortex via geniculocalcarine fibers; other efferent fibers synapse in the pulvinar.

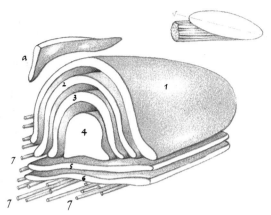

Figure 33–4 The lateral geniculate body with its stratified structure (according to Clara).

a   pregeniculate nucleus
1,2,3,4   concentric layers
5,6   horizontal layers
7   optic tract fibers

THALAMIC NUCLEI INVOLVED IN MOTOR ACTIVITY

The *ventral anterior (VA) nucleus* (Fig. 33–1) comprises large and medium-size multipolar cells arranged in irregular groups, between which the fibers of the mamillothalamic tract extend. The nucleus is an essential component of regulatory circuits, which ensure that the cerebral cortex receives feedback from various subcortical structures. Moreover, the AV nucleus has numerous connections with other intrathalamic nuclei, nonspecific as well as specific. This makes the nucleus a junction of supply routes, as demonstrated by the fiber projections. The VA nucleus is involved in the following regulatory circuits:

(a) cerebral cortex → cerebellum → ventral anterior nucleus → cerebral cortex;

(b) cerebral cortex → basal ganglia → ventral anterior nucleus → cerebral cortex;

(c) cerebral cortex → striatum → reticular part of substantia nigra → ventral anterior nucleus → cerebral cortex.

Impulses from the reticular formation reach the VA nucleus via the nonspecific thalamic nuclei and are transmitted to the cerebral cortex.

Little is known about the efferent fibers of the VA nucleus. Mention has been made of a projection to area 6 and projections to the orbito-

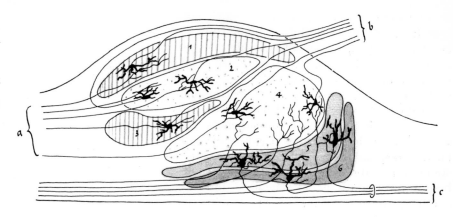

Figure 33–5 Afferent and efferent fibers of the lateral geniculate body (according to Clara).

  a optic tract fibers
  b geniculocalcarine tract
  c geniculotectal tract
  1,4,6 layers where nasal fibers synapse
  2,3,5 layers where temporal fibers synapse

frontal cortex. The latter projections seem to be very important for the production of the so-called recruiting response, for lesions of the VA nucleus block this response.

The *ventral lateral (VL) nucleus* is a synaptic station in the cerebellocortical regulatory circuit. The afferent fibers mostly originate directly from the dentate nucleus of the cerebellum. Other fibers come from the pallidum. The VL nucleus projects to areas 4 and 6 of the cerebral cortex.

THALAMIC NUCLEI INVOLVED IN THE LIMBIC SYSTEM

The *dorsomedial (DM) nucleus* is situated between the medial medullary lamina and the periventricular gray matter (Fig. 33–1). The nucleus can be divided into a magnocellular rostral and a parvicellular dorsolateral part. The DM nucleus is connected with numerous intrathalamic nuclei. Afferent fibers from outside the thalamus originate from the amygdala and the temporal cortex via the peduncular loop (inferior thalamic peduncle), from the hypothalamus via the periventricular system, and from the mesencephalic reticular formation.

Efferent fibers from the DM nucleus constitute an important part of the anterior thalamic peduncle and synapse mainly in the orbitofrontal cortex (areas 8, 9, 10, 45, and 46).

The *anterior nucleus* consists of three nuclei located in the most rostral part of the thalamus (Fig. 33–1). Afferent fibers to the anterior nucleus originate from the medial mamillary nucleus via the mamillothalamic tract, from the postcommissural fornix (see hippocampus) and from the presubiculum and parasubiculum.

Efferent fibers extend via the anterior peduncle to the gyrus cinguli (areas 23, 24, and 32). The nuclei constitute a link between hippocampus, hypothalamus, and cortical areas of the limbic system.

ASSOCIATIVE THALAMIC NUCLEI

These nuclei receive few afferent fibers from brain stem or spinal cord; they are connected with other thalamic nuclei and with certain associative areas of the cerebral cortex.

The *pulvinar* is the largest and least known nucleus of the thalamus. It is a phylogenetically young nucleus, which attains its maximal development in humans. The nucleus constitutes the very extensive dorsal pole of the thalamus.

Afferent fibers originate from many other thalamic nuclei (medial and lateral geniculate body, VPL nucleus, etc.), the tectum (superior colliculus), the lentiform and the sublentiform nuclei (pretectum), and from the cerebral cortex.

Efferent fibers extend for the most part to the cerebral cortex (areas 37, 38, 19, etc.).

THALAMIC CELL TYPES

Studies using the Golgi technique have demonstrated four principal cell types in the specific sensory nuclei of the thalamus; thalamocortical

Figure 33–6 Thalamic cell types (according to Scheibel, Scheibel, and Davis).

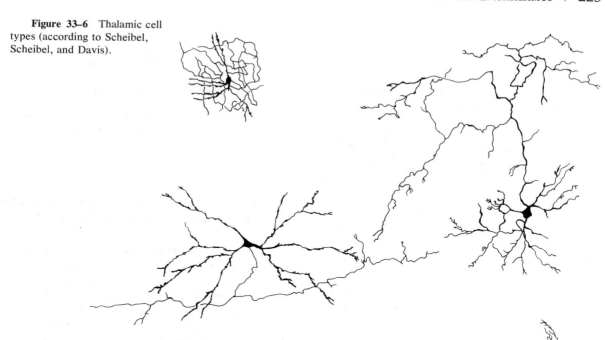

relay cells (TR-cells), long integrator cells (I-cells), Golgi-II interneurons (L-cells), and the axonless (amacrinal) neurons (A-cells; Fig. 33–6). The TR-cells are of medium size and possess four to ten fairly smooth primary dendrites; the axon joins the thalamocortical fibers and usually has no collaterals. The I-cells resemble the neurons of the reticular formation (Fig. 29–1) and have an axon with a T-shaped division into a rostral and a caudal branch. The L-cells are numerous (about 30 per cent of all cells of the VPL nucleus in a mature cat). The perikaryon has two to six primary dendrites that often end in claw-like swellings and show dendrodentritic synapses. The A-cells are exceptionally small (3 to 5 μm) and resemble the granule cells of the cerebellum (the difference being that they have no axon).

THALAMIC CIRCUITS

It is extremely difficult to study intrathalamic connections. Numerous dendrodendritic synapses between L-cells have been demonstrated in the VPL and the VPM nuclei. The network of L-cells in the thalamus is held responsible for the pacemaker function of the thalamus in relation to the cerebral cortex. The term "pacemak-

er" indicates a small, morphologically well defined area where impulses are generated that are distributed over the surrounding area and make this area follow. In the thalamocortical system the thalamus functions as pacemaker and the cortex follows.

The thalamus comprises groups of neurons so connected as to tend to act synchronously. This applies to the TR-cells of the ventrobasal nuclei (VPL and VPM nuclei) and to the intralaminar thalamic nuclei. The rhythmic discharges of the cells of the ventrobasal nuclei produce in the cortex the so-called augmenting response, while the rhythmic discharges of the intralaminar nuclei cause the so-called recruiting response.

The morphologic substrate of the rhythmic oscillation of the thalamic cell populations lies in the numerous dendrodendritic synapses between the L-cells. These synapses often have no polarity, and consequently information can be transmitted in two directions. By virtue of the characteristics of these dendrodendritic synapses, the L-cells form a kind of extensive dendritic matrix that extends throughout the thalamus.

Figure 33–7 represents a thalamic circuit with pacemaker properties; one row of L-cells has synaptic contacts with TR-cells and mutual synaptic contacts. Axons of the reticular nucleus synapse (negative feedback) with TR-cells and L-cells, the modulating impulse transmission in the TR-cells. The (inhibitory) L-cells inhibit the TR-cells synchronously, and consequently the TR-cells are unlikely to fire during about 100 msec.

FUNCTION OF THE
THALAMUS — SUMMARY

The thalamus can function in the following ways:

(a) As a synaptic and filtering station for incoming sensory impulses (VPL and VPM nuclei, lateral and medial geniculate bodies). By virtue of the synapses of the large ascending and sensory systems, the thalamus can influence impulses arriving from the periphery (skin, joints, muscles, sense organs), for example, to attenuate or suppress certain impulses so that only firing patterns rich in information reach the cerebral cortex;

(b) As a relay station for information from the striatum and the cerebellum (VA) and VL nuclei;

(c) As a center of integration for impulses arriving from the cortex (pulvinar);

(d) As a center of activation for the electrical activity of the cortex (thalamic pacemaker); and

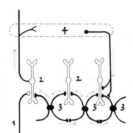

Figure 33–7 Thalamic circuits: pacemaker function of the thalamus (according to Scheibel, Arnold, and Scheibel).

1 lemniscal fiber
2 TR-cell
3 L-cells (Golgi-II interneurons)
4 reticular nucleus

(e) As a link between the limbic system and the neocortex (anterior and dorsal medial nuclei).

Thalamic lesions give rise to the so-called thalamic syndrome, which is characterized by contralateral hemianesthesia, continuing as hemiparesis. Superficial sensibility (temperature and pressure) gradually returns, but finely discriminative sensibility is lastingly disturbed. Moreover, pain sensibility is increased so that quite harmless superficial stimuli (the touch of cottonwool, for example) are perceived as disagreeably painful.

The Epithalamus

The epithalamus comprises the habenular nucleus, the pineal body, and the habenular and posterior commissures. This area is viewed by modern investigators as a synaptic system via which impulses from the striatum gain access to the limbic system.

HABENULAR NUCLEUS

The habenular nucleus is an accumulation of cells that bounds the superior colliculus of the mesencephalon (see Fig. 27–5); it constitutes the wall of the dorsal part of the third ventricle at its transition to the cerebral aqueduct. This nucleus is usually divided into two cell groups: the medial and the lateral habenular nuclei. On the basis of their structure and fiber projections, however, these two nuclei are separate entities.

Medial Habenular Nucleus

Using the Golgi technique, neurons of two different types can be distinguished: a small piriform type and a slightly larger fusiform type. The dendrites do not extend beyond the medial habenular nucleus.

Afferent Fibers. Afferent fibers originate from the septum and Broca's diagonal nucleus. These fibers extend via the stria medullaris.

Efferent Fibers. Efferent fibers extend via Meynert's fasciculus retroflexus and synapse in the interpeduncular nucleus.

Lateral Habenular Nucleus

The cells of the lateral habenular nucleus are generally larger, and four different types can be distinguished (Iwahori, 1977). Types I, II, and III are large, medium-size, and small projection cells, respectively, while type IV can be counted among the neurons with short axons.

Afferent Fibers. Afferent fibers arrive from the pallidum and the central part of the mesencephalic tegmentum, via Meynert's fasciculus retroflexus, and from the preoptic area via the stria medullaris (see Fig. 39–9).

Efferent Fibers. Efferent fibers run through the fasciculus retroflexus and synapse in the substantia nigra, the dorsal raphe nucleus, and the mesencephalic reticular formation.

Functional Aspects

The nuclei of the habenula are functionally involved in the limbic system and influence behavior patterns like food intake and certain forms of sexual behavior.

The stria medullaris, habenular nuclei, and fasciculus retroflexus are synaptic junctions of a dorsal part of the limbic system through which impulses from the septum and preoptic area travel to the mesencephalon. The striatum can exert its influence on the limbic system via the pallidohabenular projections.

Chapter 34

The Visual System

The visual system comprises all the structures that provide information on visible shapes, colors, and spatial relations in the environment. Together with hearing, vision is specialized in perception at a distance. It performs a mainly spatial analysis of the environment and is without doubt the richest source of information. About one-third of all afferent fibers that transmit information to the CNS are located in the two optic nerves.

Light of a certain frequency is required in order to obtain optical information. Moreover, the object perceived must remain outside a certain distance from the eye if it is to be sharply depicted on the retina. For a healthy eye, this minimal distance is about 8 cm. Light rays are partly absorbed and partly reflected by all solid matter. Visible light encompasses a small segment of the electromagnetic spectrum (400 to 600 nm). Most of the visible objects in the environment function as indirect light sources in that they reflect solar light.

Organization of the Visual System

In the visual system we distinguish a peripheral apparatus of reception and integration (retina) and an afferent fiber system (optic nerve, chiasm, optic tract), via which already processed retinal impulses are transmitted to central areas of the CNS. At the level of the lateral geniculate body the fibers of the optic tract diverge and then synapse in three different areas.

There are, therefore, three main routes that the retinal impulses can travel: two connect the retina with the cerebral cortex, and the third is a subcortical route. These three routes can be described as the retinogeniculocalcarine system (first visual system), the retinotectothalamocortical system (second visual system), and the retinomesencephalic system (third visual system).

The first visual system is involved in discriminative sensory functions like spatial analysis of the environment, interpretation of shapes, visual acuity, and color vision. About 80 per cent of the optic fibers synapse in the lateral geniculate body and belong to this system.

The second visual system is phylogenetically older. In birds, reptiles, etc., the superior colliculus plays the role of the highest visual center, but in mammals the perceptive aspects of vision have been "transported" to the newly developed geniculocalcarine system. The second visual system remains in charge of important motor aspects of the visual function: for example, tracking movements of the eye in order to

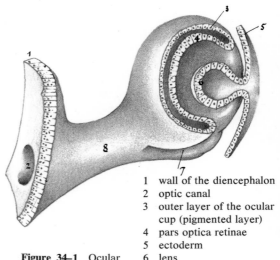

Figure 34–1 Ocular cup and ocular stalk in a human embryo of 7.5 mm (according to Hamilton).

1 wall of the diencephalon
2 optic canal
3 outer layer of the ocular cup (pigmented layer)
4 pars optica retinae
5 ectoderm
6 lens
7 choroid fissure
8 ocular stalk (primordium of the optic nerve)

228

follow the chosen object (fixation) even when it moves and automatic averting movements in relation to objects that abruptly enter the field of vision. Lesions of the superior colliculus in animals cause defects in discrimination of patterns and diminished alertness to stimuli that originate from the contralateral field of vision.

The third visual system is involved mainly in the production of subcortical optical reflexes like the light reflex (see pages 167 and 218).

Retina

EMBRYOLOGY

In spite of its peripheral position, the retina should be regarded as a component of the CNS. It develops as part of a bilateral evagination of the lateral wall of the prosencephalon (Fig. 34–1). The lateral aspect of the ocular vesicle invaginates to form the ocular cup. The ocular stalk later forms the optic nerve. The ocular cup differentiates to an inner, light-sensitive part (pars optica retinae), which anteriorly continues as a pigmented, light-insensitive part (pars ceca retinae). The ora serrata marks the boundary between pars optica and pars ceca. The outer part of the ocular cup becomes the pigmented layer. The space between the two parts (optic ventricle) becomes narrower until contact between the outer and the inner part of the ocular cup causes obliteration of the optic ventricle.

The invagination of the lateral side of the ocular vesicle continues on the ventral side (choroid fissure), even in the ocular stalk (Fig. 34–1). Through this fissure, mesenchyma with blood vessels enters the eye; one of the blood vessels (hyaloid artery) is later to vascularize the central part of the retina (central retinal artery).

MORPHOLOGIC CHARACTERISTICS

The pars optica retinae is the actual visuosensory part of the eye. It is a transparent membrane, 0.2 mm thick, which occupies about

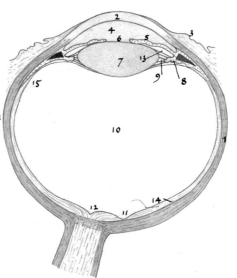

Figure 34–2 Horizontal section through the eye with the optic nerve.

1 sclera
2 cornea
3 conjunctiva
4 anterior chamber
5 iris
6 pupil
7 lens
8 ciliary body (ciliary muscle [black], ciliary processes, ciliary part of retina)
9 ciliary zonule
10 vitreous chamber
11 fovea centralis
12 optic disk (papilla of optic nerve)
13 posterior chamber
14 pars optica retinae
15 ora serrata

two-thirds of the eyeball (Fig. 34–2). At examination of the fundus, the retina has a bright red color caused by the numerous capillaries. Characteristic details of the fundus picture are the disk (papilla of the optic nerve) and the central fovea. The disk marks the site at which the optic nerve leaves the eyeball. It appears as a small, whitish, oval elevation with a diameter of about 1.5 mm. The apex of the elevation is slightly excavated and is known as the optic cup. This part of the retina consists exclusively of nerve fibers. Since light-sensitive receptors are absent here, the disk forms the blind spot in the field of vision.

About 4 mm lateral to the disk is a small, oval, yellow area (macula lutea), which has a transverse diameter of about 3 mm (Fig. 34–3).

Figure 34–3 Back of the eye (fundus). The veins are darker than the arteries.

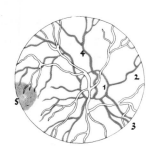

1 optic disk (papilla of optic nerve)
2 superior nasal venule
3 inferior nasal venules
4 superior temporal venules
5 macula

The pit in its center is called the fovea centralis; this is the area of maximal visual acuity. In the fovea centralis, the retina is thinner than elsewhere because layers 5 through 9 are absent (see below); layers 2 and 4, however, are thick. Three concentric areas can be distinguished in the macula: foveal, parafoveal, and a perifoveal region.

MICROSCOPIC STRUCTURE

The retina consists in principle of a chain of three successive neurons linked by synapses (Fig. 34–4). The first neurons (rods or cones) are the actual photoreceptors; their external segments contain photopigment, which assists in converting a light stimulus to a receptor potential. The photoreceptors are located in the periphery, facing out. The light must therefore pass all layers of the retina before it is caught by the external segments of the photoreceptors. This is why the term "inverted retina" is used.

The middle neurons are bipolar and their peripheral processes synapse with the bases of the rods and cones, while their central processes (axons) synapse with the ganglion cells. The middle neurons are divided into horizontal, dwarf bipolar, and flat bipolar neurons.

The ganglion cells constitute the inner cellular layers of the retina. Their axons converge toward the disk, where they form a thick bundle (optic nerve). Through most of the retina, the ganglion cells form a single layer except on the temporal side, where two layers are found. In the region of the macula there are eight to ten layers that diminish rapidly toward the fovea, where they are absent. Morphologically, dwarf ganglion cells and diffuse ganglion cells can be distinguished.

Stratification of the Retina

Apart from the ora serrata, optic disk, and central fovea, the mature retina comprises ten layers. From the outside in, they are:
1 pigmented layer
2 photosensitive layer (layer of rods and cones)
3 external limiting layer (formerly external limiting membrane)
4 outer nuclear layer
5 outer plexiform layer
6 inner nuclear layer
7 inner plexiform layer
8 ganglion cell layer
9 nerve fiber layer
10 internal limiting layer (internal limiting membrane).

This enumeration reveals a distinct sequence of cell layers and fiber layers. Layers 5 and 7 are rich in synapses; layer 9 comprises the radially arranged, still unmyelinated axons of the ganglion cells that are to become optic nerve fibers.

Receptor Layer

The receptor layer functionally comprises the pigmented layer and the layer of rods and cones. The pigmented layer consists of high cylindrical cells containing pigment. The cells in the part adjacent to the choroid are free of pigment; the rest of the cell contains pigment granules and has delicate extensions (microvilli). The microvilli (Fig. 34–5) are interlaced with the external segments of the receptor cells. The contact between the microvilli and the rods and cones is essential to the function of the sensory elements. The pigment within the cells can move in response to the influence of light; when ex-

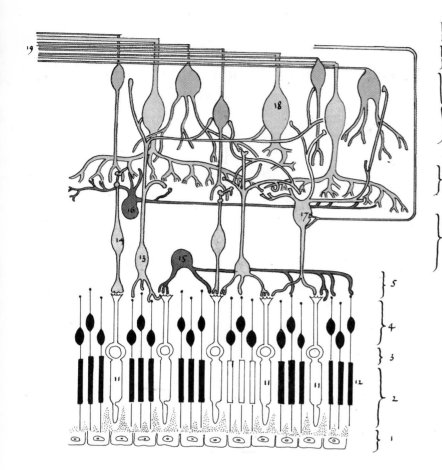

Figure 34-4 Structure of the retina. The rods are shown in black, and the cones in white, the bipolar cells in light grey and the ganglion cells in yellow (partly according to Polyak).

1 pigmented layer
2 photosensitive layer
3 external limiting layer
4 outer nuclear layer
5 outer plexiform layer
6 inner nuclear layer
7 inner plexiform layer
8 ganglion cell layer
9 nerve fiber layer
10 internal limiting layer
11 cones
12 rods
13 rod bipolar
14 dwarf bipolar
15 horizontal cell
16 amacrine cells
17 flat bipolar
18 ganglion cells
19 axons of the optic nerve

posed to intensive light, the pigment granules accumulate in the microvilli and collect the excess of light in order to prevent reflection.

The photoreceptors are oblong cells localized in layers 1 to 5. The cones are generally thicker and shorter than the rods; the central fovea has exclusively cones with a rod-like shape. Toward the periphery the number of cones diminishes and that of the rods increases. About 120 million rods and 7 million cones are found throughout the retina.

Each photoreceptor consists of an external segment, a thick internal segment connected with the previous segment by a so-called "connecting piece," a cell body, and a central process. The external segments of the rods are long and thin, while those of the cones are shorter (Fig. 34–5). Electron microscope studies have revealed a large number of "disks" arranged perpendicular to the longitudinal axis. They are formed by a membrane that encloses a central space. With the rods, the membranes are detached from the cell membrane, but with the cones they are attached to it. The so-called "connecting piece" is a bridge between the external and the internal segment, which consists of a cilium shaft. The entire external segment can be regarded as a modified cilium. The internal segment has two parts: The peripheral part (ellipsoid) contains mitochondria, while the central

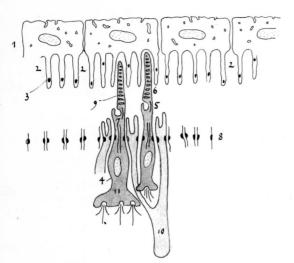

Figure 34–5 Arrangements of the rods and cones in relation to the cells of the pigmented layer of the retina (according to Noback).

1 pigmented layer
2 microvilli
3 pigment granule
4 cone
5 connecting piece
6 external segment
7 internal segment
8 external limiting layer
9 disks
10 Müller cell

part (myoid) contains the Golgi apparatus. The myoid passes through the external limiting membrane and ends in the cell body.

The rods contain the photopigment rhodopsin, which is produced in the myoid. Along the cilium shaft the rhodopsin flows to the base of the external segment, where it attaches to the cell membrane. The cell membrane invaginates to form the characteristic flat slices of the external segment. New disks with photopigment are constantly formed and push the existing disks toward the pigmented layer until the rhodopsin is released among the microvilli of the epithelial cells of the pigmented layer. Rhodopsin fades upon exposure to light. A light stimulus causes a molecular change in rhodopsin, with increased permeability of the membrane. The corresponding ion migration gives rise to a receptor potential. Rhodopsin recovers in darkness. The cones likewise contain photopigments; there are red-

sensitive, green-sensitive, and blue-sensitive cones.

The central processes of the rods and cones synapse with the bipolar neurons of layer 6. The processes of the rods are rounded, and those of the cones are broader (Fig. 35–5). The synapses are specialized ("ribbon synapses").

Bipolar Cells

There are three different types of bipolar cell: "rod bipolar," "dwarf bipolar," and "flat bipolar" cells. The rod bipolar is relatively large and has an extensive dendritic field; it synapses with a group of rods and horizontal cells in layer 5, and on the other side with large ganglion cells and amacrine cells in layer 7. The dwarf bipolar is found exclusively in the central fovea. It synapses in layer 5 with *a single cone* and on the opposite side (layer 7) with *a single ganglion cell*. The flat bipolar synapses with several cones and rods, and on the other side with large ganglion cells.

Ganglion Cell Layer

From the ganglion cells arise the axons of the optic nerve. Each dwarf bipolar synapses with a dwarf ganglion cell and thus forms a kind of "private line" to the CNS. Many other bipolar and amacrine cells synapse with the large ganglion cells. The total number of ganglion cells is about 10^6.

Other Cell Types

Apart from the already described chain of three successive neurons, the three most important cell types in the retina are the horizontal cells, the amacrine cells, and the Müller cells.

The horizontal cells are thus called because their processes are arranged in a tangential plane, that is, parallel to the optic nerve fibers. The long, thin dendrites terminate on the central processes of the rod and cone cells. The cell bodies are located in the inner nuclear layer.

The processes of the horizontal and the

Figure 34–6 Receptive fields of the retina. Each field comprises a peripheral and a central zone. The peripheral fields are larger than the central fields.

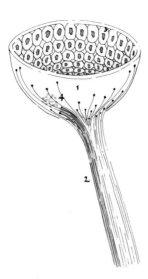

1 retina
2 optic nerve
3 receptive field of the retina
4 macula

amacrine cells are neither axonal nor dendritic and are probably able to receive as well as to transmit information. These cells undoubtedly play a role as ''crosslinks'' and afford possibilities of interaction between the radially arranged neuron chains.

The Müller cells are glia cells that, perpendicular to the internal and the external aspect, extend through the entire retina. The central process has a conical enlargement; these central processes join to form the internal limiting layer. The nucleus of these cells is located in the inner nuclear layer.

RETINAL CIRCUITS

It follows from the above description that the neuronal elements of the retina are arranged in two directions, perpendicular to each other: The neuron chains are arranged radially, while the horizontal and amacrine cells are arranged meridian-wise. The latter cells ensure interaction in transverse direction between the neuron chains and divergence of impulses from the photoreceptors.

A comparison of the number of photoreceptors (about 127×10^6) with the number of ganglion cells (10^6) warrants the expectation of a high degree of convergence in the organization of the neuronal circuits. It is evident that the axon of a ganglion cell transmits information received from a large number of receptors. Convergence can be observed in all schematic representations of the microscopic structure of the retina, which clearly show that impulses from many receptors are focused on single bipolar cells that synapse on a ganglion cell. The latter cells can be regarded as the final common pathway of the retina.

The term ''receptive field'' applies to a retinal area from which a single ganglion cell can be made to fire. The microscopic structure suggests that the size of the receptive fields varies with their situation in the retina; peripheral fields are larger than central fields. The receptive fields of adjacent ganglion cells overlap. Moreover, the size of a given field is not constant but depends on variables like the intensity of the light stimulus.

The retina can be envisaged as a curved honeycomb, with round fields that decrease in size from the periphery to the center. Each field corresponds with a ganglion cell in terms of circuitry. Moreover, these field units are not independent of each other: Horizontal and amacrine cells form crosslinks between the field units (Fig. 34–6).

FUNCTIONAL ASPECTS

The rods are the most photosensitive elements. They constitute the ''twilight sense organ'' by which shapes, contours, and shades of gray can still be seen in darkness (but not colors).

The cones need strong light intensities to be excited. Vision that exclusively involves the cones is known as ''photopic vision,'' while that which exclusively involves the rods is called ''scotopic vision.'' The cones are used to see tiny details, with the eye focused directly on the object. With markedly reduced illumination, the object can no longer be perceived by fixation; but when the eye is focused just beside the object, it becomes visible again. In that case the rods are

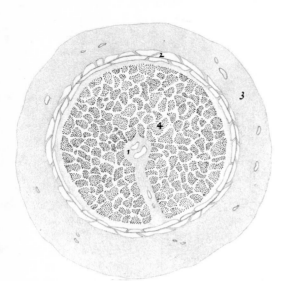

Figure 34–7 Section through the optic nerve.

1 central retinal artery and vein
2 leptomeningeal space
3 dura mater
4 optic fibers

used to see the object. In scotopic vision the resolving power is low and colors are not perceived.

Each receptive field has two functionally opposed concentric zones: the central and the peripheral zone. When stimulation of the center of a given field leads to excitation of the corresponding ganglion cell, we have a field with an "on-center." If in that case the periphery is stimulated, however, then the ganglion cell is inhibited. In fields with an "off-center" the effect is exactly opposite: Stimulation of the center causes inhibition of the ganglion cells and stimulation of the periphery causes excitation. The opposite functions of center and periphery in many cases contribute to an enhanced peripheral contrast to the retinal information.

Field of Vision

The field of vision is that portion of space that the fixed eye can see. Since the retina extends much further on the nasal than on the temporal side, the field of vision extends much farther beyond the point of fixation on the temporal than on the nasal side (Fig. 34–8). In binocular fixation, the fields of vision of the right and the left eye overlap in part. The binocular field of vision in the horizontal plane encompassed an angle of 130°, on either side of which an area remains that can only be seen with one eye (monocular half-moon).

Optic Disk

The optic disk (papilla of the optic nerve; blind spot) is an oval area to which the axons of the ganglion cells converge when they leave the eyeball. At the site of the optic disk, the retina lacks all its layers other than the optic nerve fibers. These fibers pass through the lamina cribrosa and form the optic nerve. Immediately after passing through the lamina cribrosa, the optic nerve fibers are enveloped in a thick myelin sheath, and consequently the optic nerve abruptly becomes much thicker at this point.

The fibers of the optic nerve vary in diameter from 0.2 to 6 μm. The thinnest fibers extend exclusively to the superior colliculus (W-fibers). The thicker fibers are subdivided into X-fibers, which synapse exclusively in the lateral geniculate body, and Y-fibers, which sometimes synapse in the lateral geniculate body and sometimes in the superior colliculus.

Optic Nerve, Chiasm, and Optic Tract

In its development and structure, the optic nerve is not a peripheral nerve but a central tract like, for instance, the pyramidal tract. The term *optic nerve* is used exclusively in the sense of a "grossly visible fiber bundle."

The optic nerve extends through the posterior part of the orbit and enters the base of the skull through the optic canal. The intraorbital part of the nerve shows a curving course that prevents stretching of the nerve with eye movements. About 15 mm behind the eyeball, the optic nerve is perforated by the central retinal artery and vein; from this point, these vessels extend to the optic disk. The ciliary ganglion is located between the nerve and the lateral rectus muscle. The intracranial length of the optic nerve is about 1 cm. Above the nerve, we find the olfactory tract and the gyrus rectus of the frontal lobe, with more posteriorly the anterior cerebral artery. The optic nerve is enveloped by meninges. The outer meninx is thick and strong (dura mater) and is continuous with the sclera of the eye. The inner meninx is the pia mater. From its inner surface arise septa of connective tissue that penetrate the optic nerve and divide it into many smaller bundles. Between dura mater and pia mater lies the arachnoid, separated from the pia by the subarachnoid space (Fig. 34–7).

The two optic nerves meet in front of the sella turcica and a decussation of fibers takes place (optic chiasm). The chiasm is a flat fiber plate rostral to the infundibulum; it is X-shaped. The diverging bundles that exit from the dorsal side of the chiasm form the optic tract. Between the lamina terminalis and the tuber cinereum, the chiasm forms part of the floor of the third ventricle (supraoptic recess). The upper aspects of the chiasm (anterior to the lamina terminalis) is in contact with the anterior communicating artery. The undersurface rests on the diaphragm of the sella turcica. This topography explains the fact that tumors arising from the anterior pituitary can cause compression of the optic chiasm.

The optic tract (see Fig. 14–1) appears as two flat, white bundles extending in a dorsolateral direction. Initially they form the lateral boundary of the tuber cinereum, and subsequently they extend along the ventrolateral aspect of the cerebral peduncle (Fig. 14–1). About 80 per cent of the fibers synapse in the lateral geniculate body, while the remaining 20 per cent continue through the brachium of the superior colliculus to the superior colliculus and the pretectal area, where they synapse (pages 218 and 222).

The presence of a retinohypothalamic tract has recently been definitely confirmed by autoradiographic techniques: Fibers from the retina synapse bilaterally in the suprachiasmatic nucleus of the hypothalamus (page 271).

Systematics of the Retinothalamic Fiber Projection

The fibers of the retinothalamic projection show a strict somatotopic arrangement. The exact position of the fibers from a particular area of the retina has been experimentally studied in

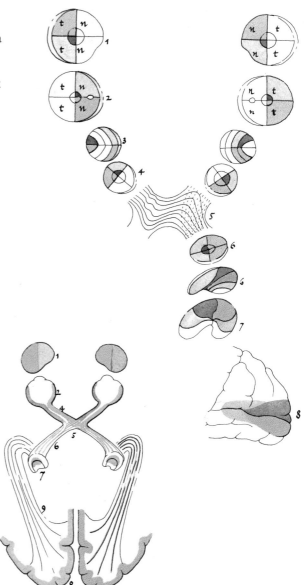

Figure 34–8 Systematics of the retinothalamic fiber projection (according to Kahle).

1 field of vision (n, nasal; t, temporal)
2 retina
3 optic nerve, proximal segment
4 optic nerve
5 optic chiasm
6 optic tract
7 lateral geniculate body
8 calcarine fissure
9 geniculocalcarine tract

monkeys. The fibers are more easily followed after dividing the retina into quadrants. A vertical line through the fovea centralis divides the retina into a nasal and a temporal half, and a second, horizontal line divides each half into an upper and a lower quadrant. Each quadrant can be further subdivided into a peripheral and a central (macular) part. The four central quadrants together form the region of maximal visual acuity.

In the initial part of the optic nerve (Fig. 34–8) the macular fibers are localized in a lateral area, while the peripheral fibers occupy the remaining, larger part of the nerve. A regrouping of fibers is observed as the bundle approaches the chiasm. The macular fibers "migrate" to the central zone of the optic nerve, while the peripheral fibers form a concentric layer around it (Fig. 34–8). At the same time the axial system rotates about 40° clockwise, so that the fibers of the two retinal halves are no longer arranged side by side but in part are stacked.

In the chiasm, fibers from the temporal and the nasal halves of the retina behave differently. Those from the temporal half extend via the lateral side of the chiasm and continue to the ipsilateral hemisphere (Fig. 34–8). Those from the nasal half cross the midline in the central part of the chiasm and continue to the contralateral hemisphere. The decussating fibers take a slightly undulating course in the chiasm before they enter the optic tract. In amphibians, fishes, and birds, all optic fibers decussate in the chiasm; in apes and humans, only 50 per cent decussate.

The arrangement of fibers in the optic tract differs from that in the optic nerve. Each tract comprises fibers from the homonymous retinal field: In the right tract, fibers from the right half of the retina extend, while in the left tract are fibers from the left half of the retina (Fig. 34–8). The partial decussation of the optic fibers causes light stimuli that for both eyes enter the left field of vision, to be projected in the right hemisphere, and vice versa. The points on both retinas on which the same part of the field of vision is projected are known as "identical points."

The fibers from the lower (temporal and nasal) quadrants extend in the lateral part of the optic tract, whereas fibers from the upper quadrants extend in the medial part. The macular fibers are similarly distributed and extend in the central part of the tract.

Lateral Geniculate Body

The lateral geniculate body is the principal final destination of the optic fibers. The contralateral fibers synapse in layers 1, 4, and 6, while the ipsilateral fibers synapse in layers 2, 3, and 5 (page 222). Each optic fiber synapses with about six cells of the corresponding layer. The macular fibers project to a fairly large wedge-shaped area at the dorsal ends of the nucleus (Fig. 34–8).

Corticothalamic fibers originating from area 17 (and perhaps from area 18) also synapse in the lateral geniculate body. The afferent impulses are processed in morphologically very complicated synaptic glomeruli, which encompass many dendrodendritic synapses.

Geniculocalcarine Tract. The principal cells of the lateral geniculate body give rise to fibers that extend along the wall of the lateral ventricle to the calcarine fissure (area 17) of the occipital lobe, where they synapse. The fibers from the dorsal part of the geniculate body take the shortest route to the retrolenticular part of the internal capsule (Fig. 34–8). Fibers from central parts of the geniculate body take a different route. First they extend laterally, in the direction of the amygdala; next, they sharply curve in a dorsal direction and continue to the occipital lobe. The geniculocalcarine fibers cross bundles of the temporopontine tract and the acoustic fibers of the geniculotemporal tract.

Visual Cortex

Of the various cortical areas involved in visual function, only areas 17, 18, and 19 of the occipital lobe and area 8 of the frontal lobe are discussed here.

AREA 17 (AREA STRIATA)

The cortex of the area striata shows a distinctly columnar organization. The fibers from the geniculate body terminate in lamina IV. The macular fibers occupy a disproportionately large part of area 17 and end up near the occipital pole. Fibers from the geniculate body that transport impulses from the upper macular quadrants terminate above the calcarine fissure; fibers that transport impulses from the lower macular quadrants terminate beneath the fissure. The geniculate fibers that conduct impulses from the retinal periphery end in the area striata rostral to the macular zone and show the same arrangement: ''Peripheral'' fibers from the upper retinal quadrants synapse above the fissure, and those from the lower retinal quadrants synapse beneath it.

Efferent fibers from area 17 synapse in the lateral geniculate body, the superior colliculus (laminae I and II), and the pretectum (lentiform nucleus).

AREAS 18 and 19

These areas are partly located on the medial surface of the occipital lobe (see Fig. 35–8). Area 18 is adjacent to area 17 and appears as a vertical strip of cortex on the lateral side; area 19 largely lies on the lateral side of the occipital lobe.

Areas 18 and 19 are essential to the interpretation of objects perceived. Disorders of area 18 cause disorders in the recognition of letters or words; disorders of area 19 cause object agnosia (objects are seen but not recognized as such). Efferent fibers from these areas synapse in the lateral geniculate body. Other efferent fibers pass between the geniculocalcarine tract and the wall of the lateral ventricle (inner sagittal layer) and reach the superior colliculus and the pretectum (lentiform nucleus). A third group of corticofugal fibers synapse in the pulvinar.

Stimulation of areas 18 and 19 causes rapid, jerky eye movements (saccades), which are produced via the corticotectal projections. These saccadic movements have proved to be very important for rapid focusing on and continued fixation of an object.

AREA 8

Part of area 8 is located in the basal part of the middle frontal gyrus (see Fig. 35–7). Cytoarchitectonically, it consists of typical frontal cortex with well developed granule cell layers. It is generally assumed that area 8 is involved in all voluntary eye movements. Electrical stimulation of this area causes contralaterally directed saccades. Derivation of the activity of neurons of area 8 during the execution of these voluntary eye movements has revealed, however, that these neurons show activity after rather than before a saccade; this is not an argument in favor of a motor role of this area.

Efferent fibers from area 8 extend (a) to other cortical areas (ipsilateral cortex of the floor of the superior temporal sulcus and the intraparietal sulcus), (b) to the striatum (caudate nucleus), (c) to the thalamus (dorsal medial nucleus, parafascicular nucleus), and (d) to the pretectum and tectum (nucleus of optic tract, superior colliculus). In the colliculus, these fibers synapse in the zonal layer and the optic layer.

Disorders of the Visual System

Lesions of the optic tract are manifested by defects in the field of vision. The nature and size of these defects are dependent on the localization and severity of the lesion. Total dysfunction of the retina or the optic nerve is manifested by total blindness (amaurosis) of the eye involved.

Lesions of the chiasm produce a variety of results. Total destruction, of course, causes total bilateral blindness. In the case of partial lesions, the resulting symptoms depend on the localization of the lesion. Lesions of the central part of the chiasm (hypophyseal tumors) cause dysfunction of the nasal, decussating retinal fibers, resulting in bitemporal hemianopia, a defect in the temporal part of the field of vision. These patients experience difficulties in seeing objects in the lateral part of the field of vision. A double lesion of the lateral part of the chiasm interrupts the temporal retinal fibers (binasal hemianopia). The patients cannot properly see objects near the midline of the field of vision. These hemianopias are heteronymous, that is, each eye loses a different part of the field of vision.

Lesions of the optic tract cause homonymous hemianopias: Of each eye, either the right or the left half of the field of vision is defective. Lesions of the optic radiation or the occipital cortex likewise give rise to homonymous hemianopias or quandrantanopias.

Chapter 35

The Cerebral Cortex

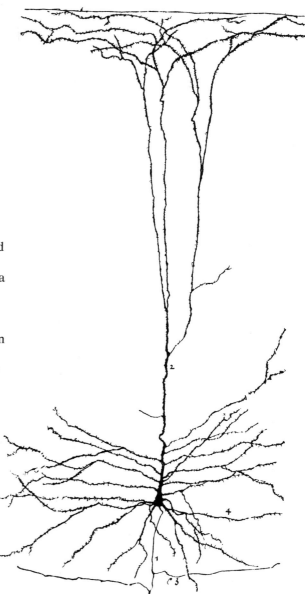

The cerebral cortex is markedly plicated and so makes optimal use of the space available within the skull. Most of the cortical surface area lies within the sulci. When flattened, the cortex would have a surface area of about 2500 cm² Its thickness varies between 1.5 and 4 mm, and its volume is about 300 ml. Owing to its thinness, an increase in cortical volume might be achieved only by more intensive plication. It is difficult to establish the number of cells with certainty, but currently it is estimated to be 2.6×10^9. The largest neuron population of the cerebrum, however, is not located in the cerebral cortex but in the cerebellum (granule cell layer).

The cortex mostly comprises six layers of cells (isocortex). In the mature brain this six-layered pattern is not always evident, but it is assumed that the entire isocortex has at least shown this pattern during embryonic development. The paleopallium (piriform area) and the archipallium (hippocampal formation), which can be regarded as phylogenetically old components of the cortex, comprise no more than two layers of cells in embryonic life. These areas are known as allocortex (page 47). Some parts of the cortex show an intermediate pattern: The meso-cortex (gyrus cinguli), for example, has no more than four or five distinguishable layers.

Figure 35–1 Pyramidal cell with numerous gemmules on the dendrites (according to Cajal).

1 axon
2 apical dendrite
3 axon collateral
4 basal dendrites
5 pia mater

Cortical Neurons

The cells of the cortex are widely diverse in type. The earlier, purely morphologic classification described a large number of cell types, many of which are now regarded as variants of two main types: pyramidal cells and stellate cells. Other, less frequently observed cell types are Martinotti cells, fusiform cells, and Cajal cells.

The pyramidal cells have a more or less triangular cell body of varying size (15 to 80 μm). The apex of the perikaryon continues in a thick apical dendrite perpendicular to the surface of the pia. Many of these dendrites reach the most superficial layer of the cortex (the molecular layer), where their terminal ramifications are located. Other dendrites (basal dendrites) extend in a horizontal direction from the base of the perikaryon (Fig. 35–1). The pyramidal cells are class I neurons; the axons of the large pyramidal cells descend to the white matter, producing several collaterals. Once they reach the white matter these axons continue as association fibers, commissural fibers, or projection fibers to the subcortical gray matter, the brain stem, or the spinal cord. Pyramidal cells can be found in all layers of the cortex except the molecular layer.

The stellate cells are class II neurons. The perikaryon is rounded or triangular, with many dendrites radiating in all directions. The axon is short and usually ramifies near the perikaryon; in other cases it ascends to the molecular layer. Stellate cells are found in all layers of the cortex except the molecular layer.

The fusiform cells (Fig. 35–2) are found mostly in the deepest layer of the cortex. The two poles of the fusiform perikaryon continue in dendrites. The axons extend to the white matter as association or projection fibers. These cells are found mostly in layer VI.

The Martinotti cells have an ascending axon that produces collaterals extending to various cortical layers; the terminal ramification is in the molecular layer.

The Cajal cells are found in the molecular layer; their processes extend parallel to the cortical surface. When mature, these cells are not readily stainable and not numerous.

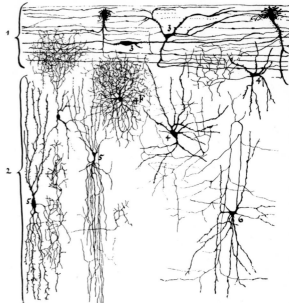

Figure 35–2 Cortical cell types (according to Cajal).

1 molecular layer
2 inner granule cell layer and pyramidal cell layer
3 Cajal's horizontal cells
4 cells with short axons (Golgi type II)
5 fusiform cells
6 small pyramidal cell of layer III

Cortical Fiber Layers

Apart from cell bodies, the cortex comprises numerous intracortical fibers, many of which are concentrated in fiber bands that extend parallel to the cortical surface. These bands are separated by layers that comprise new fibers, if any. The fiber layers are so well developed that sometimes they are grossly visible (striae of Genari in the area striata). Counting from the surface down, we see the stria of Kaes-Bechterew and the external and internal striae of Baillarger. It is assumed that most of the axons of the stria of Kaes-Bechterew originate from commissural fibers of the corpus callosum and probably from the nonspecific thalamic fibers. The external stria of Baillarger consists mainly of specific thalamic fibers on their way to their synapses in layer IV.

Baillarger's internal stria comprises axon collaterals of the pyramidal cells in layer V.

Stratification of the Cortex

Nissl-stained histologic sections show a predominantly tangential pattern of organization of the cells of the cortex, which are arranged in extensive, stacked layers. These layers are the following:

I   Molecular or Plexiform Layer.   This most superficial layer largely consists of a dense fiber plexus. Few cells (Cajal's horizontal cells) are contained in it. The fiber plexus comprises the terminal ramifications of the apical dendrites of the pyramidal cells of layers II, III, and V, and ascending axons of the nonspecific thalamocortical, association, and commissural fibers.

II   Outer Granule Cell Layer.   This comprises numerous stellate and pyramidal cells whose apical dendrites enter the molecular layer. The stria of Kaes-Bechterew marks the boundary between layers II and III.

III   Outer Pyramidal Cell Layer.   Pyramidal cells are predominant in this layer, which also comprises many granule cells and Martinotti cells. The axon collaterals of the fibers of the stria of Kaes-Bechterew, and some of the axons of Baillarger's external stria, synapse in this layer. The axons of the pyramidal cells form the association fibers (corpus callosum and long associative bundles).

During development, layers II and III are the last layers that differentiate in the cortex. These are the most highly developed layers in humans. They are regarded as associative and receptive layers in view of the fact that their axons synapse, not on the brain stem or the spinal cord, but on other parts of the cortex.

IV   Inner Granule Cell Layer.   This layer comprises many granule cells and tangentially arranged fibers (external stria). The specific thalamocortical fibers synapse with the stellate cells of this layer and, to a lesser degree, with the pyramidal cells in the lowest part of layer III. Many other axodendritic synapses connect the specific thalamic fibers with the apical dendrites of the large and medium-size pyramidal cells of layer V (Fig. 35–3).

V   Inner Pyramidal Cell Layer.   The principal components of this layer are pyramidal cells of various sizes, stellate cells, and Martinotti cells. This layer is divided into two sublayers: V_a and V_b. Sublayer V_a comprises medium-size and small pyramidal cells (corticostriatal projection fibers arise from the latter). Sublayer V_b mainly comprises large pyramidal cells, whose axons continue as projection and association fibers. The descending axons produce collaterals, some of which terminate in layers V and VI, while

Figure 35–3   Structure of the neocortex. Cell types impregnated by the Golgi technique on the left, a Nissl-stained pattern at the center, and fiber layers on the right (according to Brodman, 1909).

a   Kaes-Bechterew's stria
b   Baillarger's external stria
c   Baillarger's internal stria
1   molecular layer
2   outer granule cell layer
3   pyramidal cell layer
4   inner granule cell layer
5   ganglion cell layer
6   polymorphous layer

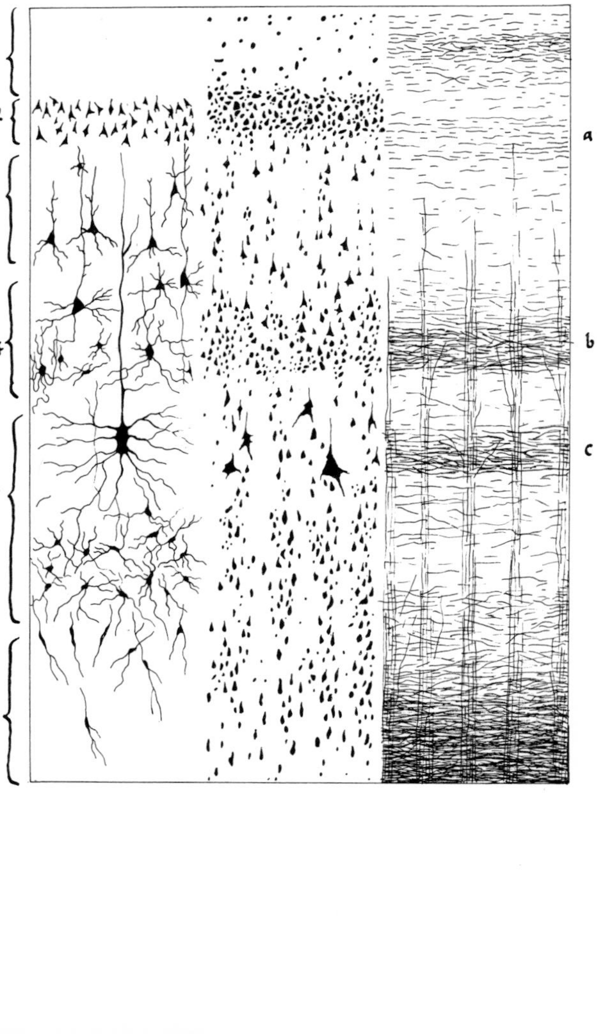

others (recurrent collaterals) ascend to the upper layers and terminate there.

VI Polymorphous Layer. This layer comprises mostly fusiform (spindle-shaped) cells, whose axons reach the white matter as corticothalamic fibers. The dendrites of the upper pole of these cells sometimes ascend to the molecular layer.

The layers of the cortex can be divided into receptor and effector layers. Afferent impulses to the cortex are distributed primarily to layers II, III, and IV (receptor layers). The cortical projection fibers to lower parts of the CNS arise mostly from layers V and VI (effector layers).

Variations in the Structural Pattern of the Isocortex

The above described six-layered structural pattern is in reality extremely variable. Areas in which the six layers are all well developed are known as homotypical cortex. In many areas, however, this pattern is less definite, and these areas are known as heterotypical cortex. In these areas the stellate cells may become predominant at the expense of the pyramidal cells; these granular cortical areas may in extreme cases be called koniocortex. On the other hand, when the pyramidal cells are predominant so that layers II and IV are hardly recognizable (if at all), the term "agranular cortex" applies. In this way, patterns of five different types are distinguished: agranular (area 4), granular (area 17), frontal (areas 8 and 9), polar (areas 10 and 38), and parietal (areas 7, 19, and 21).

In the frontal type, layers III and V are highly developed but the granule cells (small stellate cells) are readily identifiable. In the parietal type, the granule cells are highly developed (layers II and IV), but layers III and V are readily identifiable also. The polar type is characterized by a thin cortex with well developed layers.

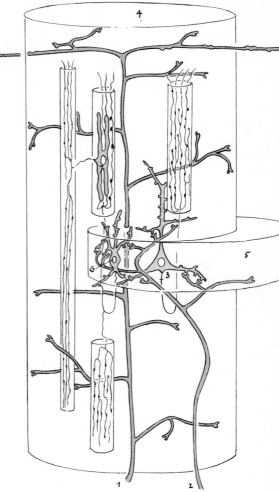

Figure 35–4 Columnar organization of the cerebral cortex. The main cylinder encompasses a cell column with a diameter of about 300 μm, arranged around a central callosal fiber. The flat cylinder comprises the terminal ramification of a specific thalamocortical fiber (according to Szentágothai, slightly simplified).

1	callosal fiber
2	specific thalamocortical fiber
3	star pyramid
4	cell column
5	area of termination of a specific thalamocortical fiber
6	spiny stellate
7	double pyramidal cell

Vertical Organization of the Cerebral Cortex

Examination of preparations of certain cortical fields impregnated by the Golgi technique reveals that a vertical organization is more evident than a horizontal one. Results of modern research indicate the existence of functional cortical units in the form of cell columns. Each colum is a virtually cylindrical "pillar" perpendicular to the brain surface, which extends right through the thickness of the cortex (Fig. 35–4). Some investigators (Szentágothai) regard the entire cortex as a mosaic of cell columns.

Most columns have a diameter of about 300 μm, and some 2500 neurons are stacked in each column. The lower layers of the column are effector layers, while the upper layers (IV, III and II) are receptor and associative layers. The dense fiber plexus of layer I probably lies outside the column.

The neuron population of a cell column comprises excitatory and inhibitory cells. Inhibitory cells are identified on the basis of the morphologic characteristics of their terminal synapses (symmetry, flattened vesicles), but this identification is somewhat uncertain. The inhibitory neurons usually synapse on the perikaryon or the initial segment of the large dendrites of the pyramidal cells. The principal inhibitory neurons are the large basket cells (Fig. 35–5), localized in layers III, IV, and V. These cells have horizontal axons that produce perpendicular collaterals so that the axon ramification is encompassed in a vertical "slice" of cortex. The terminal synapses are thus localized on the perikaryons of the neurons localized in cortical slices with a width of 50 to 100 μm (Fig. 35–5). Other, smaller inhibitory basket cells have been identified in layer II. However, a complete picture of the inhibitory circuits in the cortex is yet to be obtained.

The integration of the various layers of a cell

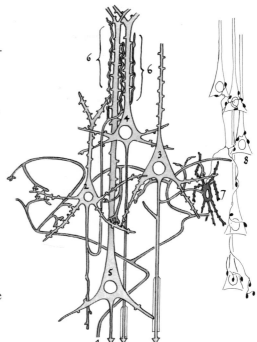

Figure 35–5 Terminal synapses of specific thalamocortical fibers and inhibitory basket cells.

1 specific thalamocortical fiber
2 spiny stellate of layer IV
3 medium-size pyramidal cell of layer IV-III
4 medium-size pyramidal cell of layer III
5 large pyramidal cell of layer V
6 complex axodendritic synapses ("cartridge synapses")
7 inhibitory basket cell
8 inhibitory axosomatic synapses on pyramidal cells

column is affected by ascending or descending intracolumnar fibers that connect the layers. These fibers are (a) ascending axon collaterals of the pyramidal cells, (b) axons of the Martinotti cells (Fig. 35–4), (c) vertical axon collaterals of the so-called double pyramidal cells, and (d) the commissural fibers of the corpus callosum, which produce collaterals to all layers and function as the axis of the cell column.

BOUNDARIES OF THE CELL COLUMNS

The term "cell column" is largely a dynamic term. In the neuronal continuum that constitutes the cortex, there are no glia layers — let alone connective tissue septa — to demarcate and separate the columns. The cell column is a functional, not a morphologic, unit. An activated column is separated from its surroundings by a zone of lateral inhibition, while inactive columns merge into the neuronal continuum. This means that the columns should not be viewed as rigid, immutable neuronal constructions but rather as units of continually changing composition. Successions of new cell columns that form in the cerebral cortex can optimally adapt to rapidly changing functional demands.

SYNAPTIC CIRCUITS

Little is known about the synaptic links between the neurons in the cortex. Research into this exceedingly difficult subject has yet to succeed in providing us with a comprehensive picture. We confine ourselves to the following partial aspects: terminations of the specific thalamocortical fibers, terminations of the associative callosal fibers, and terminations of the nonspecific thalamic fibers.

The specific thalamic fibers extend, without collaterals, as far as layer IV of the cortex. Their terminal ramifications are localized within a flattened cylindrical space of about 300 μm diameter, which extends through layer IV and the lower part of layer III. The cortical cells on which the (axodendritic) synapses are localized are variants of the stellate neurons (spiny stellates and star pyramids). Moreover, thalamic

fibers synapse on basal dendrites of pyramidal cells of layer III (Fig. 35–5). The axons of these stellate neurons ramify to form a (usually ascending) fiber bundle that ends on the apical dendrites of pyramidal cells of layer V, in series of "*synapses en passage*" (Fig. 35–5).

The associative callosal fibers extend through the entire cortex to layer I, where they show a T-shaped division. These fibers produce many collaterals to all layers of the cell column except layer IV. The terminal ramification of the callosal fibers is localized within an imaginary cylindrical column of gray matter that is 3 mm high and 300 μm wide; the callosal fibers function as the axes of the cell columns (Fig. 35–4).

Little is known about the terminations of the nonspecific thalamic fibers. According to Lorente de Nó (1949), these fibers ramify mostly in layer I, where they end in axodendritic synapses.

Cortical Fiber Connections

Afferent Fibers. Afferent fibers to the cortex originate mainly from the thalamus, basal ganglia, raphe nuclei, locus ceruleus, and other cortical areas (association and commissural fibers).

The afferent fibers from the thalamus (page 220) are very numerous and make an important contribution to the formation of the corona radiata. The terminal synapses of these fibers in the cortex have already been described. The afferents from the basal ganglia comprise thin fibers that follow the course of the corticostriatal fibers (reciprocal connections); little is known about them. The afferent fibers from the raphe nuclei comes from the medial and the dorsal raphe nucleus and reach the cortex (for example, gyrus cinguli and olfactory bulb) via the medial fasciculus of the telencephalon. The afferent fibers from the locus ceruleus likewise synapse in the gyrus cinguli and other cortical areas. The afferents from the cortex are association and commissural fibers, which can form grossly visible bundles (uncinate fasciculus, cingulum, corpus callosum, etc.). Most of them are axons from pyramidal cells in layers III and IV and axons of fusiform cells.

Efferent Fibers. Apart from the association fibers, the cortex is connected with nearly all subcortical centers except the pallidum and the vestibular nuclei. The number of efferent fibers is relatively small compared with the large number of cortical neurons. This is because most cortical cells are involved in intracortical association functions.

In the complicated stream of corticofugal fibers, six "substreams" can be distinguished:

(a) Corticothalamic fibers, which arise from layer VI and connect the cortex with many thalamic nuclei (reciprocal connections). The feedback from the cortex enables the thalamus to influence impulses arriving from the periphery (that is, to attenuate certain impulses or to suppress them completely).

(b) Corticospinal tract (pyramidal tract; see page 158 and Fig. 35–6).

(c) Corticostriatal fibers, which form one of the most important projections from the cortex. They arise mostly from prefrontal, premotor and sensorimotor parts of the cortex (areas 9, 8, 6, 4, 3 1, 2, and 5). These fibers originate from an exceedingly small group of pyramidal cells localized in layer V_a. They extend through the internal capsule and ipsilaterally enter the putamen via its dorsal aspect.

(d) Corticopontine tract, the fibers of which arise from each of the four lobes of the brain and extend via the internal capsule and the cerebral peduncle to the homolateral pontine nuclei, where they synapse. Axons from the pontine nuclei cross the midline and extend to the cerebellum via the middle cerebellar peduncle.

(e) Corticoreticulospinal tract (COEPS), which constitutes a multisynaptic link between cortex and spinal cord (page 160).

(f) Corticobulbar (corticonuclear) tract, which is morphologically indistinguishable from the corticospinal tract; its fibers terminate in the nuclei of the cranial nerves.

1 internal capsule
2 optic nerve
3 trigeminal nerve
4 middle cerebellar peduncle
5 corticospinal tract
6 restiform body (inferior cerebellar peduncle)
7 anterior limb of the internal capsule
8 posterior limb of the internal capsule

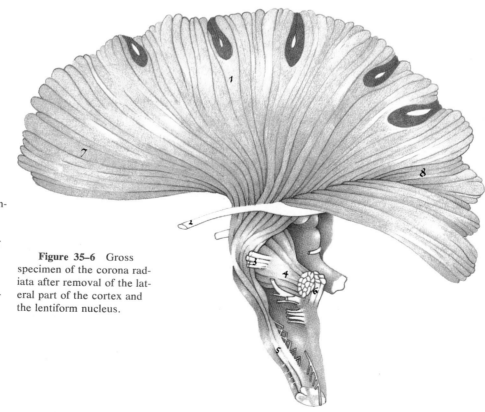

Figure 35–6 Gross specimen of the corona radiata after removal of the lateral part of the cortex and the lentiform nucleus.

Cerebral Localization: Mosaic versus Holistic Views

In the early years of the 19th century, Gall emphasized the role of the cerebral cortex in all intellectual functions. In his view, the cortical gyri were unequal because each gyrus had its own individual function. Gall maintained that, the higher the development of a particular intellectual function, the larger the corresponding gyrus. He divided the cerebral cortex into 27 fields, each with its own specific function. Although Gall's views were erroneous, the fact remains that he was the first to attempt to find the anatomic substrate of the various functions of the brain.

Modern theories on the localization of functions started with Broca's discovery (1861) that a lesion of the posterior part of the left third frontal gyrus leads to disorders of speech but does not interfere with the understanding of spoken language. This meant that a complex mental function was localized in a well defined area of the cortex. Moreover, the inequality of the left and the right hemisphere was emphasized. Subsequently studies in fact demonstrated that the language functions are located in the left hemisphere, not only in right-handed but also in 70 per cent of left-handed individuals.

In 1873 Wernicke demonstrated that lesions in the posterior part of the superior temporal gyrus (area 39) cause disturbances in the comprehension of spoken language. Many neurologists have since tried to chart a wide diversity of cerebral functions. On the basis of the relationship between clinical symptomatology and the localization of brain lesions, the *"mosaic view"* developed, which envisaged the cortex of the brain as a mosaic of more or less well defined areas, to each of which a specific "function" might be assigned. In this view, elimination of one of these areas causes a specific functional disorder.

To neuroanatomy, the great popularity of the mosaic view meant a revival of attention to research into the structure of the cerebral cortex, which led to the description of numerous cytoarchitectonic areas (page 247).

The *holistic view* (Flourens, 1824; Head, 1926; Goldstein, 1927) emphasizes the role of the totality of the cortex and refutes the functional specificity of most brain lesions. According to Goldstein, the CNS comprises numerous interlocking components and always functions as a total organ. A brain function is a dynamic process that exceeds the boundaries of each separate area and activates the entire CNS. Lashley demonstrated experimentally that whatever part of the cerebral cortex is removed, it is the size of the area removed that determines the extent to which an acquired response is lost.

The mosaic and the holistic views in their extreme forms are now both regarded as obsolete. *Peripheral and central zones* are distinguished in the cortex. The former are projection zones in which thalamocortical fibers synapse or from which long efferent pathways (pyramidal tract, COEPS) arise. These zones are characterized morphologically by a columnar organization; functionally, they have proved to be excitable. Electrical stimulation of these zones results in muscle contractions or sensory perceptions, depending on the location of stimulation. It is evident that lesions of these peripheral zones cause specific functional disorders which, in many cases, are hardly distinguishable from an interruption of the corresponding fiber projection.

The central (associative) zones are not directly connected with the periphery but are linked with other cortical areas, ipsilateral or heterolateral, or with the so-called associative thalamic nuclei. The information that comes in via the corticocortical association fibers is highly integrated. Electrical stimulation of these zones produces no response ("silent areas"). Lesions confined to the central zones cause bilateral disorders in all sensory systems (visual, auditory and tactile), such as concentric reduction of the field of vision and tactile agnosia.

According to current views, the higher psychological functions presuppose activity of interlinked parts of the central zones (analyzers). Damage to one or several of these analyzers disorganizes the totality, in a manner that depends on the partial function of the analyzer.

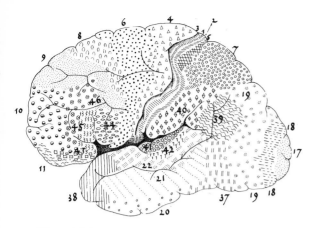

Figure 35–7 Lateral aspect of the brain: cytoarchitectonic areas (according to Brodmann).

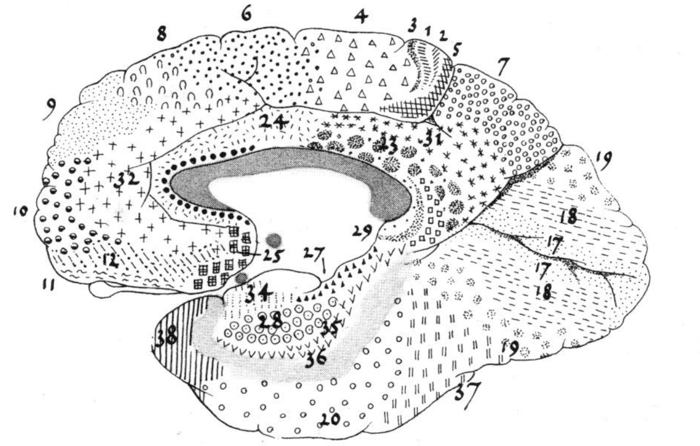

Figure 35–8 Medial aspect of the brain: cytoarchitectonic areas (according to Brodmann).

Morphologic Cartography of the Cortex

On the basis of the numerous variations in the general structural pattern of the cortex, numerous cytoarchitectonic fields have been described. The most widely used classification is that according to Brodmann (1909), who studied the cortical structure in horizontal sections stained according to Nissl. The structurally different cortical areas were numbered, and consequently cortical areas in a horizontal direction often have consecutive numbers. Brodmann described 47 areas (Fig. 35–7). Other authors (Von Economo, 1929; Vogt, 1919; Rose, 1935) distinguished a much larger number of areas, but these more detailed classifications are of doubtful use.

ORGANIZATION OF THE MOTOR CORTEX

It has long been known that electrical stimulation of the precentral gyrus causes movement in the extremities. This region was therefore called the motor cortex. In humans, this region corresponds with Brodmann's areas 4 and 6 (Fig. 35–7).

Area 4

Area 4 is located along the anterior wall of the central sulcus and the adjacent parts of the precentral sulcus; the upper part of this area is fairly wide, but descending it gradually narrows toward the anterior wall of the central sulcus. Medially on the hemisphere, it extends over the anterior part of the paracentral gyrus.

The cortex of area 4 is about 4 mm thick and is characterized by an abundance of pyramidal cells and virtual absence of stellate cells (agranular cortex). Layer V contains the so-called giant cells of Betz (about 90 μm), which numbers about 34,000 per hemisphere.

Some 30 per cent of the corticospinal fibers arise from area 4. Most of them are thin fibers; the Betz cells have thick axons but constitute only 3 per cent of the total number of corticospinal fibers.

Stimulation of area 4 causes movement of the contralateral muscles, mostly flexor muscles. Weak stimuli cause isolated muscular movements and incompletely "efficient" movements. Moreover, a somatotopic localization prevails, that is, each part of the body has its well defined site of representation in this area. It is a striking fact that the representation of the hand, upper extremity, and head occupy a much larger area than those of the trunk or the lower extremities

(Fig. 35–9). This has to do with the necessity of adequate control over the complex pattern of movements of the face and upper extremities.

Area 6

Area 6 is located rostral to area 4 (Fig. 35–7) and comprises the anterior part of the precentral gyrus and the upper part of the superior frontal gyrus. On the medial side of the hemisphere, area 6 extends into the sulcus cinguli. Areas 6 and 4 show similarities of structure, the difference being that area 6 lacks giant cells. About 28 per cent of the corticospinal fibers arise from this area.

Area 6 is electrically excitable. The results of stimulation (rotation of head and trunk to the contralateral side, flexion and extension of the extremities) are complex movements, more complex than those that occur in response to stimulation of area 4. However, the stimuli required are stronger.

Supplemental Motor Area

This area (Ms II in Woolsey's nomenclature) is located rostral to area 4, on the medial side of the frontal lobe. Stimulation of this area causes muscular contractions that enable the execution of complex movements (elevation of the contralateral arm, rotation of the head) or the assumption of a particular body posture.

Cortical Lesions of Areas 4 and 6

When the lesion is confined to area 4, as in some surgical interventions, paralysis of the contralateral extremity (extremities) follows. The distal muscles of the extremity are more severely affected than the proximal muscles. Minor cortical ablations in area 4 cause only slight spasticity.

Combined lesions of areas 4 and 6 (Ms I according to Woolsey) cause more severe paralysis, associated with spasticity and increased myotatic reflexes. The last two symptoms probably result from interruption of many COEPS fibers that arise from area 6.

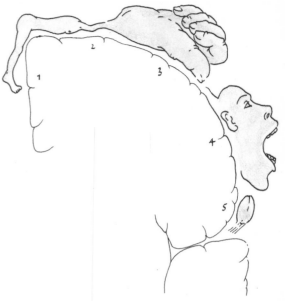

Figure 35–9 Section through the primary motor cortex; cortical areas from which movements can be elicited.

1 extremities
2 trunk
3 fingers
4 speech movements, facial expression
5 tongue

SOMATOSENSORY AREAS

The primary somatosensory area (Sm I) comprises three narrow strips in the postcentral gyrus (areas 3, 1 and 2) and extends from the depth of the central sulcus over the entire postcentral gyrus (Fig. 35–7). Cytoarchitectonically it belongs to the granular cortex. The afferent fibers originate from the thalamus (ventral posterolateral and ventral mediolateral nuclei). The area shows an exact somatotopic localization, the lower extremity being represented superiorly by the face in its inferior part.

Analogous to the situation in the motor cortex, the cortical representations of the body parts in this area differ considerably in size. Hands and head are privileged, with very extensive and detailed representations, whereas the sites of representation of the trunk and the proximal parts of the extremities are much smaller (Fig. 35–10).

Most of the cell columns in area 2 probably

receive impulses from the receptors in the joints; the columns in area 1 are believed to be involved in assimilating the information supplied by skin stimuli (touch and pressure). There is hardly any lateral spreading of incoming impulses over adjacent columns; this greatly enhances perception contrast and facilitates exact location of the source of the impulses.

The sensory cortex enriches perception with delicate discriminatory qualities, for example, recognition of spatial relations and awareness of minor differences in intensity. Pain impulses are conducted to Sm II (areas 40 and 43).

Cortical Lesions of the Postcentral Gyrus

Lesions of this gyrus reduce in particular the mechanical discriminatory capacities, both in the perception of delicate tactile stimuli and in the ability to determine the positions of fingers and extremities. Pain and temperature sensibility is hardly disturbed. Upon recovery, the pain sense is the first to return, and kinesthesia the last.

SENSORIMOTOR CORTEX

It can be deduced from the above that the central sulcus marks the boundary between the motor cortex (anterior to it) and the sensory cortex (posterior to it). However, it has been found in recent years that: (a) motor effects can be produced also by stimulation of the sensory cortex; and (b) sensory impulses from the thalamus produce action potentials not only in the sensory but also in the motor cortex. The recent discovery that fibers from the ventral posterolateral nucleus also terminate in area 4 has explained the anatomic substrate of this phenomenon.

This has led to the introduction of the term ''sensorimotor cortex'' (SM), which encompasses the cytoarchitectonic areas 6, 4, 3, 1, and 2. The predominantly motor areas are collectively known as Ms I, while the supplemental motor area is called Ms II. The predominantly sensory areas are known as Sm I (areas 3, 1, and 2), while the supplemental sensory area is Sm II.

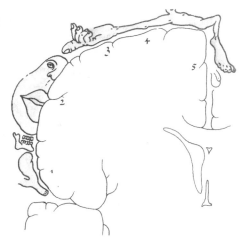

Figure 35–10 Frontal section through the primary somatosensory cortex; localization of the sensory areas.

1	teeth, larynx, abdomen
2	face
3	hand
4	arm and trunk
5	leg and genitals

SUPPLEMENTAL SENSORY AREA (Sm II)

This small area lies hidden in the lateral cerebral fissure, and constitutes its upper wall. The projection from the periphery is bilateral, with some predominance of contralateral impulses. Some cortical neurons in this area respond to pain impulses that originate from the posterior nucleus of the thalamus; impulses arriving from the periphery via the spinothalamic system probably synapse in Sm II.

Visual Cortex (Area Striata)

The area striata (Brodmann's area 17) is located in the posterior part of the cortex on the medial side of the occipital lobe, on either side of the calcarine fissure, and for a small part on the lateral surface. Cytoarchitectonically the area is of the granular type (koniocortex). Layer IV is exceptionally thick and can be subdivided into three sublayers (IV_a, IV_b, and IV_c). Sublayer IV_b has a markedly thickened external stria of Baillarger, which is here called Gennari's stria.

The fibers of the geniculocalcarine tract terminate, for the most part, on the granular cells of layer IV. The area striata is to be regarded as a primarily optic area (peripheral cortex); it is surrounded by association areas (Brodmann's areas 18 and 19; Fig. 35–7), which are essential to eye movements, psychologic interpretation of optic impressions, and integration of optic impressions with other types of information.

Auditory Area

The auditory area (Brodmann's areas 41 and 42) lies in the cortex of the superior temporal gyrus, in the depth of the lateral cerebral fissure. The afferent projection fibers (geniculotemporal tract) originate either from the medial geniculate body or directly from the inferior colliculus. This area is structurally a typically granular cortex (koniocortex).

A tonotopic localization has been demonstrated in the auditory area in animals. The basal cochlear winding (high frequencies) projects on the anterior part of area 41, while the apical cochlear turn (low frequencies) is represented in the posterior part of this area. Each cochlea is bilaterally represented in the auditory area, although there are left/right differences.

Psychologic Cortical Areas

Apart from the areas directly involved in processing sensory information, there are extensive areas in which no response occurs after stimulation (central areas). They include the prefrontal cortex (areas 9, 10, 11, and 45) of the frontal lobe, and areas 28, 21, and 22 of the temporal lobe. These areas are the anatomic substrate of higher psychologic functions.

Areas 9 and 10 are connected with the thalamus (dorsal medial nucleus) by fibers that extend in the anterior thalamic peduncle. Efferent fibers from the prefrontal cortex extend to areas 21, 22, and 38 of the temporal lobe (via the uncinate fasciculus) and to areas 39 and 40 of the parietal lobe (via the arcuate fasciculus), where they synapse.

Bilateral lesions of the prefrontal cortex cause defects in intelligence and in personality.

The patients show a diminished ability to think in abstract terms and to concentrate. The personality change is very conspicuous: The patient loses stability, self-criticism, and initiative, and his sense of decorum is reduced. Feelings of self-satisfaction and "well being" are common.

Surgical severance of the fiber projections of the prefrontal cortex has important psychologic consequences. One of the most interesting phenomena is the patient's changed attitude to pain; this is why this operation is sometimes performed on patients suffering from severe, intractable pain. They cease to complain after the operation, although the pain impulses persist.

Areas 39 and 40, in the lower part of the parietal lobe, are indispensable for the integration of the entire exteroceptive and proprioceptive input required for recognition of one's own body parts as such and their position in space. This area is involved in the maintenance of the so-called body schema. It is remarkable that lesions in the nondominant (usually right) parietal lobe lead to disturbances in the body schema, while lesions in the contralateral parietal lobe usually give rise to aphasia (language disorders).

Concept of "Cerebral Dominance"

Functionally the extremities, and particularly the hands, are not entirely equivalent. Humans show a pronounced tendency to differentiate in the assignment of task to the hands. In the case of complex actions there is always one hand that executes the principal movement, while the other hand plays a more supportive and static role. About 90 per cent of people are right-handed, and in these individuals muscular strength is most pronounced on the right side. In right-handed people, therefore, the right hand can be said to "dominate." Since this hand is controlled by the left hemisphere, we conclude that — at least in terms of motor activity — the left hemisphere plays a leading role.

Broca's description of a patient with speech disorders after a hemorrhage in the left hemisphere, revealed the importance of this hemisphere in language functions. Subsequent clinical studies disclosed that an intact left hemisphere is indispensable for normal language functions. In view of the importance of the left hemisphere for these language functions and for the control of the right hand, this hemisphere came to be called the "dominant hemisphere."

The speech center proves to be localized in the right hemisphere in about 30 per cent of all left-handed people. In view of the predilection for the left hemisphere, language disorders are of unmistakable significance in locating cerebral lesions.

Functional Differences between the Cerebral Hemispheres

The functional inequality of the right and the left hemispheres is apparent from numerous clinical studies. In 96 per cent of all cases the left hemisphere encompasses the speech center. Moreover, this hemisphere functions analytically and sequentially and is, therefore, particularly well suited to the execution of mathematical calculations. Finally, it is possible that conscious awareness is also localized in the left hemisphere.

However, the dominance of the left hemisphere does not mean that the right hemisphere is not important, let alone that it is superfluous. In some respects the right hemisphere is superior to the left: in recognizing abstract forms and spatial relations, in non-verbal expression (that is, drawing), and in enjoying music. The left hemisphere functions mostly analytically, while the right has a better grasp of totalities. The problem of the right hemisphere is that it is unable to "speak for itself." Without the left hemisphere, the right is doomed to silence, and in view of the close relationship between speaking and thinking, the question is whether the right hemisphere by itself is capable of conceptual thinking.

Function of the Corpus Callosum

The corpus callosum, with about 200 million fibers, is the largest commissure of the neocor-

tex. These fibers connect homologous cortical areas in such a manner as to enable the two hemispheres to function as a unit. Very few cortical areas (some areas of the temporal lobe) have no callosal fibers.

Until recently, the function of the corpus callosum was a mystery. It was known, however, that patients in whom the corpus callosum had failed to develop (agenesis) or had been surgically severed showed no neurologic abnormalities. Recent research has revealed that this commissure plays an essential role in the transfer of information from one hemisphere to the other. Humans show marked lateralization of cortical functions, that is, many functions are represented not bilaterally but unilaterally. The other hemisphere gains access to the neuronal substrate of such functions via the fibers of the corpus callosum and other commissures.

The role of the corpus callosum was first demonstrated by Sperry in experiments with blindfolded cats. After sagittal severance of the optic chiasm, the optic impulses from each eye are transferred exclusively to the ipsilateral visual cortex. Cats with a blindfolded right eye can be taught to distinguish certain geometric patterns. When subsequently the left eye is blindfolded and the same patterns are offered to the right eye, the cat can distinguish them just as well as it could with the trained left eye. This implies that a transfer of information has taken place between the two hemispheres.

When the experiment is repeated after severance of the corpus callosum, however, the cat can no longer distinguish the patterns with the eye that was blindfolded during training. The information received by one hemisphere is no longer transferred to the other. Animals thus treated are therefore known as split-brain animals. The transfer of information in these experiments takes place via the commissural fibers that connect the visual cortical areas.

Severance of the corpus callosum has no consequences for intelligence, behavior, and emotions. This operation is sometimes performed on epileptic patients in order to prevent expansion of epileptic seizures from one hemisphere to the other. It was found in such cases that perceptions effected in the right hemisphere via the left hand or via the left field of vision could not be verbally expressed and that the patient was not aware of them. When the patient was given an object in his right hand while his eyes were closed, he could name the object, but he was unable to do so when the object was placed in his left hand. However, he was able to *point out* what he held in his left hand when the same object was offered to him among a variety of other objects.

Chapter 36

Basal Ganglia

The basal ganglia consist of three large nuclei: the caudate nucleus, the putamen, and the globus pallidus, collectively known as the corpus striatum. Modern investigators also include other nuclei like the substantia nigra. The caudate nucleus and the putamen together form the neostriatum and function as a unit. The pallidum is divided by a layer of fibers (internal medullary lamina) into an external pallidum and an internal pallidum. The basal ganglia are separated from the thalamus by fibers of the internal capsule (see Fig. 26–2).

Histologic Structure of the Neostriatum

The caudate nucleus and the putamen show structural similarities. Both nuclei contain an abundance of blood capillaries and bundles of unmyelinated fibers. They mainly have small neurons, with a few scattered multipolar neurons among them (one large neuron for every 30 to 40 small neurons). The nuclei show a homogeneous structure without regional differences.

The small cells have dendrites that radiate in all directions. The dendritic field of such a neuron is conical in shape, with a diameter of about 400 μm. The dendrites have numerous gemmules. The axon is short (Golgi II cells).

These small neurons can be regarded as receptor cells or associative cells.

The larger neurons can be divided into two types. The first type has an oval nucleus, long smooth dendrites, and a myelinated axon with collaterals; these cells are the source of the efferent neostriatal fibers. The second type has a round nucleus and dendrites with gemmules; little is known about this type.

Structure of the Paleostriatum (Pallidum)

The globus pallidus derives its name from the numerous myelinated fibers that traverse it. The cells of the pallidum are fairly large, fusiform neurons with long smooth dendrites (Fig. 36–1) and thick myelinated axons. With the electron microscope, synapses have been demonstrated on the dendrites and sometimes on perikaryons of the striatal cells, particularly axodendritic synapses on the gemmules. The corticostriatal and thalamostriatal fibers terminate in asymmetric synapses; intrastriatal fibers end in symmetric or asymmetric synapses. Many axodendritic synapses in the caudate nucleus and the putamen contain dopamine (nigrostriatal fibers).

Fiber Connections

In the basal ganglia we distinguish a receptor and an effector part. The receptor part is extensive and comprises the caudate nucleus and the putamen; the effector part is almost entirely confined to the pallidum, to which many fibers from receptor areas converge.

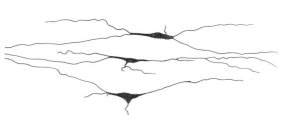

Figure 36–1 Neurons of the pallidum (according to Clara).

Figure 36–2 Frontal section through thalamus and striatum; fiber connections of the neostriatum.

1 caudate nucleus
2 dorsomedial (DM) nucleus
3 ventral posterolateral (VPL) nucleus
4 ventral posteromedial (VPM) nucleus
5 central nucleus (centrum medianum)
6 putamen
7 pallidum
8 substantia nigra
9 red nucleus
10 pyramidal fibers

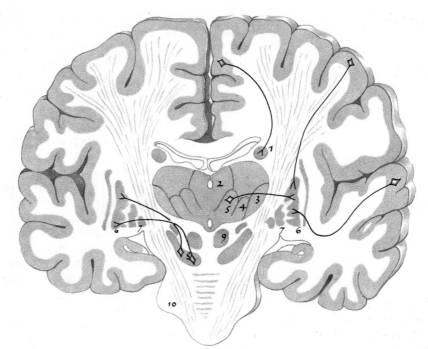

NEOSTRIATUM

Afferent Fibers. Afferent fibers come from the cerebral cortex, the thalamus, and the substantia nigra (Fig. 36–2). Large parts of the cerebral cortex project to the caudate nucleus and putamen, this projection being largely ipsilateral. Cortical fibers for the putamen reach the nucleus via the external capsule. Fibers for the caudate nucleus extend through the white matter of the hemisphere.

The fibers from the thalamus originate from the nonspecific thalamic nuclei. The intralaminar nuclei (central nucleus or centrum medianum, and parafascicular nucleus) project to the putamen via fibers that cross the internal capsule; the fibers for the caudate nucleus come from other, smaller intralaminar nuclei (paracentral nucleus and medial ventral nucleus).

Fibers from the substantia nigra arise from the pars compacta, cross the internal capsule and the pallidum, and synapse with the small striatal neurons. Caudal parts of the substantia nigra project to the putamen, and rostral parts to the caudate nucleus. The nigrostriatal fibers contain dopamine.

Efferent Fibers. Efferent fibers project to the pallidum and the substantia nigra. The striopallidal fibers are very numerous; they reach the pallidum via the internal and the external medullary laminae. The fibers from the caudate nucleus cross the internal capsule. The strionigral projection synapses in the pars reticulata and is topically organized (page 214). These fibers probably contain GABA as the neurotransmitter.

PALEOSTRIATUM (PALLIDUM)

Afferent Fibers. Afferent fibers converging on the globus pallidus come from the neostriatum, thalamus, red nucleus, substantia nigra, and the subthalamic nucleus. Apart from the neostriatal fibers, the principal afferent fibers come from the subthalamic nucleus. These fibers cross the internal capsule and synapse on the medial part of the globus pallidus.

Efferent Fibers. The basal ganglia exert their influence on other regions of the CNS via the pallidofugal fibers. From the internal pallidum arise the lenticular loop (ansa of the lenticular nucleus) and the lenticular fasciculus. The

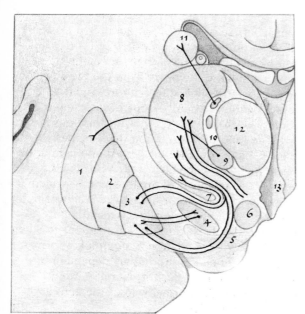

Figure 36–3 Lenticular loop (ansa of lenticular nucleus), lenticular fasciculus, and thalamic fasciculus (according to Carpenter).

1 putamen
2 external pallidum
3 internal pallidum
4 subthalamic nucleus
5 substantia nigra
6 red nucleus
7 zona incerta
8 thalamus (VA and VL nucleus)
9 central nucleus (centromedian)
10 internal medullary lamina
11 caudate nucleus
12 dorsal medial nucleus
13 third ventricle

The fibers of the subthalamic fasciculus originate in the external pallidum; they cross the caudal part of the internal capsule and synapse on the subthalamic nucleus (reciprocal connection). The subthalamopallidal fibers, however, synapse on the internal pallidum (Fig. 36–3). Other pallidofugal fibers project via the tegmental central fasciculus to the pedunculopontine tegmental nucleus, the red nucleus, and the inferior olive. Recent research has shown that the pallidum projects also to the lateral habenular nucleus. These projections give the striatum access to the limbic system.

It follows from the above described projections that the basal ganglia as a whole project mainly to the thalamus and, via this, to the premotor and the orbitofrontal cortex. Descending pallidofugal fibers do not extend beyond the level of the inferior olive.

The basal ganglia are unable to exert a direct influence on the motoneurons; the pyramidal tract and the COEPS are the principal routes via which the activity of the basal ganglia is expressed.

STRIATAL REGULATORY CIRCUITS

The projections of the basal ganglia are organized according to the principle of a regulatory circuit: The efferent striatal fibers project, via the thalamus or otherwise, to the same centers from which the afferent fibers originate. There are three interwoven regulatory circuits:

(a) cerebral cortex → neostriatum → pallidum → thalamus (VA and VL) → cerebral cortex (area 6 and orbitofrontal cortex);

(b) thalamus (CM + PF) → other intralaminar nuclei → neostriatum → pallidum → thalamus;

(c) neostriatum → substantia nigra → neostriatum.

SUBTHALAMIC REGION

The subthalamic region is localized lateral to the hypothalamus and ventral to the thalamus; it is an area of transition to the tegmentum of the

fibers of the lenticular loop (Fig. 36–3) leave the rounded apex of the pallidum, curve around the posterior limb of the internal capsule and, via the outside of the fornix, reach the so-called tegmental field H of Forel. The fibers of the lenticular fasciculus (Forel field H2) arise from the dorsomedial part of the internal pallidum, traverse the internal capsule, and finally reach Forel field H via a detour between the zona incerta and subthalamic nucleus (Fig. 36–3). From Forel field H the pallidofugal fibers continue to the thalamus, where they synapse on the ventral anterior (VA) and the ventral lateral (VL) nuclei (Fig. 36–4).

mesencephalon. The region is traversed by important fiber bundles (lenticular loop, lenticular fasciculus, thalamic fasciculus). Its best known nuclei are the zona incerta and the subthalamic nucleus. The zona incerta is a fairly diffuse layer of neurons that continues as the reticular nucleus of the thalamus (Fig. 36–3). This zone lies between the lenticular fasciculus and the thalamic fasciculus. The projections of the zona incerta are unknown. The subthalamic nucleus is located medial to the internal capsule (Fig. 36–3). In frontal sections this nucleus has an oval shape. It contains numerous fusiform or pyramidal neurons.

Afferent fibers to the subthalamic nucleus arise from the external pallidum and extend via the subthalamic fasciculus (Fig. 36–3).

Efferent fibers from the subthalamic nucleus synapse on the internal pallidum; these fibers likewise run in the subthalamic fasciculus.

Functional Significance of the Basal Ganglia

The function of the basal ganglia is still obscure. Current knowledge about the structure and projections and more recent insight into the neuropharmacology of the region give no clear information on function. Moreover, interpretation of results of animal experiments is by no means simple, quite apart from the technical problems inherent to elimination of particular centers without simultaneous destruction of fibers "on their way to other destinations."

The kind of information that reaches the basal ganglia is highly integrated and cannot be easily defined. The cortical afferent fibers come from extensive cortical areas, some of which are characterized as motor areas whereas others are considered to be sensory or associative areas. Afferent impulses from the intralaminar thalamic nuclei likewise contain very complex information; these impulses are in part dependent on activity in the reticular formation. Little is known about the normal role of the activity of the substantia nigra.

On the basis of comparative anatomic data it is assumed that the basal ganglia are involved in motor activity. In reptiles and birds, the basal ganglia function as the highest motor center that regulates the delicate coordination of the highly developed motor activities of these animals. In

Figure 36–4 Parasagittal section; projections of the basal ganglia (according to Carpenter).

1 caudate nucleus
2 putamen
3 thalamus (VA nucleus)
4 thalamus (VA and VL nuclei)
5 external pallidum
6 internal pallidum
7 zona incerta
8 central nucleus (centromedian)
9 ventral posteromedial (VPM) nucleus
10 subthalamic nucleus
11 substantia nigra
12 optic tract
13 superior colliculus
14 medial lemniscus
15 pedunculopontine reticular nucleus

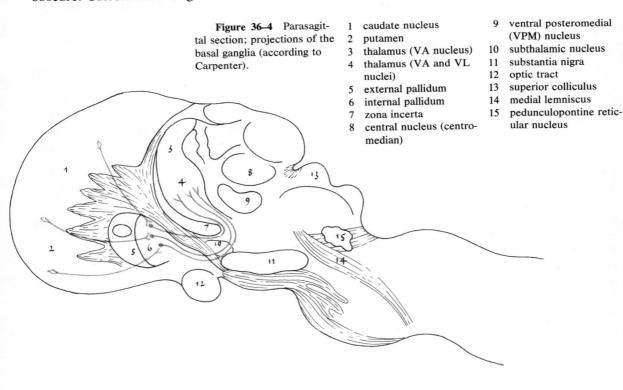

higher mammals, and particularly in humans, the cerebral cortex has taken over numerous functions originally carried out by the basal ganglia. In these cases the nuclei might perhaps function as the seat of numerous motor programs for automatic and trained movements.

Automatic movements play an important role in day-to-day life and help determine characteristic personality traits: facial expression, general posture, the movements of the arms in walking, etc. As regards the trained movements, it is possible that these complex recurrent movements (walking, writing, swimming, cycling, dancing) are automated in fixed motor patterns that are stored in the striatum.

The basal ganglia are involved also in regulating muscle tone, particularly the tone of the muscles subservient to body posture.

Experimental Results

Attempts to analyze the function of the striatum in experiments have so far failed to provide a comprehensive picture of the function of these nuclei. Repeated high-frequency stimulation of the caudate nucleus in active, freely moving cats results in averting movements of the head to the contralateral side. Other experiments with low frequency of stimulation, however, have demonstrated inhibition of movements activated by the cortex.

Bilateral elimination of the pallidum in test animals causes lack of activity and enables them to persist in uncomfortable body postures for hours. Bilateral elimination of the putamen leads to increased activity: The animals are constantly in motion.

Lesions of the basal ganglia, in particular, lead to dyskinesia, that is, the occurrence of involuntary movements of the face, trunk, or extremities at intervals of varying duration (hyperkinetic syndrome). Other patients show hypokinesia (abnormally decreased mobility and lack of associated movements), tremor, and rigidity. The tremor is unintentional and disappears after a purposeful movement. The muscles offer considerable resistance to passive stretch (increased muscle tone).

Neurosurgical procedures have revealed that rigidity in Parkinson's disease can be alleviated by partial elimination of the pallidum and that the tremor can be reduced by elimination of the ventral anterior (VA) nucleus of the thalamus, the site at which most of the pallidofugal fibers synapse. The operations are performed under stereotactic guidance. The development of a tremor seems to result from rhythmic discharges in the VA nucleus of the thalamus. Dysfunction of the inhibitory dopaminergic nigrostriatal fibers causes hyperactivity of the pallidum, which results in overstimulation of the VA nucleus. The consequence is oscillation of the thalamic neurons (frequency: 4 to 6 per second), and these impulses reach the α-neurons and γ-neurons of the spinal cord via the corticospinal tract.

Chapter 37

The Hippocampal Formation

The hippocampal formation is the largest structure of the allocortex. With the cerebellum, it is among the best known areas of the CNS. Newly discovered facts on fiber projections, the nature of the hippocampal transmitters, and the topographic distribution of certain chemical substances have supplemented the classic studies of Cajal (1893, 1901) and Lorente de Nó (1933, 1934) to provide a more profound knowledge of the structure of this region. The function of the hippocampal formation, however, is less well understood. The clinical observations and exper-

imental findings are too incoherent to permit definite conclusions on the functional role of this region.

The hippocampal formation has been characterized on page 69 as a ring of cerebral cortex around the choroid fissure (see Fig. 9–3). Here, we confine ourselves to the morphology of its highly developed retrocommissural part. This retrocommissural part comprises two concentric rings (Fig. 9–3). The inner ring (archicortex) comprises the dentate gyrus, the hippocampus (horn of Ammon), and the subiculum; the latter constitutes the transition to the outer ring (periallocortex), which comprises the presubiculum (area 27), the retrosplenial area (area 29e), the parasubiculum (area 49), and the entorhinal area (area 28). The periallocortical area extends laterally to the rhinal sulcus (Fig. 37–1), beyond which the isocortex of the fusiform gyrus (areas 35 and 36) is located.

The archicortex is characterized by the fact that the six-layered cytoarchitectonic pattern of the isocortex is replaced by a two-layered pattern. Counting the fiber layers as well, one finds a six-layered structure. This applies in particular

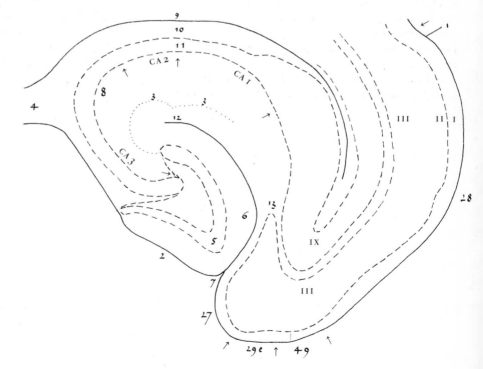

Figure 37–1 Horizontal section through the hippocampal formation and periallocortex (schematically, according to Angevine).

1   rhinal sulcus
2   dentate gyrus
3   hippocampus
4   fimbria
5   stratum granulosum
6   stratum moleculare
7   hippocampal fissure
8   stratum radiatum
9   alveus
10 stratum oriens
11 stratum pyramidale
12 stratum moleculare
13 subiculum
27 area 27
28 area 28
29e area 29e
49 area 49

to the hippocampus; the stratification of the dentate gyrus is less well-defined.

Dentate Gyrus

In the dentate gyrus we distinguish (counting down from the surface) three layers: molecular layer, granule cell layer, and a polymorphous layer (Fig. 37–1). The molecular layer consists of a dense fiber plexus in which the dendrites of the granule cells are located (Fig. 37–2); the fibers of the so-called perforating fasciculus (see below) synapse on these dendrites. The granule cell layer is a layer of closely packed granule cells, whose dendrites ramify in the molecular layer; the axons (mossy fibers) extend to the hippocampus, where they synapse on the proximal part of the apical dendrites of the pyramidal cells (Fig. 37–2). The polymorphous layer is an area of transition between dentate gyrus and hippocampus. The cells in this layer are pyramidal or fusiform; the axons extend either to the molecular layer or to the alveus of the hippocampus.

Hippocampus (Horn of Ammon)

Pyramidal cells and basket cells are the most characteristic cell types of the horn of Ammon. The cell body of the pyramidal cells is spindle-shaped and shows two dendrite ramifications in opposite directions, perpendicular to the wall of the hippocampal fissure (Fig. 37–2). These dendrites run parallel to each other and traverse the entire thickness of the hippocampus. In the transverse plane, the pyramidal cell layer extends from the border of the subiculum as far as the hilus of the dentate gyrus (polymorphous layer).

The basket cells are smaller neurons localized in the stratum oriens and have an ascending axon that synapses on the cell body of the pyramidal cells.

LAYERS OF THE HIPPOCAMPUS

As a component of the allocortex, the hippocampus has two layers of cells and a few layers

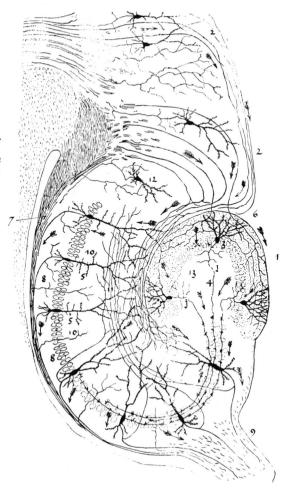

Figure 37–2 Structure and projections of the hippocampus. Golgi technique (according to Cajal).

1 stratum moleculare
2 perforating fasciculus
3 granule cells (stratum granulosum)
4 mossy fiber
5 pyramidal cell
6 hippocampal fissure
7 alveus
8 stratum oriens
9 fimbria
10 stratum radiatum
11 Schaffer collaterals
12 cell of the subiculum
13 fascia dentata

of fibers, with some scattered neurons between them. The length of the dendrites of the pyramidal cells and the abundance of afferent fibers explain the fact that the hippocampus has more fiber layers than the dentate gyrus. Counting up from the depth (wall of the lateral ventricle) to the surface (hippocampal fissure), the following layers are encountered:

Alveus. This is a thin layer of myelinated fibers localized directly against the ependymal lining of the lateral ventricle. Some of the fibers of the alveus are axons of the pyramidal cells (efferent hippocampal fibers). Afferent (septo-hippocampal) fibers are also found.

Stratum Oriens. This layer is localized between the alveus and the pyramidal cell layer (Fig. 37–2) and comprises neurons with ascending axons (basket cells), the ramifications of the basal dendrites of the pyramidal cells, and their axon collaterals. The axons of the basket cells terminate in axosomatic synapses on the cell body of the pyramidal cells.

Stratum Pyramidale. The dendrite ramifications of the cells in this layer extend from the stratum oriens to the stratum moleculare (Fig. 37–3). The axons arise from the cell body or from a thick dendrite, traverse the stratum oriens, and enter the alveus. The axon collaterals synapse with the basket cells of the stratum oriens (among other cells).

The afferent fibers to the pyramidal cells are systematically distributed over the receptive surface. On each receptive dendritic field (apical and basal), a specific group of afferent fibers synapses. The axodendritic synapses are excitatory, while the axosomatic synapses (basket cells) are inhibitory. As in the Purkinje cells of the cerebellum, most of the afferent fibers run parallel to each other.

The axons of the pyramidal cells of the hippocampal fields CA4 and CA3 (see below) give rise to a fairly thick collateral branch that ascends in the stratum oriens and traverses the wall of the hippocampus to the stratum lacunosum, where it runs horizontally. During their course through the stratum lacunosum, these fibers have numerous exodendritic synapses with pyramidal cells of CA3, CA2, and CA1. According to Cajal (1904), these *"Schaffer collaterals"* extend as far as the subiculum (Fig. 37–2).

Stratum Radiatum. This layer owes its name to the parallel arrangement of the apical dendrites of the pyramidal cells, on which the moss fibers of the dentate gyrus synapse.

Stratum Lacunosum. A dense fiber plexus is the principal component of this layer. In it, we distinguish Schaffer collaterals, axons ascending from the alveus, and axons and collaterals ascending from neurons of the stratum oriens.

Stratum Moleculare. The apical dendrites of the pyramidal cells end in this layer. Most of the fibers of this layer originate from the entorhinal area (perforating fibers). Stellate or fusiform cells are found scattered among the fibers.

REGIONAL DIFFERENCES IN THE HIPPOCAMPUS

In view of local differences in the structure of the hippocampus (size of pyramidal cells, presence or absence of Schaffer collaterals, distribution of the afferent fibers), it has been subdivided into so-called CA fields (Lorente de Nó, 1934). Field CA4 is localized in the transition between hippocampus and dentate gyrus and corresponds with the latter's polymorphous layer; field CA3 encompasses a large part of the hippocampus and is characterized by large pyramidal cells that give rise to Schaffer collaterals; field CA2, however, is narrow (Fig. 37–1); field CA1 is adjacent to the subiculum, and the superposed stratum oriens shows an increasing abundance of neurons.

Subiculum

The subiculum constitutes the transition between the hippocampus and the laterally localized periallocortex. This region (Fig. 37–1) is characterized by a thick superficial layer (stratum moleculare), which continues in the homonymous layer of the hippocampus. Embedded in this layer are islands of neurons separated by small bundles of ascending fibers (Fig. 37–4). The following layers are distinguished in the subiculum (Cajal, 1904):

Stratum Moleculare. Many of the fibers in this layer extend to the hippocampus or dentate gyrus (perforating fibers), where they synapse (see below).

Stratum Pyramidale. The neurons of this

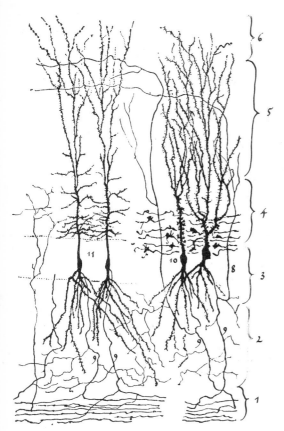

Figure 37–3 Pyramidal cells of the hippocampus; Schaffer collaterals (according to Cajal).

1   alveus
2   stratum oriens
3   stratum pyramidale
4   stratum radiatum
5   stratum lacunosum
6   stratum moleculare
7   mossy fibers
8   Schaffer collaterals
9   axons of the pyramidal cells
10 large pyramidal cells of CA3 and CA4
11 small pyramidal cells of CA1

layer are of medium size; the apical dendrites extend between the neuronal islands of the stratum moleculare.

Stratum Multiforme. This layer marks the inferior boundary of the previous layer and comprises scattered triangular cells with ascending axons that synapse with the pyramidal cells.

Periallocortex

The periallocortex comprises a number of concentrically arranged cortical areas that structurally belong to the allocortex or the mesocortex. These areas are the presubiculum (area 27), the retrosplenial area (area 29e), the parasubiculum (area 49), and the entorhinal area (area 28). The last area extends as far as the rhinal sulcus (Fig. 37–1), which marks the boundary between the entorhinal area and the neocortex of the fusiform gyrus.

The structure of the periallocortex is much more complex than that of the hippocampus. Its principal characteristic is the so-called lamina dissecans, an acellular zone between cell layers II and III on the one hand and IV on the other. We confine ourselves to a few items on the structure of the entorhinal area.

The entorhinal area is part of the "piriform lobe" (paleopallium). Grossly it constitutes the largest part of the parahippocampal gyrus, with the gyrus ambiens above (prepiriform area), and the rhinal sulcus below (see Fig. 11–2).

The layers distinguished in the entorhinal area are as follows: (a) *stratum moleculare*, which consists of a rich plexus of tangentially arranged fibers, (b) *external principal lamina*, which is a thick layer of large stellate or pyramidal cells, (c) *lamina dissecans*, which comprises one of the richest and most delicate fiber plexuses of the entire CNS (Cajal, 1904), and (d) *internal principal lamina*, which comprises small neurons with ascending axons that synapse in the external principal lamina.

The axons of the cells of the external principal lamina collect in the underlying white matter and form three bundles: commissural fibers for the psalterium (commissure of the fornix), the perforating fasciculus, and the alvear fasciculus. The last two bundles connect the entorhinal area with the hippocampus and dentate gyrus.

Fiber Connections

AFFERENT FIBERS

The afferent fibers to the hippocampal formation can be divided into three categories:

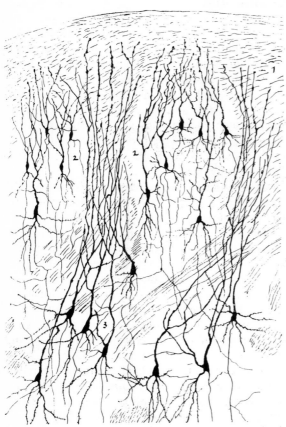

Figure 37–4 Structure of the subiculum; Golgi technique (according to Cajal).

1 stratum moleculare
2 islands of small pyramidal cells
3 medium-size pyramidal cells of the stratum pyramidale

the superficial system from the prepiriform area. With the exception of the fornix, these fibers converge on the entorhinal area and the parasubiculum, where they synapse.

The uncinate fasciculus comprises fibers from the orbitofrontal cortex (areas 10 and 11). The cingulum comprises fibers from the anterior nucleus (AN) of the thalamus and from the cortex of the gyrus cinguli. The fornix comprises fibers from the septum: These fibers synapse in the hilus of the dentate gyrus and in the stratum oriens of CA3, CA2, CA1, and the subiculum.

Fibers from the prepiriform area descend through the surface of the uncus and synapse in the lateral portion of the entorhinal area.

Commissural Fibers. Commissural fibers originate from the contralateral hippocampus (or the subiculum) and traverse the psalterium (hippocampal commissure); they connect symmetric areas of both hippocampi and synapse in the stratum oriens.

Intrinsic Fibers. The principal bundles of afferent fibers *within* the hippocampal formation are the perforating fasciculus, the alvear fasciculus, the mossy fibers, the Schaffer collaterals, and fibers that connect CA1 with the subiculum.

The perforating fasciculus arises from the medial portion of the entorhinal area. The fibers first extend to the white matter and then traverse the parasubiculum and presubiculum (Fig. 37–5), until they reach the stratum moleculare of the subiculum. Their further course is superficial. The terminal synapses are in the molecular layer of the hippocampus and dentate gyrus. These fibers are the principal afferents for the dentate gyrus.

The alvear fasciculus probably also arises from the entorhinal area; its fibers traverse the alveus and terminate in CA1.

The mossy fibers are axons of the cells of the stratum granulosum of the dentate gyrus. They synapse with the proximal part of the apical dendrites of the pyramidal cells.

The Schaffer collaterals connect CA4 and CA3 with CA1; from CA1, axons extend to the subiculum via the alveus.

extrinsic, commissural, and intrinsic fibers. The extrinsic fibers originate from other cerebral areas and mostly synapse in the periallocortex; the commissural fibers originate from the contralateral hippocampus, and the intrinsic fibers connect parts of the hippocampal formation with each other.

Extrinsic Fibers. The course of the extrinsic afferent fibers to the hippocampal formation is determined by the partly intraventricular position of this region. The principal routes of access are uncinate fasciculus, cingulum, fornix, and

EFFERENT FIBERS

Most of the efferent fibers of the hippocampal formation extend to the fornix via the fimbria (Fig. 37–6). At the decussation of the fornix and anterior commissure, the fornix divides into a precommissural part (which passes in front of the anterior commissure to the septal area) and a postcommissural part (which passes behind the anterior commissure and disappears in the wall of the third ventricle on its way to the mamillary bodies). Recent studies have shown that the actual hippocampal fibers synapse exclusively in the septal area, including the nucleus accumbens and the nucleus of the diagonal band. The entire postcommissural fornix is believed to originate from the subiculum.

From the Hippocampus. The efferent fibers from the hippocampus arise mainly from CA3 and CA1. According to Siegel and Tassoni (1971), these fibers extend to the septum: fibers from the dorsal (posterior) part of the hippocampus synapse in the medial part, while those from the ventral (anterior) part synapse in the lateral part of the septum. Most of the fibers of the hippocampus project to the lateral nucleus of the septum.

From the Subiculum. The subiculum projects to the lateral nuclei of the septal area (nucleus accumbens, lateral nucleus of septum, Broca's diagonal nucleus), to the medial mamillary nucleus, and to the entorhinal area and other areas of the limbic cortex.

From the Presubiculum and Parasubiculum. Fibers from these areas synapse in the anterior nucleus of the thalamus. They extend via the postcommissural fornix.

INTERNAL CIRCUITS

The pyramidal cells are the principal cells of the internal circuits of the hippocampus. The apical and basal dendrite systems of these cells are traversed by thousands of parallel afferent fibers. Ascending axons of cells of the stratum oriens, ascending axon collaterals of the pyramidal cells (Andersen, 1971), Schaffer collaterals, afferent septohippocampal fibers, and mossy fibers synapse with the apical dendrites. The basket cells of the stratum oriens synapse with the perikaryon (inhibitory synapses). Fibers of the alvear fasciculus, commissural fibers, and

Figure 37–5 Horizontal section through the entorhinal area and the hippocampal formation (according to Cajal).

1 dentate gyrus
2 subiculum
3 hippocampus
4 entorhinal area
5 perforating fasciculus
6 alvear fasciculus
7 stratum lacunosum

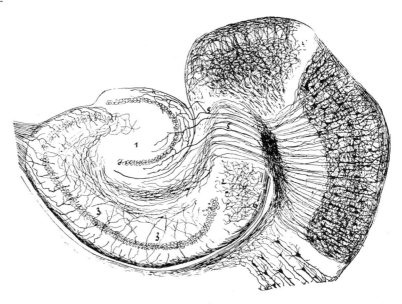

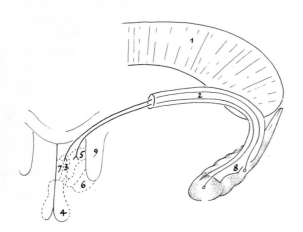

Figure 37–6 Efferent projections of the hippocampus. The ventral part of the hippocampus projects to the lateral part of the septum, and the dorsal part of the hippocampus to the medial part of the septum (according to House, Pansky and Siegel).

1	corpus callosum
2	fornix
3	medial septal nucleus
4	nucleus of Broca's diagonal band
5	lateral nucleus of the septum
6	nucleus of accumbens
7	dorsal septal nucleus
8	hippocampus
9	lateral ventricle

some of the afferent fibers of the septum synapse with the basal dendrites.

Schematically, the elementary circuit of the hippocampus can be envisaged as a chain of four neurons (Fig. 37–2). The axons of all four neurons are arranged in parallel bands so that each elementary circuit is encompassed in a transverse ''slice of the hippocampus'' that is about 400 μm thick. The totality of a large number of such slices, in parallel connection, determines the functional architecture of the hippocampus.

Function of the Hippocampus

The function of the hippocampal formation is not fully known. Experimental findings indicate that it is involved in a wide diversity of partial functions. A theory that might explain the function of the hippocampus as a whole on the basis of these partial functions has yet to be advanced.

The hippocampus seems to exert a strong influence in modulation of aggressive *behavior patterns* (of hypothalamic origin). Stimulation of ventral areas facilitates the development of ag-gressive reactions, and stimulation of dorsal areas has the opposite effect. This functional difference may be related to the unequal projection of these areas to the septum. Lesions of the hippocampus in experimental animals cause a tendency to persist in a given behavior pattern although the original reason for this behavior has disappeared. These lesions cannot suppress a trained behavior pattern.

It has recently been established that the pyramidal cells of the hippocampus are able to bind certain *hormones* (estradiol, corticosterone) in a relatively high concentration. Thus the hippocampus is believed to be capable of measuring the serum hormone level and transmitting information to the hypothalamohypophyseal system via the precommissural fornix and the septohypothalamic projections. This feedback mechanism could contribute to the regulation of the release of these hormones. Clinical findings are suggestive of a *mnemonic function* (short-term memory). Bilateral ablation of the basal temporal cortex and hippocampus causes amnesia for recent events. The patient is quite capable of following a conversation but loses the drift of it as soon as a subject is changed.

Chapter 38

Septum and Amygdala

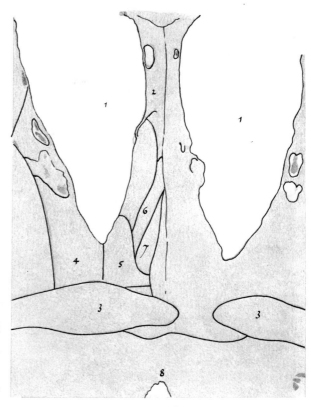

Figure 38–2 Frontal section through the human septum; arrangement of nuclei (according to Andy and Stephan).

1 lateral ventricle
2 septum pellucidum
3 anterior commissure
4 "bed nucleus of the stria terminalis"
5 lateral septal nucleus
6 medial septal nucleus
7 nucleus of Broca's diagonal band
8 median preoptic nucleus

Septal Area (Septum)

The term "septal area" covers that part of the hemispheres that is localized rostral to the anterior commissure. In humans, a distinction is made between the septum pellucidum and the true septum. The former consists of glia cells and fibers, while the latter comprises neurons and fiber bundles.

The septal area develops from the commissural plate and extends over a small distance into the medial wall of the hemisphere (Fig. 38–1). The boundary between the septal area and the cerebral cortex proper is marked by the posterior parolfactory sulcus. The septal area thus comprises a *cortical* part (subcallosal gyrus and parolfactory area) and a *subcortical* part (various cell agglomerations like the medial septal nucleus, lateral septal nucleus, etc.).

BOUNDARIES

The septal area is localized rostral to the anterior commissure; it is bounded superiorly by the rostrum of the corpus callosum and continues in the septum pellucidum. Ventrally it is bounded by the nucleus accumbens and the olfactory tubercle; rostrally it continues in the subcallosal gyrus. Owing to the marked development of the corpus callosum, the human septal area has a narrow, oblong shape.

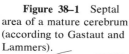

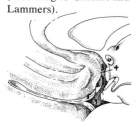

Figure 38–1 Septal area of a mature cerebrum (according to Gastaut and Lammers).

1 anterior perforated substance
2 olfactory tubercle
3 subcallosal gyrus
4 posterior parolfactory sulcus
5 medial olfactory stria
6 anterior commissure
7 optic chiasm

Figure 38-3 Nuclei of the septal area in apes (according to Powell and Hines).

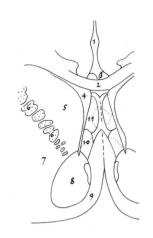

1 longitudinal cerebral fissure
2 corpus callosum
3 indusium griseum
4 lateral ventricle
5 caudate nucleus
6 internal capsule
7 putamen
8 nucleus of accumbens
9 nucleus of Broca's diagonal band
10 lateral septal nucleus
11 dorsomedial septal nucleus

SEPTAL NUCLEI

The septal nuclei can be divided into four groups: a dorsal group (dorsal septal nucleus), a ventral group (lateral septal nucleus), a medial group (medial septal nucleus, nucleus of Broca's diagonal band), and a caudal group (nucleus of the anterior commissure and nucleus of the stria terminalis). Of these nuclei, the lateral septal nucleus and the medial septal nucleus are of particular interest (Figs. 38-2 and 38-3). The former is found in a ventrolateral position and is bounded by the lateral ventricle and anterior commissure. Small, not readily stainable cells constitute this nucleus. The cells of the medial septal nucleus are heterogeneous: Some are large, readily stainable cells with long dendrites that exceed the boundaries of this nucleus.

FIBER PROJECTIONS

The septal area is one of the principal links in the limbic system. It occupies a central position between the hippocampus on the one hand, and the hypothalamus and habenula on the other.

Afferent fibers to the septum originate from:

(a) hippocampus (CA3, CA1); these fibers mainly synapse in the lateral septal nucleus;

(b) so-called ventral tegmental area (Tsai), which is localized in the mesencephalon, medial to the substantia nigra and lateral to the interpeduncular nucleus (see Fig. 30-7); the axons extend through the lateral hypothalamus via the telencephalic medial fasciculus and synapse in the nucleus of the stria terminalis and the nucleus accumbens; these fibers contain dopamine; and

(c) the amygdala, the fibers of which extend via the stria terminalis and synapse in the homonymous nucleus.

Efferent fibers extend in the fornix, the telencephalic medial fasciculus, and the stria medullaris of the thalamus. Efferent fibers in the fornix originate from the medial septal nucleus and the nucleus of the diagonal band, and synapse in the hippocampus (CA4, CA3, and CA1), the subiculum, and the entorhinal area.

In the telencephalic medial fasciculus, fibers extend from the septum (lateral septal nucleus and nucleus of the diagonal band) to the preoptic area, the lateral part of the hypothalamus, and the mesencephalic tegmentum. Via the septal area, the hippocampus can transmit information to the preoptic area and the hypothalamic continuum.

The septum is connected with the habenular trigone by fibers that extend in the stria medullaris. The latter is a fiber bundle that marks the superior boundary of the third ventricle; the rudimentary roof of the third ventricle (choroid lamina) attaches to it. The stria medullaris comprises fibers from the septal area, from the preoptic area of the hypothalamus, and from the anterior nuclei of the thalamus. The stria medullaris is among the principal efferent pathways of the limbic system.

FUNCTION

It is difficult to distinguish the functional activity of the septal area from that of the hippocampus; this could be expected in view of the fiber connections between the two structures and the connection "in series" of the septal area within the hippocampohypothalamic circuit. Some of the most interesting functional aspects are discussed in the following paragraphs.

Drinking Behavior. Increased water uptake is demonstrable in animals with septal lesions. This increase results not from diminished release of antidiuretic hormone (ADH), but from dysregulation of the hypothalamic drinking center.

Septal Area as a Reward Center. When electrodes are placed at certain brain sites and the test animal can apply a weak stimulus to these sites by depressing a lever, self-stimulation is sometimes observed. Whether the animal does or does not depress the lever depends on the location of the electrode. A high frequency of self-stimulation is observed when an electrode is placed in the septal area. In view of these experiments (Olds and Milner, 1954), the area has been named the ''reward center'' or ''pleasure center.'' In humans, too, electrical stimulation of the septal area elicits feelings of well-being and joy.

Amygdaloid Body (Amygdala)

The amygdala is a nuclear complex located immediately beneath the cortex of the uncus (see Fig. 40–3). This complex is bounded superiorly by the substantia innominata, the anterior commissure and the claustrum; in an anterior direction it continues as the anterior perforated substance and prepiriform cortex; in a posterior direction it gradually merges with the tail of the caudate nucleus. Ontogenetically, the amygdala and the tail of the caudate nucleus develop from the inferior part of the lateral ridge of the corpus striatum. The persistent contact between the two structures indicates their common origin.

NUCLEI OF THE AMYGDALA

Structurally, two groups of nuclei are distinguished in the amygdala (Johnston, 1923): the corticomedial and the basolateral groups. These nuclei consist of irregular agglomerates of pyramidal cells and granule cells. The corticomedial group encompasses the cortical nucleus, medial nucleus, and central nucleus. The last-mentioned nucleus is characterized by a high concentration of dopamine. The corticomedial group is localized in the dorsomedial part of the amygdala. The basolateral group encompasses the lateral nucleus, basal nucleus, and the accessory basal nucleus. These nuclei have many pyramidal cells with irregularly arranged apical dendrite ramifications. The neurons in these nuclei are not very homogeneous in size or shape.

FIBER PROJECTIONS

The amygdala is connected with other areas by the stria terminalis and the ventral amygdalofugal fiber (VAF) system.

The stria terminalis arises from the dorsomedial aspect of the amygdala (Fig. 38–4) and extends on the medial aspect of the caudate nucleus, which it joins as far as the level of the anterior commissure. At this level the stria terminalis divides into three components: a precommissural component, which passes in front of the anterior commissure and enters the septal area; a commissural component, which continues in the anterior commissure; and a postcommissural component, which passes behind the anterior commissure and reaches the preoptic area and the supraoptic region of the hypothalamus. The stria terminalis takes an arcuate course that parallels that of the fornix.

The VAF is a relatively diffuse fiber system that arises mainly from the basolateral nuclear complex. The fibers fan out in a plane perpendicular to the stria terminalis. They initially extend through the substantia innominata and anterior perforated substance, and then diverge to the preoptic area, the lateral hypothalamic area, and the peduncular loop of the thalamus.

Corticomedial Nuclear Complex

Afferent fibers arise from the olfactory bulb (via the lateral olfactory stria), from the preoptic area (via the stria terminalis), and from the parabrachial nucleus (pontine reticular formation).

Efferent fibers extend in the stria terminalis to the preoptic area, the tuberal region of the hypothalamus, and the entorhinal area.

Basolateral Nuclear Complex

Afferent fibers to the basolateral group originate from the prepiriform area, the orbitofrontal cortex (via stria terminalis and the internal capsule), the cortex of the temporal lobe, and the ventromedial nucleus of the hypothalamus.

Efferent fibers take a dual route: Some extend via the postcommissural component of the stria terminalis to the so-called bed nucleus of

Figure 38–4 Schematic representation of the components of the limbic system; fiber projections of the amygdala (according to Krieg).

1 hippocampus
2 dentate gyrus
3 fornix
4 precommissural component of the fornix
5 postcommissural component of the fornix
6 mamillary body
7 interpeduncular nucleus
8 habenular nucleus
9 septal area
10 stria medullaris
11 stria terminalis
12 indusium griseum
13 amygdala
14 uncus
15 lateral olfactory stria
16 gyrus cinguli
17 olfactory tubercle
18 anterior commissure

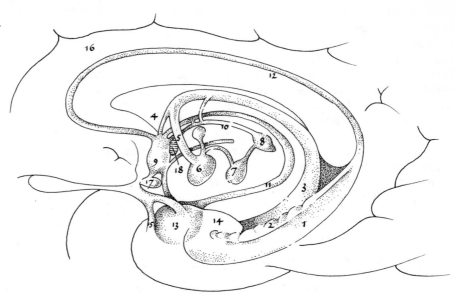

this stria, while other fibers extend via the VAF and project to extensive regions of the brain (septal area, areas 25 and 32 of the frontal lobe, area 35 of the temporal lobe, the tuberal region of the hypothalamus, and the thalamus). The projection to the thalamus is via the peduncular loop.

In view of the difference in fiber projections between the individual nuclei, it seems justifiable to conclude that the amygdala is a conglomerate of heterogeneous nuclei that have been brought under a common denominator. The corticomedial nuclear complex is, in a way, part of the olfactory brain; the basolateral complex, however, seems to be an important link in the mechanism by which the limbic system controls the hypothalamus. The axis between the amygdala and the ventromedial nucleus of the hypothalamus plays a role in this respect.

INTERACTION BETWEEN AMYGDALA AND VENTROMEDIAL NUCLEUS

The amygdala exerts its influence on the hypothalamus chiefly via the fiber connections with the ventromedial nucleus. These fibers take two routes: stria terminalis and VAF. Both pathways converge on the outer fiber capsule of the ventromedial nucleus, which can be regarded as a junction in the projection of the amygdala to the hypothalamus. The fibers of the stria terminalis synapse on the dendrites of the peripheral (bipolar) neurons of the nucleus, whereas the fibers of the VAF terminate on the central bipolar and multipolar neurons. Physiologic experiments have revealed that the peripheral neurons are inhibitory neurons.

FUNCTIONAL ASPECTS

Stimulation of the amygdala with the aid of delicate electrodes gives rise to a diversity of reactions, depending on the location and intensity of the stimulus. The principal phenomena are arrest reaction (a movement already in progress ceases abruptly), arousal phenomenon with cortical desynchronization, flight and fear reactions, visceral phenomena (tachycardia or bradycardia, swallowing, biting, licking), changes in the metabolism of food and water, and changes in sexual behavior. Stimulation of the human amygdala sometimes produces feelings of rage and anxiety but may also cause a sense of restful calmness. The patient may feel he is in a different (better?) world. These differences in effect depend not only on the location of the electrode but also on the emotional state that preceded stimulation.

Experimental interruption of the two pathways also leads to different results. The VAF fibers prove to be indispensable for the development of the "defense reaction" (in cats), while interruption of the stria terminalis suppresses the ovulation that otherwise follows stimulation of the corticomedial nuclei. Destruction of the amygdala has a "taming" effect. Animals thus treated show fewer interactions with other individuals of their species and tend to seek an isolated, group-independent position.

Chapter 39

The Hypothalamus

The hypothalamus is that portion of the diencephalon that lies beneath the hypothalamic sulcus. Anteriorly it extends as far as the preoptic region, lamina terminalis, and anterior perforated substance; superiorly and posteriorly it continues as subthalamus, and laterally it reaches as far as the optic tract and the lower part of the internal capsule.

Despite its limited dimensions, the hypothalamus functions as the highest regulatory center of many homeostatic and endocrine mechanisms. Anatomically, it occupies a strategic position as principal link between the higher centers of the CNS (hippocampus, amygdala, septal area) and the reticular formation. This situation, combined with its close relation to the hypophysis, characterizes the hypothalamus as a junction where normal synaptic mechanisms are associated with phenomena of active hormonal synthesis and where the CNS is directly informed about physical and chemical changes in the composition of the internal environment. The following points are of importance in this context: (a) Hypothalamic neurons can function as nerve cells and as endocrine cells. (b) Several fiber bundles that are part of the limbic system converge on the hypothalamus. (c) Many hypothalamic neurons are directly susceptible to physical (temperature, osmotic pressure) and chemical (blood pH, hormone level) characteristics of the internal environment. (d) The hypothalamus controls the distal portion of the hypophysis by the neurohormonal route.

External Configuration

In view of the anatomic configuration of the basal surface of the hypothalamus, the tuber cinereum and the mamillary bodies are distinguishable. The tuber cinereum is a gray elevation between the posterior margin of the optic chiasm and the mamillary bodies. In the tuber is found the attachment of the infundibulum, the paired lateral eminences, and the postinfundibular eminence. The lateral eminences are outpouchings of the surface on either side of the tuber, caused by the marked development of the lateral tuberal nuclei. The mamillary bodies are two pronounced round, white elevations that mark the boundary from the mesencephalon (see Fig. 14–1).

Morphologic Characteristics

Histologic sections through the human hypothalamus reveal a diffuse, poorly differentiated pattern. Two nuclei — the supraoptic nucleus and paraventricular nucleus — are an exception; they comprise large, multipolar, readily stainable nerve cells. As regards the fiber composition of the area, we can distinguish a lateral, highly myelinated part from a medial area adjacent to the ventricle, where most fibers are unmyelinated.

The hypothalamic nuclei can be classified on the basis of either topographic or cytoarchitectonic criteria. Topographic classifications make use of local variations in the arrangement of the neurons, in sections stained according to Nissl or by a variant of this technique. Cytoarchitectonic classifications are based on morphologic differences between the cell nuclei of the hypothalamic neurons. According to cytoarchitectonic criteria, a distinction is made between isomorphous nuclei, which comprise neurons of a single type, and anisomorphous nuclei, which comprise neurons of several types.

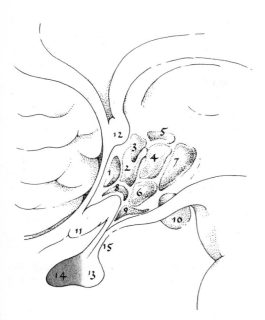

Figure 39–1 The position of the hypothalamic nuclei in the wall of the ventricle (according to Carpenter).

1 preoptic nucleus
2 anterior nucleus
3 paraventricular nucleus
4 dorsomedial nucleus
5 dorsal hypothalamic area
6 ventromedial nucleus
7 posterior nucleus
8 supraoptic nucleus
9 arcuate nucleus
10 mamillary body
11 optic chiasm
12 anterior commissure
13 neurohypophysis
14 adenohypophysis
15 infundibulum

Topographic Classification

Of the existing classifications, that of Le Gros Clark (1938) is the most widely known. It divides the hypothalamus into:

(a) Preoptic area: This comprises the medial preoptic nucleus and the periventricular preoptic nucleus;

(b) Hypothalamus in the restricted sense, which is subdivided into: *1*, a supraoptic portion, with the supraoptic nucleus, paraventricular nucleus, and suprachiasmatic nucleus; *2*, a tuberal portion, with the arcuate nucleus, ventromedial

nucleus, and dorsomedial nucleus; and *3*, a mamillary portion, with the medial, lateral, intermediate mamillary nuclei, etc.

Another classification divides the hypothalamus into three longitudinal zones: periventricular zone, medial lamina, and lateral lamina. The last two laminae are separated by a plane that extends through the fornix and the mamillothalamic tract.

The hypothalamic nuclei can also be classified on the basis of their projections to the hypophysis: into "hypophyseal" and "nonhypophyseal" nuclei. The former extend axons to the neurohypophysis, while the latter do not or hardly do. This classification is used in the following paragraphs.

NONHYPOPHYSEAL NUCLEI

Preoptic Area

This area extends between the supraoptic and the paraventricular nuclei on the one hand, and the lamina terminalis on the other. The area is dorsally bounded by the anterior commissure, and laterally by Broca's diagonal band (Fig. 39–1). The principal nuclei of the preoptic area are the medial preoptic nucleus (Fig. 39–2), the median preoptic nucleus (unpaired), and the periventricular preoptic nucleus. The preoptic nuclei are of fairly diffuse structure and comprise small to very small neurons.

Little is known about the fiber projections of the preoptic area. Afferent fibers come from the ventromedial hypothalamic nucleus, from the septum, from the amygdala via the ventral amygdalofugal (VAF) fibers, and from olfactory areas via the telencephalic medial fasciculus.

Efferent fibers extend (likewise in the telencephalic medial fasciculus) to the lateral hypothalamus and the reticular formation of the mesencephalon. Other, shorter fibers extend to the septum.

Medial Hypothalamic Zone (Medial Lamina)

Suprachiasmatic Nucleus. This nucleus consists of a group of small neurons, localized

Figure 39–2 Transverse section through the human hypothalamus at the level of the optic chiasm.

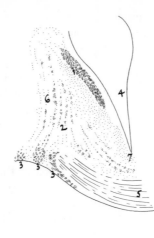

1 paraventricular nucleus
2 anterior hypothalamic area
3 supraoptic nucleus
4 third ventricle
5 optic chiasm
6 medial preoptic nucleus
7 suprachiasmatic nucleus

Figure 39–3 Transverse section through the hypothalamus at the level of the infundibulum.

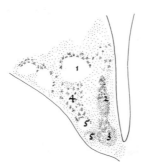

1 fornix
2 dorsomedial nucleus
3 ventromedial nucleus
4 lateral tuberal nucleus
5 fibers of the telencephalic medial fasciculus

immediately above the optic chiasm (Fig. 39–2). This nucleus is connected with the retina via the so-called retinohypothalamic tract, with the amygdala via the stria terminalis, and with the septum via the telencephalic medial fasciculus. Efferent fibers from the suprachiasmatic nucleus synapse in the ventromedial nucleus, dorsomedial nucleus, and arcuate nucleus (infundibular nucleus). Functionally, the suprachiasmatic nucleus is regarded by modern investigators as a kind of pacemaker that ensures the characteristic rhythmic quality of many hypothalamic activities.

Ventromedial Nucleus. This is the largest nucleus of the tuber cinereum. It comprises small to medium-size cells and is separated from adjacent structures by a narrow, fiber-dense zone (capsule). Cajal (1904) distinguished bipolar neurons at the periphery and stellate neurons at the center of the nucleus.

Afferent fibers to the ventromedial nucleus ramify in the capsule and synapse with the peripheral bipolar neurons (axodendritic synapses). The axons of the bipolar neurons extend to deeper regions of the nucleus and synapse with the stellate neurons. These cells give rise to the efferent fibers of the ventromedial nucleus. The bipolar cells are probably inhibitory neurons. Afferent fibers to the ventromedial nucleus originate from the amygdala (via stria terminalis and VAF), from the preoptic area (via the telencephalic medial fasciculus), from the subiculum (via the fornix), and from the lenticular fasciculus.

Efferent fibers from the ventromedial nucleus extend to the thalamus (periventricular nucleus) and to the preoptic area, the amygdala, the capsule of the mamillary bodies, and the central gray matter of the mesencephalon.

Dorsomedial Nucleus. This nucleus lies in a position dorsomedial to that of the previous nucleus and is bounded by the ependymal lining of the third ventricle. A layer of glia fibers is located between this nucleus and the ependyma. Laterally, the nucleus merges into the perifornical nucleus (Fig. 39–3).

Dorsal Hypothalamic Area. This area is located immediately beside the ventricular wall, dorsal to the dorsomedial nucleus (Fig. 39–3). In a caudal direction this area extends as far as the central gray matter of the mesencephalon; it is laterally bounded by the zona incerta. The area shows a decidedly anisomorphous structure. In addition to small and medium-size cells, conspicuously large neurons are found scattered in this area.

The dorsal hypothalamic area is the source of numerous delicate fibers which, extending along the ventricular wall, form a rather diffuse bundle known as the dorsal longitudinal fasciculus of Schütz. This bundle descends in the central gray matter of the mesencephalon and rhombencephalon and innervates the nuclei of the cranial nerves and the reticular formation.

Mamillary Bodies. Owing to their characteristic abundance of myelinated fibers, the mamillary bodies occupy a special position within

Figure 39–4 Transverse section through the mamillary bodies (according to Le Gros Clark).

1 mamillothalamic tract
2 posterior hypothalamic nucleus
3 medial mamillary nucleus
4 lateral mamillary nucleus
5 intermediate nucleus

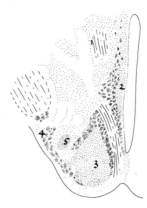

the hypothalamus. They comprise two principal nuclei: the medial and the lateral mamillary nuclei. The former is the larger nucleus (Fig. 39–4); its neurons are relatively small and it is enclosed in a capsule of myelinated fibers. The lateral mamillary nucleus is much smaller and may be difficult to identify. Its neurons are larger than those of the medial mamillary nucleus and stain more readily.

Afferent fibers originate from the subiculum of the hippocampus, via the postcommissural fornix, from the ventromedial nucleus, and from the mesencephalon via the mamillary peduncle. The fornical fibers are numerous (about 10^6) and terminate in the medial mamillary nucleus. Some extend past the mamillary body and synapse in the tegmentum of the mesencephalon or in its central gray matter. Afferents from the mesencephalon come via the mamillary peduncle from the central gray matter and from the cuneiform nucleus (reticular formation).

The efferent fibers of the mamillary bodies are an essential component of the limbic system. Fibers from the medial mamillary nucleus form a strong ascending bundle, the principal mamillary fasciculus. This bundle divides into a rostrodorsal component (mamillothalamic tract) and a smaller caudal component (mamillotegmental fasciculus). The fibers of the mamillothalamic tract arise mostly from the medial mamillary nucleus and synapse in the anterior thalamic group (anterior nucleus). The latter nucleus gives rise to fibers that extend to the gyrus cinguli,

where they synapse. The circuit hippocampus → fornix→mamillary body→anterior thalamic nucleus→gyrus cinguli is known to be a central circuit in the limbic system (Papez' "emotional circuit"). The efferent fibers of the mamillotegmental fasciculus arise from the dorsal portion of the medial mamillary nucleus and synapse in the mesencephalic tegmentum.

Hypothalamic Commissures. Hypothalamic fiber bundles that cross the midline have long been known. They are probably not always true commissures but rather decussations of fibers. The following decussations are distinguished: dorsal supraoptic decussation (Ganser), ventral supraoptic decussation (Gudden and Meynert), and supramamillary decussation. The origin of the fibers of the two supraoptic decussations is obscure. Those of the dorsal supraoptic decussation seem to come from the subthalamic nucleus, among other sites, and synapse in the contralateral globus pallidus. The fibers of the ventral supraoptic decussation lie snugly against the dorsal surface of the optic chiasm. Many fibers are believed to originate from the lateral geniculate body and the superior colliculus. The fibers of the supramamillary decussation take a course dorsocaudal to the mamillary body. These fibers probably originate from the fornix and the telencephalic medial fasciculus. Where they synapse is not known with certainty.

Lateral Hypothalamic Zone (Lateral Lamina)

The hypothalamic region lateral to the fornix comprises larger but less closely packed neurons. The lateral zone shows an anisomorphous structure, with a wide variety of cell types.

Lateral Tuberal Nuclei. These nuclei are most highly developed in humans; they comprise three oblong, horizontal cell columns beneath the superficially visible lateral eminences (Fig. 39–3). The medium-size triangular neurons are not readily stainable. Fiber projections of the lateral tuberal nuclei are virtually unknown.

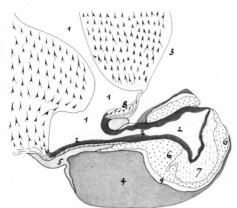

Figure 39-5 Sagittal secretion through the hypothalamus and the hypophysis of the mature cat. The infundibular recess reaches as far as the posterior lobe. The wall of the infundibulum is shown in heavy black.

1	third ventricle
2	infundibular recess
3	mamillary body
4	distal portion
5	infundibular portion
6	intermediate portion
7	posterior lobe
8	caudal part of the tuber
9	lumen of Rathke's pouch

HYPOPHYSEAL NUCLEI

The hypophyseal nuclei are connected with the hypophysis via long or short axons. The principal hypophyseal nuclei are the supraoptic nucleus, the paraventricular nucleus, and the infundibular (arcuate) nucleus.

Supraoptic Nucleus

The rostral portion of the nucleus is located in front of and above the optic chiasm, on either side of the midline. Most of the nucleus, however, extends along the optic tract (Fig. 39-1). This part can be divided into a rostral and a caudal area. The nucleus is isomorphous, with fairly large (25 to 30 μm) multipolar cells, and is abundantly vascularized. The cytoplasm of the neurons contains inclusions that readily stain with the Gomori technique (neurosecretion granules); these inclusions are found in the axons as well. The axons of the supraoptic nucleus (supraopticohypophyseal tract) extend through the infundibulum to the posterior hypophyseal lobe, where they end around the capillaries.

Paraventricular Nucleus

This nucleus is localized against the wall of the third ventricle and, like the previous nucleus, is among the ''Gomori-positive'' hypothalamic nuclei (Fig. 39-2). The nucleus is anisomorphous and comprises a population of large, medium, and small neurons. Some of the axons of the paraventricular nucleus join the supraoptic fibers, with which they enter the infundibulum. Modern studies have shown that these axons terminate in the palisade zone of the infundibulum (Silverman, 1976), where high concentrations of neurophysins have been demonstrated. Most of the axons of the paraventricular nucleus, however, terminate in the supraoptic nucleus (Fig. 39-6).

The neurons of the Gomori-positive hypophyseal nuclei secrete certain chemical substances in the Golgi apparatus (neurohypophyseal hormones). These migrate along the axons as secretion granules. The supraoptic nucleus contains vasopressin (ADH) in its ventromedial portion, and oxytocin in its dorsolateral portion. The rostral portion of the paraventricular nucleus contains mostly oxytocin, while the dorsal portion is rich in vasopressin. In humans the amount of vasopressin in the magnocellular neurosecretory system significantly exceeds the amount of oxytocin.

The neurohypophyseal hormones and their ''vehicles'' (neurophysins I and II) are transported by the axons of the supraopticohypophyseal tract and released into the perivascular space of the capillaries of the posterior hypophyseal lobe (see below).

Infundibular Nucleus

The infundibular (arcuate) nucleus comprises small, fusiform, Gomori-negative cells that are arranged in a ring around the attachment of the infundibulum. The nucleus has close relations with the wall of the third ventricle — in such a way that locally the characteristically high ependyma is replaced by flat ependymal cells with irregular perikaryons, with tanycytes scattered between. Some of the subependymal neurons are probably in direct contact with the CSF.

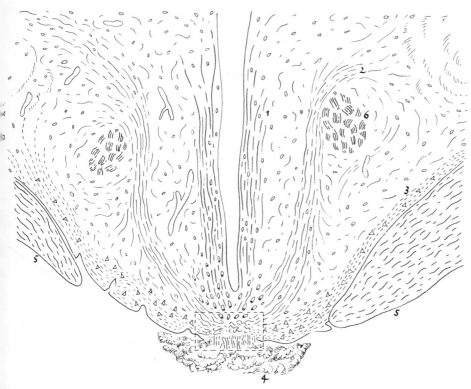

Figure 39–6 Transverse section through the feline hypothalamus. The hypothalamic fibers "on their way" to the neurohypophysis converge on the ventral lip of the infundibulum.

1 periventricular tract
2 perifornical tract
3 supraoptic tract (fasciculus)
4 infundibular portion
5 optic tract
6 fornix

Some 20 per cent of the axons of the infundibular nucleus join the tuberohypophyseal tract and reach the poorly cellularized superficial zone of the infundibulum (palisade zone), where they terminate against the wall of the short capillary loops of the "mantle plexus."

Structure of the Hypophysis

The hypophysis comprises the adenohypophysis, which originates from the ectoderm of the roof of the mouth (Rathke's pouch), and the neurohypophysis, which belongs to the floor of the diencephalon. Contrary to generally accepted views, these two parts have always been in close contact. In the course of development, the adenohypophysis differentiates into a distal portion (anterior lobe), an infundibular portion (tuberal part), and an intermediate portion.

The neurohypophysis ultimately differentiates into a proximal portion (infundibulum) and a distinctly enlarged distal portion (infundibular process, "posterior lobe"). The adenohypophysis grows around the neurohypophysis in such a way that the infundibulum is enveloped by its tuberal portion and the infundubular process by its intermediate portion. Its distal portion is the only part of the adenohypophysis that is not in direct contact with the neurohypophysis (Fig. 39–5).

MICROSCOPIC STRUCTURE OF THE INFUNDIBULUM

In many mammals, the following three layers are distinguishable in the infundibulum (Fig. 39–7):

(a) Ependymal zone, which comprises the ependymal layer that lines the cavity of the infundibular recess, and a subependymal layer of nerve fibers;

(b) Fibrillar zone (middle layer), which com-

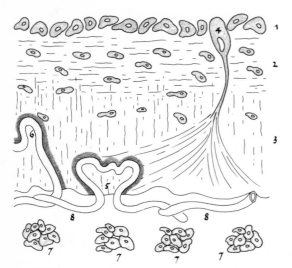

Figure 39–7 The layers in the wall of the infundibulum. The long capillary loops perforate farther than the figure shows.

1 ependymal zone
2 fibrillar zone
3 palisade zone
4 tanycyte
5 short capillary loop
6 long capillary loop
7 cells of the infundibular portion
8 mantle plexus

prises sagittally arranged nerve fibers (supraopticohypophyseal tract) and numerous glia cells; and

(c) Palisade zone (superficial layer), already in contact with the tuberal part of the adenohypophysis. This layer is characterized by low cellularity and a high density of fibers (nerve, glia and ependymal fibers) and nerve endings. The nerve fibers of this zone belong to the tuberohypophyseal tract.

"Radix Infundibuli." At the boundary between tuber cinereum and infundibulum is an area of transition that contains structures of the tuber as well as of the neurohypophysis. A wedge of nerve cells that are part of the infundibular nucleus forces itself between the fibrillar zone and the ependymal zone and separates these layers. This wedge of nerve cells does not extend very deep but ends at a short distance from the infundibular sulcus. This area of transition is called the "radix infundibuli" (Nowakowski, 1951).

Tanycytes. Tanycytes (Horstmann, 1956) are special ependymal cells found in the infundibular recess and the inferior part of the third ventricle. The cytoplasm of these cells has a long peripheral process that extends over the entire thickness of the infundibular wall and ends on the perivascular sheath of the short or the long capillary loops.

Hypophyseal Circulation

The hypophysis is vascularized by the superior hypophyseal arteries and the inferior hypophyseal artery (Fig. 39–8). The former ramify into a network of arterioles (mantle plexus) between the infundibular portion of the adenohypophysis and the palisade zone. The mantle plexus gives rise to many branches that perforate the wall of the infundibulum. Some of them reach the subependymal zone (long capillary loops) and come close to the CSF; other branches do not perforate beyond the palisade zone (short capillary loops). An ascending and a descending branch can be distinguished in all capillary loops (Fig. 39–7). In the long loops the transition between these two tends to expand, and this results in a vascular tangle immediately beneath the ependyma. The descending branch of the long loops is characterized by its larger luminal width and its direct anastomosis with the portal veins. The short loops, however, return into the capillary network of the mantle plexus.

The capillary loops are surrounded by a special, dense zone of processes of the tanycytes and neuroglia cells. Numerous nerve endings laden with granules are localized among these processes. The actual *perivascular space* is found between the capillary endothelium and the nerve fibers and glia fibers; this space contains collagenous bundles and fibroblasts and is bounded by basal membranes.

Numerous venules from the mantle plexus unite to form larger vessels that traverse the length of the infundibulum as far as the anterior lobe. These are the *portal veins* which, in the anterior lobe of the hypophysis, ramify into a capillary network that is in close contact with the cells of the distal portion of the adenohypophysis (Fig. 39–8).

Figure 39–8 Blood vessels of the infundibulum (rat) after injection of Indian ink followed by tissue clearing. The afferent arteries ramify into a capillary network (mantle plexus), from which the portal veins arise (center of figure). The sinusoids of the distal portion are shown at the bottom.

1   superior hypophyseal arteries
2   portal veins (hypophyseoportal veins)
3   sinusoids of the distal portion

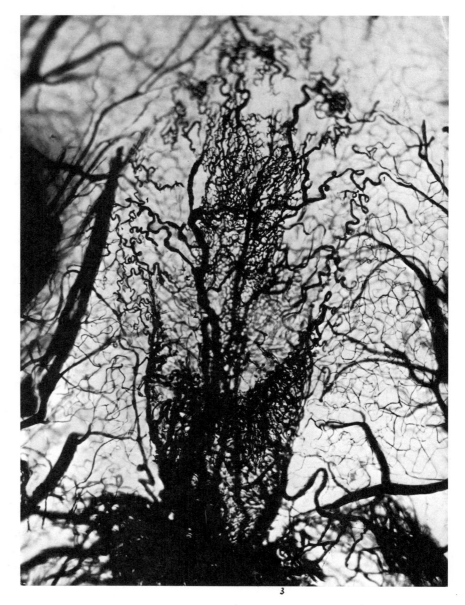

Fiber Connections of the Hypothalamus

The fibers that connect the hypothalamus with other parts of the CNS often form large, sometimes grossly visible bundles, for example, the postcommissural fornix and the mamillothalamic tract. Other projections, however, are fairly diffuse and cannot be readily followed by classic neuroanatomic methods. The principal fiber connections are localized in one of the following systems (Fig. 39–9).

Telencephalic Medial Fasciculus. This bundle is known by various names like "median forebrain bundle," olfactomesencephalic tract," and "basal olfactory bundle" ("basales Riechbündel"). It consists of relatively thin fibers of variable length that connect olfactory

Figure 39–9 Some hypothalamic fiber connections, more specifically those with the diencephalon and mesencephalon (according to Carpenter).

1 fasciculus retroflexus
2 mamillothalamic tract
3 mamillotegmental fasciculus (black lines); mamillary peduncle (brown lines)
4 telencephalic medial fasciculus
5 stria medullaris
6 superior colliculus
7 superior central nucleus
8 septum
9 habenula
10 interpeduncular nucleus
11 Tsai's ventral tegmental area
12 anterior commissure

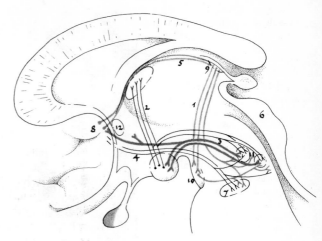

and nonolfactory areas of the hemisphere with the hypothalamus and the mesencephalic tegmentum. The telencephalic medial fasciculus extends through the lateral hypothalamic zone (lateral to the fornix) and has ascending and descending components. The principal descending fibers arise from the septum and synapse in the preoptic area of the hypothalamus (short fibers) or in the tegmentum of the mesencephalon (Tsai's ventral tegmental area, reticular formation, etc.). Other descending fibers arise from the preoptic area of the hypothalamus and synapse in the hypophyseal nuclei, the nucleus of the dorsal raphe of the mesencephalon, and the central gray matter. The ascending fibers connect the reticular formation of the mesencephalon with the lateral hypothalamic zone, extending into the lateral part of the septum.

Postcommissural Fornix. This bundle connects the subiculum of the hippocampal formation with various hypothalamic nuclei (ventromedial and medial mamillary nucleus).

Stria Terminalis. This bundle arises from the amygdala and extends parallel to the fornix. Some of its fibers synapse in the preoptic area and the ventromedial nucleus.

Mamillothalamic Tract. This is a large, grossly visible bundle that connects the medial mamillary nucleus with the nuclei of the anterior thalamus (Fig. 39–9).

Mamillotegmental Fasciculus. This connects the medial mamillary nucleus with the tegmentum of the mesencephalon and constitutes a route via which the hypothalamus can exert influence on the reticular formation. The fibers terminate in the dorsal tegmental nucleus.

Dorsal Longitudinal Fasciculus of Schütz. This is a diffuse, not readily stainable bundle found in a central position immediately beneath the central sulcus. The bundle comprises ascending and descending fibers of varying length. Descending fibers arise from the dorsal hypothalamic area and can be followed as far as the lower boundary of the medulla oblongata. The fibers synapse with cells of the central gray matter of the brain stem and nuclei of the cranial nerves. Ascending fibers in this bundle arise from the nucleus of the solitary tract and the dorsal tegmental nucleus, and end mostly in the periventricular areas of the hypothalamus.

AFFERENT FIBERS TO THE HYPOTHALAMUS

Many fibers from structures of the limbic system converge on the hypothalamus. This is one reason for regarding this region as the final common pathway for impulses from the limbic system. Afferent fibers originate from the septum (lateral septal nucleus and nucleus of the diagonal band) via the telencephalic medial fasciculus; from the amygdala, via the stria terminalis and VAF system; from the subiculum, via the fornix; and from the reticular formation, via the telencephalic medial fasciculus.

EFFERENT FIBERS

Hypophyseal and nonhypophyseal connections are distinguished.

Hypophyseal Connections. The hypothalamic fibers extending to the hypophysis converge to the midline on the way to the attachment of the infundibulum to the tuber cinereum (radix infundibuli). In cross-section, the radix infundibuli has the shape of a ring, in which four "lips" are distinguished. The hypothalamic fibers enter the infundibulum through all four lips (Fig. 39–6). The hypothalamic fibers destined for the hypophysis extend in three main bundles:

(a) The periventricular tract extends parallel and close to the wall of the third ventricle. Its axons originate from the paraventricular nucleus, the dorsomedial nucleus, and the infundibular nucleus.

(b) The perifornical tract originates from areas near the fornix. Its axons arise from the paraventricular nucleus, the perifornical nucleus, the fornix, and the zona incerta. Some of the fibers may originate from the mesencephalic tegmentum (via the telencephalic medial fasciculus).

(c) The supraoptic tract largely originates from the homonymous nucleus and, to a lesser extent, from the suprachiasmatic nucleus. Its fibers are localized entirely in the lateral and superficial part of the hypophyseal peduncle (hypothalamic infundibulum).

Immediately above the attachment of the infundibulum to the tuber, the perifornical and the periventricular tracts unite to form the tuberohypophyseal tract. These fibers cross the superficially localized fibers of the supraoptic

tract (Fig. 39–6) and thus reach the superificial zone of the infundibulum (palisade zone), where they end against the wall of the short capillary loops.

Monoaminergic Innervation of the Infundibulum

Falck and Hillarp's fluorescence studies have demonstrated numerous catecholamine-bearing fibers in the infundibulum of the neurohypophysis. The distribution of dopamine and norepinephrine terminals has likewise been studied by the immunofluorescence technique. The dopamine-bearing neurons of the hypothalamus form two systems: the ventrally localized tuberoinfundibular fiber system and the dorsal incertohypothalamic system. The terminals of the ventral system are for the most part localized in the palisade zone of the infundibulum, and particularly in its lateral portion. The dorsal system's fibers synapse in the dorsomedial nucleus and the anterior hypothalamic area.

Noradrenergic fibers originate from the brain stem (locus ceruleus) and innervate the paraventricular, the dorsomedial, and the infundibular nuclei. In the infundibulum, noradrenergic terminals are localized in the fibrillar zone.

Little is known about the functional significance of the catecholaminergic terminals. The dopamine in the lateral portion of the palisade zone is believed to inhibit the release of LRH to the portal veins via axo-axonic synapses. In this way, dopamine inhibits the hypophyseal release of LH. The hypothalamic monoamines might therefore play a role in the regulation of the release of "releasing factors" to the distal portion of the hypophysis.

Nonhypophyseal Efferent Fibers. Efferent impulses from the hypothalamus travel via the telencephalic medial fasciculus to the reticular formation of the brain stem, via the mamillotegmental fasciculus to the tegmentum of the mesencephalon, and via the dorsal longitudinal fasciculus of Schütz to the central gray matter and the nuclei of the cranial nerves. Many shorter projections extend between the various hypothalamic nuclei.

Functional Aspects

The hypothalamus is involved in the maintenance of the normal composition of the internal environment; it also plays a role in the expression of emotional reactions (palpitations, dilatation of the pupils, secretion of "cold sweat"). Even after decortication and ablation of the dorsal thalamus, rage reactions are possible ("sham rage"). Finally, the hypothalamus is involved in somatic maturation processes (growth, sexual maturation). Lesions of the hypothalamus can, therefore, lead to extensive and remarkable combinations of endocrine, metabolic, and behavioral (emotional) disorders.

The hypothalamus can influence the internal environment via the hypophyseal hormones but also via the reticular formation and the autonomic nervous system (ANS). For its information the hypothalamus is dependent not only on the normal afferent channels, but its neurons are susceptible also to physical and chemical stimuli (such as temperature of the blood) from the internal environment. The control centers of some vegetative functions are localized in the hypothalamus proper; in other functions, its role is restricted to that of a modulator superimposed on lower centers (respiration and heart action).

HYPOTHALAMIC CONTROL OF THE HYPOPHYSIS

Recent research has shown that hypothalamic neurons are able to synthesize hormones. This applies not only to vasopressin and oxytocin but also to other substances known as releasing factors or releasing hormones. These are substances that can activate the endocrine cells of the distal portion of the hypophysis to increased synthesis and/or release of hypophyseal hormones. The releasing factors are transported to the palisade zone of the infundibulum via the axons of the tuberohypophyseal tract. Having passed through the wall of the short capillary loops, the releasing factors are transported to the distal portion of the hypophysis via the blood in the portal veins of the mantle plexus. Since the neurohormones are released in the capillary loops, their concentration in the portal sinusoids of the distal portion is still fairly high. It is here that the hypothalamic neurohormones (TRF, LRH, GRH, etc.) exert a direct influence on the release of the well known hypophyseal hormones.

Modern investigators assume that the neurohormones are synthesized in specific hypothalamic areas; many current studies aim at demarcation of these areas.

The tanycytes likewise seem to play a role as an access route to the distal portion. On the basis of biochemical assays it is assumed that some of the hypothalamic hormones are released into the third ventricle. The tanycytes absorb minute amounts of CSF, and the resulting pinocytotic vesicles are transported via the tanycyte cytoplasm to the perivascular space of the capillary loops of the infundibulum. Dopaminergic fibers are believed to be capable of inhibiting this hormone transport.

REGULATION OF WATER BALANCE

Lesions of the supraopticohypophyseal tract or of the supraoptic nucleus give rise to diabetes insipidus, a condition characterized by the voiding of large amounts of highly dilute urine due to lack of antidiuretic hormone (ADH). This ADH acts mainly on the distal segment of the renal tubules and so regulates water absorption that the blood water level is held constant within narrow limits. The neurons of the supraoptic nucleus are sensitive to changes in the osmotic pressure of the arterial blood (osmoreceptors).

FOOD INTAKE

Lesions of the ventromedial nucleus cause an excessive increase in food ingestion (hyperphagia), while lesions of the lateral hypothalamic area have the opposite effect, markedly reduced food ingestion (hypophagia). These phenomena involve two linked reciprocal centers ("food thermostat").

HEAT REGULATION

The preoptic area of the hypothalamus comprises a zone that is sensitive to any increase in body temperature. Relevant information reaches the preoptic area via nerve pathways that transport impulses from peripheral thermoreceptors. This area also comprises neurons that are sensitive to an increased blood temperature. Lesions in this area cause hyperthermia.

An area dorsal to the mamillary bodies is sensitive to a decrease in blood temperature. Lesions in this area lead to an inability to maintain the proper body temperature in a cold environment.

REPRODUCTION

The hypothalamus also influences gametogenesis, the ovarian cycle, and the secondary sex characteristics. This is a result of the control exercised by the neurohormones on the gonadotrophic hormones in the distal portion of the hypophysis.

BIOLOGIC RHYTHMS

A certain periodicity is discernible in the function of many organs. This applies to such factors as body temperature, serum glucose level, and eosinophil count. The period involved is about 24 hours. The sleep-wake rhythm is a good example. Particularly for these rhythms, a normally functioning hypothalamus is required.

Chapter 40

The Rhinencephalon

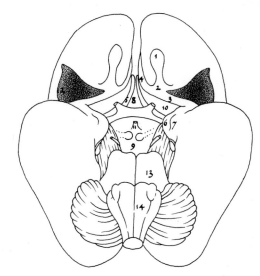

Figure 40–1 Schematic representation of the rhinencephalon in a human fetus of six months (according to Villinger).

1	olfactory bulb
2	olfactory trigone
3	lateral olfactory stria
4	medial olfactory stria
5	Broca's diagonal band
6	semilunar gyrus
7	ambient gyrus
8	lamina terminalis
9	interpeduncular fossa
10	anterior perforated substance
11	infundibulum (cut end)
12	Reil's insula
13	pons
14	medulla oblongata

The term rhinencephalon has caused confusion and prompted discussion. This is partly explained by the marked differences in the size of this area between macrosmatic and microsmatic mammals. Extensive areas of the medial aspect of the hemispheres (gyrus cinguli, hippocampus, septum) used to be included in the olfactory region of the brain, but modern investigators tend to restrict the rhinencephalon more and more.

We define the rhinencephalon as the olfactory bulb together with all other areas where efferent fibers from the bulb synapse. The efferent fibers from the bulb are called secondary olfactory fibers.

The totality of the rhinencephalic structures is divided into an anterior and a posterior olfactory lobe. The boundary between the two lobes is still debated. Gastaut and Lammers (1963) hold that the boundary is marked by the olfactory fissure in the depth of the lateral fossa (sylvian sulcus).

The anterior olfactory lobe comprises the olfactory bulb, anterior olfactory nucleus (retrobulbar region), olfactory trigone, anterior perforated substance, olfactory tubercle, lateral olfactory stria, and Broca's diagonal band (Fig. 40–1).

The posterior olfactory lobe (piriform lobe) comprises cortical areas of the temporal lobe. In the piriform lobe we distinguish the prepiriform area, periamygdaloid area, and entorhinal area.

The termination of secondary olfactory fibers in the endorhinal area, however, is doubtful.

Olfactory Bulb

In humans the olfactory bulb is relatively smaller than in macrosmatic mammals. During embryonic development the bulb has a lumen, which in maturity is replaced with an accumulation of glia cells.

Several structural layers can be distinguished in the bulb. From the surface in, we encounter the glomerular, the mitral, and the granular layers (Fig. 40–2). The glomerular layer can be compared with the molecular layer of the allocortex. The mitral and the granular layer compare with the pyramidal and the polymorphous layers of the allocortex, respectively.

The glomerular layer is a superficial layer that consists of a dense plexus of unmyelinated fibers. Its characteristic feature is the so-called olfactory glomerulus. The term ''glomerulus'' indicates a complex of synapses within a well defined area, which consists of interlaced nerve processes. In the olfactory glomeruli one finds not only axodendritic synapses between the dendrites of the mitral cells and the axons of the olfactory nerves (Fig. 40–2) but also dendrodendritic synapses between the dendrites of the mitral cells and those of the preglomerular cells. The olfactory bulb comprises about 2000 glomeruli and some 50 million olfactory axons. These figures give an impression of the degree of convergence of the olfactory axons on each glomerulus.

The mitral layer has the fairly large, triangular mitral cells (Fig. 40–2) arranged in a row. They have a thick dendrite that extends to the glomerular layer where it ends in a short, brush-like arborization.

The granular layer consists of alternate rows of cells and fibers. The cells (granule cells) have long dendrites (Fig. 40–2) that synapse with the axon collaterals of the mitral cells. The axons of the mitral cells enter the granular layer, divide in a T-shaped division and constitute the largest part of the olfactory tract.

Afferent Fibers. The processes of the neuroepithelial cells of the olfactory mucosa are exceptionally thin (about 0.2 μm) and form 15 to 20 small bundles (olfactory nerves or fila olfactoria) that enter the cranial cavity via the corresponding foramina in the lamina cribrosa. The olfactory fibers synapse in the olfactory bulb, which is localized immediately above the lamina cribrosa.

Olfactory Tract

The olfactory tract is a fiber bundle that extends from the olfactory bulb to the olfactory trigone. Some of its fibers synapse with the neurons of an oblong nucleus that accompanies

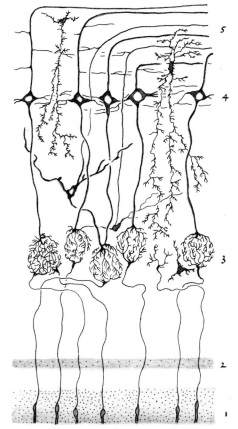

Figure 40–2 Structure of the olfactory bulb (according to Clara).

1	olfactory epithelium
2	lamina cribrosa
3	glomerular layer
4	mitral layer
5	granular layer

the olfactory tract, the anterior olfactory nucleus. The olfactory tract thus comprises secondary olfactory fibers and the neurons of the anterior olfactory nucleus (Fig. 40–3). The entire structure might be described as an ''olfactory peduncle.''

The boundaries of the anterior olfactory nucleus are variable. Its rostral portion extends as far as the posterior aspect of the bulb. In a caudal direction, the nucleus reaches as far as the olfactory trigone. The axons of the anterior olfactory nucleus extend in the anterior commissure and in the telencephalic medial fasciculus. The fibers in the anterior commissure synapse in the contralateral homonymous nucleus and the contralateral olfactory bulb. The fibers in the telencephalic medial fasciculus synapse in the preoptic area.

Olfactory Trigone

The olfactory trigone is formed by the bifurcation of the olfactory tract into medial and lateral olfactory striae (Fig. 40–1). The two striae are separated from Broca's diagonal band by the anterior perforated substance, an area of the paleocortex where secondary olfactory fibers synapse. In macrosmatic animals, the rostral portion of the perforated substance shows a distinct elevation (olfactory tubercle).

Lateral Olfactory Stria

The secondary olfactory fibers extend exclusively through the lateral olfactory stria and follow this until it ends in the anterior portion of the uncus (semilunar gyrus). The lateral olfactory stria thus comprises all the secondary fibers on their way to the uncus, and the neurons of the lateral olfactory gyrus. The latter is markedly reduced in size in humans.

Lateral to the lateral olfactory gyrus is another cortical area where secondary olfactory fibers synapse. This is the ambient gyrus which, together with the lateral olfactory gyrus, constitutes the prepiriform area.

Secondary olfactory fibers synapse in the following areas: anterior olfactory nucleus, anterior perforated substance, lateral olfactory gyrus, ambient gyrus, semilunar gyrus (periamygdaloid area), and the corticomedial nuclear complex of the amygdala (Fig. 40–3). The entorhinal area probably receives no secondary olfactory fibers. The fibers of the lateral stria thus constitute the olfactory projection to the primary olfactory cortex. The central processing of olfactory impulses is done primarily outside the thalamus. A high degree of integration is already ensured in the olfactory bulb.

The fibers in the medial olfactory stria are

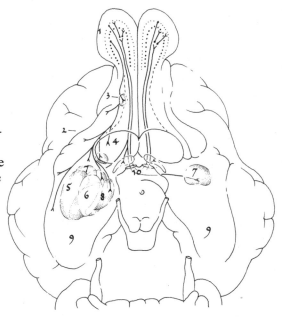

Figure 40–3 Fiber projections of the rhinencephalon and the amygdala.

1 olfactory bulb
2 rhinal sulcus
3 anterior olfactory nucleus
4 olfactory tubercle
5 lateral nucleus of amygdala
6 basal nucleus of amygdala
7 central nucleus of amygdala
8 medial nucleus of amygdala
9 piriform lobe
10 anterior commissure

not secondary olfactory fibers but tertiary fibers that arise from scattered nerve cells of the olfactory peduncle. These short fibers synapse in Broca's diagonal band and in the subcallosal gyrus.

Efferent Projection from the Primary Olfactory Cortex

In view of the marked influence of olfactory stimuli on instinctive behavior patterns, the rhinencephalon can be regarded as an important input channel for the limbic system. The efferent projection from the primary olfactory cortex to limbic areas is currently being studied with the aid of tracer techniques.

Many efferent fibers extend from this area to the entorhinal area. Other fibers synapse in the thalamus (dorsomedial nucleus), which they reach via the telencephalic medial fasciculus and the inferior thalamic peduncle. The existence of possible connections with the septum and the mesencephalic reticular formation still awaits confirmation.

Bibliography

Parts I and II

Addison, W. H. G.: The development of the Purkinje cells and of the layers in the cerebellum of the albino rat. J. Comp. Neurol., *21*:459–488, 1911.

Andres, K. H.: Über die Feinstruktur der Arachnoidea und Dura mater von Mammalia. Z. Zellforsch., *79*:272–295, 1967.

Bergh, R. van den: De Subcorticale Angioarchitectuur van het Menselijk Telencephalon. Proefschrift Leuven. Arscia Uitgaven, Brussels, 1960.

Berry, M., and Rogers, A. W.: The migration of neuroblasts in the developing cerebral cortex. J. Anat., *99*:691–709, 1965.

Bolk, L.: De Segmentale Innervatie van Romp en Ledematen bij den Mensch. Haarlem, De Erven F. Bohn, 1910.

Carpenter, M. B.: Human Neuroanatomy. Baltimore, Williams & Wilkins, 1976.

Clara, M.: Das Nervensystem des Menschen. Leipzig, Johan Ambrosius Barth, 1959.

Chorobski, I., and Penfield, W.: Cerebral vasodilator nerves and their pathway from the medulla oblongata. Arch. Neurol. Psychiatr., *28*:1257–1289, 1933.

Cooper, E. R. A.: Development of the human red nucleus and corpus striatum. Brain, *69*:34–44, 1946.

Duvernoy, H., Koritké, J. G., and Monnier, G.: Sur la vascularisation de la lame terminale humaine. Z. Zellforsch., *102*:49–77, 1969.

Duvernoy, H. M.: Human Brain Stem Vessels. New York, Springer, 1978.

Eayrs, J. T.: Endocrine influence on cerebral development. Arch. Biol., *75*:561–595, 1965.

Eecken, H. M. van den: Signification morfologique des anastomoses lepto-meningées aux confins du territoire des artères cérébrales. Acta Neurol. Psychiat. Belgica, *54*:525–533, 1954.

Eecken, H. M. van den: Anastomoses between the leptomeningeal arteries of the brain: Their morphological, pathological and clinical significance. Springfield, Illinois, Charles C Thomas, 1959.

Ellenberger, C., Hanaway, J., and Netsky, M. G.: Embryogenesis of the inferior olivary nucleus in the rat: A radioautographic study and a reevaluation of the rhombic lip. J. Comp. Neurol., *137*:71–88, 1969.

Elliot Smith, G.: A preliminary note on the morphology of the corpus striatum and the origin of the neopallium. J. Anat., *53*:271–291, 1919.

Essick, C. R.: On the embryology of the corpus pontobulbare and its relationship to the development of the pons. Anat. Rec., *3*:254–257, 1909.

Essick, C. R.: The development of the nuclei pontis and the nucleus arcuatus in man. Am. J. Anat., *13*:25–54, 1912.

Gaskell, W. H.: On the relation between the structure, function, distribution and origin of the cranial nerves, together with a theory of the origin of the nervous system of vertebrata. J. Physiol., *7*:153–211, 1889.

Gilbert, M. S.: The early development of the human diencephalon. J. Comp. Neurol., *62*:81–117, 1935.

Harkmark, W.: Cell migrations from the rhombic lip to the inferior olive, the nucleus raphe and the pons: A morphological and experimental investigation on chick embryos. J. Comp. Neurol., *100*:115–210, 1954.

Hicks, S. P., and D'Amato, C. J.: Cell migrations to the isocortex in the rat. Anat. Rec., *160*:619–634, 1968.

Hines, M.: Studies in the growth and differentiation of the telencephalon in man. J. Comp. Neurol., *34*:73–171, 1922.

Hayashi, M.: Einige wichtige Tatsachen aus der ontogenetische Entwicklung des menschlichen Kleinhirns. Dtsch. Z. Nervenheilk., *81*:74–82, 1924.

Hochstetter, F.: Beiträge zur Entwicklungsgeschichte des menschlichen Gehirns. II: Die Entwicklung des Mittel- und Rautengehirns. Vienna, Franz Deuticke, 1929.

Hörstadius, S.: The neural crest. London, Oxford University Press, 1950.

Howard, E.: Reductions in size and total DNA of cerebrum and cerebellum in adult mice after corticosterone treatment in infancy. Exp. Neurol., *22*:191–208, 1968.

Hugosson, R.: Studien über die Entwicklung der longitudinalen Zellsäulen und der Anlagen der Gehirnnervenkerne in der Medulla oblongata der verschiedenen Vertebraten. Z. Anat. Entwicklungsgesch., *118*:543–566, 1955.

Humphrey, T.: The development of the human amygdala during early embryonic life. J. Comp. Neurol., *132*:135–167, 1968.

Ikeda, J.: Beiträge zur normalen und abnormalen Entwicklungsgeschichte des kaudalen Abschnittes des Rückenmarks bei menschlichen Embryonen. Z. Anat. Entwicklungsgesch., *92*:380–491, 1930.

Jacobs, M. J.: The development of the human motor trigeminal complex and accessory facial nucleus and their topographic relations with the facial and abducens nuclei. J. Comp. Neurol., *138*:161–195, 1970.

Jacobson, M.: Developmental Neurobiology. New York, Plenum Press, 1978.

Krayenbühl, H. A., and Yasargil, M. G.: Cerebral Angiography. London, Butterworths, 1968.

Langman, J., Guerrard, R. L., and Feeman, B. G.: Behavior of neuro-epithelial cells during closure of the neural tube. J. Comp. Neurol., *127*:339–412, 1966.

Langman, J., and Haden, C. C.: Formation and migration of neuroblasts in the spinal end of the chick embryo. J. Comp. Neurol., *138*:419–433, 1970.

Larsell, O.: The development of the cerebellum in man in relation to its comparative anatomy. J. Comp. Neurol., 87:85–129, 1947.

Lazorthes, G., and Gouazé, A.: Les voies anastomotiques de suppléance de la vascularisation artérielle de l'axe cérebromédullaire. C. R. Ass. Anat., 140:1–230, 1968.

Lazorthes, G., Lacomme, Y., and Lazorthes, Y.: Innervation vasculaire et vasomotricité de l'extrémité céphalique. Acta Otorhinolaryngol. Belg., 20:173–294, 1965.

Legrand, J.: Variations en function de l'âge de la réponse du cervelet à l'action morphogénétique de la thyroide chez le rat. Arch. Anat. Microsc. Morphol. Exp., 56:291–307, 1967.

Lopéz Antúnez: Anatomia funcional del sistema nervioso. Editorial, Limusa, Mexico, 1980.

Marin-Padilla, M.: Prenatal and early postnatal ontogenesis of the human motor cortex: A Golgi study. I: The sequential development of the cortical layers. Brain Res., 23:167–183, 1970.

Marin-Padilla, M.: Early prenatal ontogenesis of the cerebral cortex (neocortex) of the cat (Felix domestica): A Golgi study. I: The primordial neocortical organization. Z. Anat. Entwicklungsgesch., 134:117–145, 1971.

Noback, C. R., and Demarest, R. J.: The Human Nervous System. Tokyo, McGraw-Hill, 1975.

Pigache, R. M.: The anatomy of "paleocortex." A critical review. Ergeb. Anat. Entwicklungsgesch., 43:1–59, 1970.

Rakić, P.: Guidance of neurons migrating to the fetal monkey neocortex. Brain Res., 33:471–476, 1971.

Rakić, P.: Mode of cell migration to the superficial layers of the fetal monkey neocortex. J. Comp. Neurol., 145:61–84, 1972.

Rakić, P.: Embryonic development of the LP-pulvinar complex in man. In Cooper, J. S., Riklan, M., and Rakić, P.: Pulvinar-LP Complex. Springfield, Illinois, Charles C Thomas, 1973.

Rakić, P., and Sidman, R. L.: Histogenesis of cortical layers in human cerebellum, particularly the lamina dissecans. J. Comp. Neurol., 139:473–500, 1970.

Rakić, P., and Yakovlev, P. I.: Development of the corpus callosum and cavum septi in man. J. Comp. Neurol., 132:45–72, 1968.

Rebière, A., and Legrand, J.: Effets comparés de la sousalimentation, de l'hypothyroïdisme et de l'hyperthyroïdisme sur la maturation histologique de la zone moléculaire du cortex cérébelleux chez le jeune rat. Arch. Anat. Microsc. Morphol. Exp., 61:105–126, 1972.

Richter, E.: Die Entwicklung des Globus Pallidus und des Corpus subthalamicus. Monografien aus dem Gesamtgebietes der Neurologie und Psychiatrie, No. 108. Berlin, Springer, 1965.

Rio-Hortega, P. del: El "tercer elemento" de los centros nerviosos. Histogénesis y evolución normal; éxodo y distribución regional de la microglia. Mem. Soc. Esp. Hist. Natural, 11:213–268, 1921.

Rose, J. E.: The ontogenetic development of the rabbit's diencephalon. J. Comp. Neurol., 77:61–131, 1942.

Sauer, F. C.: Mitosis in the neural tube. J. Comp. Neurol., 62:377–405, 1935a.

Sauer, F. C.: The cellular structure of the neural tube. J. Comp. Neurol., 63:557–560, 1935b.

Sharp, J. A.: The junctional region of the cerebral hemisphere and the third ventricle in mammalian embryos. J. Anat., 93:159–168, 1959.

Sidman, R. L., Miale, I. L., and Feder, N.: Cell proliferation in the primitive ependymal zone: An autoradiographic study of histogenesis in the nervous system. Exp. Neurol., 1:322–333, 1959.

Sidman, R. L., and Rakić, P.: Neuronal migration with special reference to developing human brain: A review. Brain Res., 62:1–35, 1973.

Sotelo, C., and Changeux, I. P.: Bergmann fibres and granular cell migration in the cerebellum of homozygous weaver mutant mouse. Brain Res., 77:484–491, 1974.

Taber-Pierce, E.: Histogenesis of the nuclei griseum pontis, corporis pontobulbaris and reticularis tegmenti pontis (Bechterew) in the mouse. J. Comp. Neurol., 126:219–240, 1966.

Toole, J. F., and Tucker, S. H.: Influence of head position upon cerebral circulation. Arch. Neurol., 2:616–623, 1960.

Windle, W. F., and Fitzgerald, J. E.: Development of the human mesencephalic trigeminal root and related neurons. J. Comp. Neurol., 77:597–608, 1942.

Part III

Aghajanian, G. K., and Wang, R. S.: Habenular and other midbrain raphe afferents demonstrated by a modified retrograde tracing technique. Brain Res., 122:229–242, 1977.

Angevine, J. B.: Development of the hippocampal region. In Isaacson, R. L., and Pribram, K. (eds.): The Hippocampus. Volume I. New York, Plenum Press, 1975.

Armstrong, D. M.: Functional significance of connections in the inferior olive. Physiol. Rev., 54:358–417, 1974.

Beal, J. A., and Fox, C. L.: Afferent fibres in the substantia gelatinosa of the adult monkey: A Golgi study. J. Comp. Neurol., 168:113–145, 1976.

Björklund, A., Falck, B., Hromek, F., et al.: Identification and terminal distribution of the tubero-hypophyseal monoamine fibre systems in the rat by means of stereotaxic and microspectrofluorimetric techniques. Brain Res., 17:1–23, 1970.

Boesten, A. J. P., and Voogd, J.: Projections of the dorsal column nuclei and the spinal cord on the inferior olive in the cat. J. Comp. Neurol., 161:215–238, 1975.

Bremer, F., and Terzuolo, C.: Contribution à l'étude des mécanismes physiologiques du maintien de l'activité vigile du cerveau. Interaction de la formation réticulée et de l'écorce cérébrale dans le processus du réveil. Arch. Int. Physiol. Biochem., *62*:157–178, 1954.

Broca, P.: Anatomie comparée des circumvolutions cérébrales: Le grand lobe limbique et la scissure limbique dans la série des mammifères. Rev. Anthropol., *1*(3s):385–498, 1978b.

Brodal, A.: Neurological Anatomy in Relation to Clinical Medicine. New York, Oxford University Press, 1969.

Brodmann, K.: Vergleichende Lokalisationslehre der Grosshirnrinde in ihren Prinzipien dargestellt auf Grund des Zellenbaues. Leipzig, J. A. Barth, 1909.

Carpenter, M. B.: Human Neuroanatomy. Baltimore, Williams & Wilkins, 1976.

Carpenter, M. B., Nakano, K., and Kim, R.: Nigrothalamic projections in the monkey demonstrated by autoradiographic technics. J. Comp. Neurol., *165*:401–416, 1976.

Carpenter, M. B., and Pierson, R. J.: Pretectal region and the pupillary light reflex. An anatomical analysis in the monkey. J. Comp. Neurol., *149*:271–300, 1973.

Dahlström, A., and Fuxe, K.: Evidence for the existence of monoamine neurons in the central nervous system. Acta Physiol. Scand., *62*[Suppl. 232]: 1–55, 1965.

Dow, R. S., and Moruzzi, G.: The physiology and pathology of the cerebellum. Minneapolis, Univ. of Minnesota Press, 1958.

Eccles, J. C., Ito, M., and Szentágothai, I.: The cerebellum as a neuronal machine. New York, Springer, 1967.

Gastaut, H., and Lammers, H. J.: Anatomie du rhinencéphale: Les grandes activités du rhinencéphale. Paris, Masson, 1961.

Gerebtzoff, M. A.: Contribution à l'étude des voies afférentes de l'olive inférieure. J. Belge Neurol. Psychiat., *10*:719–728, 1939.

Geren, B. B.: The formation from the Schwann cell surface of the myelin in peripheral nerves of chick embryos. Exp. Cell Res., *7*:558–562, 1954.

Goldstein, K.: Die Lokalisation in der Grosshirnrinde. *In* Bethe, A., et al. (eds.): Handbuch der normale und Pathologischen Physiologie. Vol. 10. Berlin, Springer, 1927.

Groenewegen, H. J., and Voogd, I.: The longitudinal management of the olivocerebellar, climbing fiber projection in the cat: An autoradiographic and degeneration study. Exp. Brain Res. [Suppl. 1], 65–71, 1976.

Hardy, M.: Observations on the innervation of the macula sacculi in man. Anat. Rec., *59*:403–418, 1935.

Head, H.: Aphasia and Kindred Disorders of Speech. Cambridge, Cambridge University Press, 1926.

Hernández-Peón, R.: Reticular mechanisms of sensory control in sensory communication. *In* Rosenblith, W. A. (ed.): Processing Neuroelectric Data. London, MIT Press, 1959.

Hubel, D. H., and Wiesel, T. N.: Shape and arrangements of columns in cat's striate cortex. J. Physiol., *165*:559–568, 1963.

Jones, E. G.: Some aspects of the organization of the thalamic reticular complex. J. Comp. Neurol., *162*:285–308, 1975.

Jones, E. G., and Leavitt, R. J.: Retrograde axonal transport and the demonstration of non-specific projections to the cerebral cortex and striatum from thalamic intralaminar nuclei in the cat, rat and monkey. J. Comp. Neurol., *154*:349–378, 1974.

Kemp, J.: An electron microscopic study of the termination of afferent fibres in the caudate nucleus. Brain. Res., *11*:464–467, 1968.

Kuhlenbeck, H., and Miller, R. N.: The pretectal region of the human brain. J. Comp. Neurol., *91*:369–408, 1949.

Kuypers, H. G. J. M.: Corticobulbar connections to the pons and lower brain stem in man. Brain Res., *81*:364–388, 1954.

Kuypers, H. G. J. M.: The anatomical organization of the descending pathways and their contributions to motor control, especially in primates. *In* Desmedt, J. E. (ed.): New Developments in EMG and Clinical Neurophysiology. Vol. 3. Basel, Karger, 1973.

Kuypers, H. G. J. M., and Tueerk, J. D.: The distribution of cortical fibres within the nucleus cuneatus and gracilis in the cat. J. Anat., *98*:143–162, 1964.

Leichnetz, G. R., and Astruc, J.: The course of some prefrontal corticofugals to the pallidum, substantia innominata and amygdaloid complex in monkeys. Exp. Neurol., *54*:104–109, 1977.

Lorente de Nó, R.: The area entorhinalis. J. Psychol. Neurol., *45*:381–438, 1933.

Maeda, T., Pin, C., Salvert, D., et al.: Les neurones conténant des catecholamines du tegmentum pontique et leurs voies de projection chez le chat. Brain Res., *57*:119–152, 1973.

Martinez-Martinez, P. F.A.: The structure of the pituitary stalk and the innervation of the neurohypophysis in the cat. Thesis. Leiden, Luctor et Emergo, 1960.

Nauta, W. J. H.: Hippocampal projections and related neural pathways to the midbrain in the cat. Brain, *81*:319–340, 1958.

Nauta, W. J. H., and Kuypers, H. G. J. M.: Some ascending pathways in the brain stem reticular formation. *In* Jasper, H. H., and Proctor, L. D. (eds.): Reticular Formation of the Brain. Toronto, Little and Brown, 1958.

Nieuwenhuys, R.: Comparative anatomy of the cerebellum. Prog. Brain Res., *25*:1–93, 1964.

Palay, S. L., Sotelo, C. I., Peters, A., et al.: The axonhillock and the initial segment. J. Cell Biol., *38*:193–201, 1968.

Polyak, S.: The retina. Chicago, University of Chicago Press, 1941.

Powell, T. P. S., Cowan, W. M., and Raisman, G.: The central olfactory connections. J. Anat., *99*:791–813, 1965.

Ralston, H. J.: The organization of the substantia gelatinosa Rolandi in the cat lumbosacral cord. Z. Zell., 1965, 671–723.

Réthelyi, M., and Szentágothai, J.: The large complexes of the substantia gelatinosa. Exp. Brain Res., *7*:258–274, 1969.

Rexed, B.: A cytoarchitectonic atlas of the spinal cord in the cat. J. Comp. Neurol., *100*:297–379, 1954.

Rinvik, E.: Demonstration of nigrothalamic connections in the cat by retrograde axonal transport of horseradish peroxidase. Brain Res., *90*:313–318, 1975.

Rivera-Dominguez, M., Mettler, F. A., and Noback, C. R.: Origins of cerebellar climbing fibres in the rhesus monkey. J. Comp. Neurol., *155*:331–342, 1973.

de Robertis, E.: Submicroscopic morphology and function of the synapse. Exp. Cell Res. Suppl., *5*:347–369.

Scheibel, M. E., Davies, T., and Scheibel, A. B.: On dendrodendritic relations in the dorsal thalamus of the adult cat. Exp. Neurol., *36*:519–529, 1972.

Siegel, A., and Edinger, H.: A comparative neuroanatomical analysis of the differential projections of the hippocampus to the septum. *In* Proceedings of the Society of Neuroscience, San Diego, 1973.

Siegel, A., and Tassoni, J. P.: Differential efferent projections from the ventral and dorsal hippocampus of the cat. Brain, Behav. Evol., *4*:185–200, 1971a.

Snider, R. S., and Stowell, A.: Receiving areas of the tactile, auditory, and visual systems in the cerebellum. J. Neurophysiol., *7*:331–357, 1944.

Sotelo, C., Llinás, R., and Baker, R.: Structural study of inferior olivary nucleus of the cat: Morphological correlates of electrotonic coupling. J. Neurophysiol., *37*:541–599, 1974.

Sperry, R. W.: Brain bisection and mechanisms of consciousness. *In* Eccles, J. C. (ed.): Brain and Conscious Experience. Berlin, Springer, 1966.

Sperry, R. W., Gazzaniga, M. S., and Bogen, J. E.: Interhemispheric relationship: the neocortical commissures; syndromes of hemisphere disconnection. *In* Vinken, P. J., and Bruyn, G. W. (eds.): Handbook of Clinical Neurology. Amsterdam, North-Holland Publishing Company, 1969.

Swanson, L. W., Connelly, M. A., and Hartman, B. K.: Ultrastructural evidence for central monoaminergic innervation of blood vessels in the paraventricular nucleus of the hypothalamus. Brain. Res., *136*:166–173, 1977.

Szabo, J.: Projections from the body of the caudate nucleus in the rhesus monkey. Exp. Neurol., *27*:1–15, 1970.

Szentágothai, I.: The neuron network of the cerebral cortex: A functional interpretation. Proc. Roy. Soc. Lond. [Biol.], 219–248, 1978.

Szentágothai, I.: The module concept in cerebral cortex architecture. Brain Res., *95*:475–496, 1975.

Taber, E.: The cytoarchitecture of the brain stem of the cat. J. Comp. Neurol., *116*:27–70, 1971.

Voogd, J.: The cerebellum of the cat: Structure and fibre connections. Thesis. Assen, van Gorcum, 1964.

Woolsey, C. N.: Organization of somatic sensory and motor areas of the cerebral cortex. *In* Harlow, C. F., and Woolsey, C. N. (eds.): Biological and Biochemical Bases of Behavior. Madison, University of Wisconsin, 1958.

Index

Note: Page numbers in *italics* refer to illustrations; page numbers followed by (t) refer to tables.